FUNCTIONAL BANDAGING

in Orthopedic and Sports Traumatology

Claudio Zimaglia

FUNCTIONAL BANDAGING
in Orthopedic and Sports Traumatology

edi·ermes

FUNCTIONAL BANDAGING IN ORTHOPEDIC AND SPORTS TRAUMATOLOGY
Claudio Zimaglia

ISBN 978-88-7051-523-7 - Print edition
ISBN 978-88-7051-463-6 - Digital edition

A book is the final product of a very specific series of operations that requires numerous verifications of the text and images. It is nearly impossible to publish a volume without errors.
We would be grateful to those who notify us of the presence of any errors.
For indications or suggestions regarding this volume, please use the following address:

Public relations - Edi.Ermes srl - Viale Enrico Forlanini, 65 - 20134 Milan (Italy)

Phone +39.02.70.21.121 - Fax +39.02.70.21.12.83

The Publisher is available for intellectual property owners with whom it was not possible to communicate, as well as for any inadvertent omissions and inaccuracies in the quotation of sources presented in this volume.

Printed in November 2017 by Faenza Printing Industries SpA
for Edi.Ermes - viale Enrico Forlanini, 65 - 20134 Milan (Italy)
http://www.ediermes.com - Phone +39.02.70.21.121 - Fax +39.02.70.21.12.83

Preface

Functional bandaging finds its applications in the prevention, treatment, and rehabilitation in the field of so-called minor musculoskeletal traumatology in more than just the realm of athletics, and carries out an intermediate role between simple compressive bandaging and rigid plaster casting.

The primary objective of functional bandaging is to treat traumatic injuries with spontaneous benign evolution, such as the aftereffects of muscular injuries from indirect trauma (pulled muscles, sprains, contractures) or direct trauma (light contusions), traumatic capsuloligamentous injuries, or myotendinous injuries.

The applied technique requires a good understanding of muscular anatomy and basic joint biomechanics, and requires the use of both elastic and inelastic (rigid inextensible) adhesive bandages as well as both elastic and inelastic cohesive bandages, and of the latest generation of bandages, which allow for combined bandaging with high retention capacity.

Today, the modern direction is moving toward the functional treatment of trauma. This entails the need to look at retention systems that use partial immobilization configurations or dynamic bandaging that allows for the protection of the injured motor structures, the reduction of strain on the compromised area, and the preservation of normal functionality of the other areas, as well as the elimination of the inconveniences of inactivity. The total immobilization caused by plaster casting actually slows posttraumatic recovery and impedes the performance of not only strictly therapeutic actions, but also and prevalently those of musculoskeletal rehabilitation.

In this book, we describe the application methods for bandages that fully satisfy these demands, which are particularly relevant in the world of sports. Described herein are methods of retention bandaging using adhesive elastic and inelastic bandages, and combined bandaging methods using the latest materials for effective preventive and athletic use.

Acknowledgements

I would like to sincerely thank those who have collaborated on the draft of this book, and those who have made themselves available for the application of the various bandages; particular thanks to Sergio Cravero and Franco Demarin for the photographs, to Laura Ardissone as an ex-athlete of international status in the 100-meter dash, and to Giorgio Barberis, Monica Melis, Luca Seoni, Alessio Donadon, and surgeon Davide Delicio for being of help in the application of bandages.

Table of contents

THEORETICAL ELEMENTS OF FUNCTIONAL BANDAGING 1
Basic techniques 2
Indications, precautions, contraindications 4
Materials 6
Pre-tape 7
Non-adhesive elastic bandage . 7
Adhesive elastic bandage 7
Cohesive fixation bandage. 7
High-resistance cohesive bandage 8
Inelastic adhesive tape 8
Inelastic cohesive tape 9
Foam rubber bandage 9
Hydrating cream 9
Razor blade 9
Lister scissors 10

UPPER LIMB 11
Acromioclavicular joint 12
Stabilization for “piano key” injury 13
Glenohumeral joint 14
Base bandaging with elastic adhesive bandage 15
Base bandaging with elastic adhesive tape 19
Tape-based stabilization and reinforcement of base bandaging. 23
Crossing stabilization and reinforcement of base bandaging. 27
Stabilization and reinforcement of tape base bandaging 29
Unloading, retention, and guidance of movement . 31
Limitation of outward rotation and abduction 35
Stabilization and limitation of outward rotation 37
Elbow joint. 46
Unloading and limitation of extension 47
Stabilization and limitation of extension 51
Stabilization, limitation of extension and supination 55
Muscular and tendinous unloading 57
Supinator muscle 60
Muscular unloading 61
Radiocarpal joint 64
Base bandaging 65
Limitation of extension on base bandaging 69
Support and limitation of extension 71
Limitation of flexion on base bandaging 79

Limitation of flexion on tape base bandaging 81
Limitation of flexion 85
Metacarpophalangeal joints 88
Unloading and protection of the thumb 89
Stabilization of the thumb 93
Limitation and stabilization of abduction and extension of the thumb 97
Stabilization of the fingers 109
Limitation of the extension and flexion of the fingers .. 111
Proximal interphalangeal joints ... 112
Lateral stabilization 113
Stabilization and limitation of flexion 115

Lower limb 117
Medial muscles of the thigh 118
Unloading and limitation of abduction, extension, and outward rotation....... 119
Quadriceps femoris 120
Muscular unloading via compressive bandaging 121
Rectus femoris 124
Unloading, support, and guidance of movement . 125
Posterior muscles of the thigh 128
Muscular unloading via compressive bandaging 129
Unloading, support, and guidance of movement .. 135
Posterior muscles and joint of the knee 138
Muscular unloading with bandage in X-shape, taking on of the satellite joint...... 139
Knee joint 140
Base bandaging 141
Base bandaging with cohesive bandage 145
Stabilization of the collateral ligament on the base bandaging...... 147
Unloading and stabilization with reinforcement of the collateral ligaments... 149
Limitation of extension, support for collateral ligaments 153
Support of the anterior cruciate ligament 159
Limitation of extension 161
Recentering of the patella 163
Unloading of the patellar tendon with a pad................ 165
Unloading of the patellar tendon with inelastic adhesive tape . 167
Unloading of the patellar tendon with elastic adhesive tape ... 169
Support of the patellar tendon 171
Posterior muscles of the lower leg.. 172
Muscular unloading via compressive bandaging 173
Tibiotarsal joint 178
Base bandaging 179
Retention base bandaging 183
Base bandaging with cohesive elastic bandage 185
Fast bandaging with stabilization of the hindfoot 187
Stabilization of the hindfoot and support at the lateral space 191
Support via inelastic bandage.. 199
Stabilization of the hindfoot... 205
Stabilization of the hindfoot reinforced with tape........ 207

Retention of the lateral space . . 209
Stabilization of the lateral space 211
Stabilization of the lateral space with reinforcement . . . 215
Limitation of inversion and eversion 223
Unloading and limitation of plantar flexion 229
Achilles tendon 230
Preventative bandaging 231
Unloading with X-shaped bandage, limitation of dorsal flexion 233
Musculotendinous unloading, limitation of dorsal flexion . 235
Unloading bandaging 237
Unloading with stabilization of the hindfoot 239
Musculotendinous unloading with stabilization of the hindfoot 243
Unloading and support with elastic bandage 251
Unloading, support, and stabilization with inelastic bandage 255
Plantar aponeurosis 258
Unloading with elastic adhesive tape 259
Unloading with reinforcement . 261
Support of the foot and the plantar arch 267
Metatarsophalangeal joints 270
Unloading with pad 271
Stabilization of the joint of the great toe 273
Unloading of the metatarsophalangeal joint of the great toe 277
Support of the great toe, limitation of hyperextension and abduction 283

Theoretical elements of functional bandaging

The term *functional bandaging* refers to a means of dynamic retention with partial immobilization, capable of sustaining and stabilizing the components of a joint among one another, by reinforcing, relieving, and supporting a functional biomechanical unity of the locomotor apparatus. This bandaging technique is based on knowledge of functional anatomy, and is practiced primarily by implementing retention with elastic and inelastic adhesive or cohesive bandages.

Dynamic-retention bandaging employs the tensile-elastic properties of bandages to produce an effect that is both *compressive* with the aim of aiding decongestion of muscular edema and hematomas or joint effusions, and *preventative* to ensure the proper functioning of individual motor units while stabilizing them. The primary action of this type of bandaging is thus essentially that of *mechanical retention*.

The materials and techniques of application that involve joint and muscle biomechanics allow us to offer functional unloading and support, reducing the demands placed on the wounded area and keeping the healthy parts active and functional. This function is performed via *active and passive joint stabilization*.

The patching effect of *adhesive bandaging* on exteroceptive cutaneous afferents provides a neuromuscular facilitation stimulus in response to cutaneous stress, thus avoiding abnormal levels of mobility that could bring the joint beyond its physiological limits. Analogous results may be obtained through the use of the latest breathable high-resistance *cohesive bandages*; these are capable of improving the bandage's mechanical capacity for retention and stabilization, additionally reducing problems that may arise from the application of the adhesive to the skin, especially for people with sensitive skin or who have skin allergies related to the adhesive.

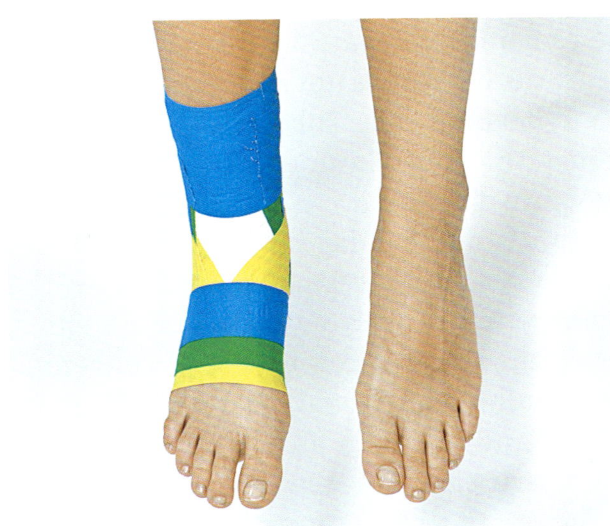

In many cases, dynamic-retention functional bandaging facilitates the healing process and provides significant advantages over total-immobilization bandaging.

One of the most significant objectives of functional bandaging is to inhibit the movement that caused the trauma. By limiting joint excursion and overextension of the capsuloligamentous tissues, we may avoid causing pain and/or incurring new trauma, while simultaneously maintaining free movement and guiding it in a physiological way. In cases of posttraumatic joint instability, the adoption of dynamic-retention partial-immobilization bandaging also encourages the functional recovery of muscles that can compensate for the laxity of the ligaments during movement. In fact, the muscles, with their tendinous insertions, actively contribute to the maintenance of balanced joint action, and within certain limits, in synergy with the passive capsuloligamentous joint elements, may perform their functions. This form of bandaging is thus recommended in all cases of wounds or alterations that do not require complete immobilization. However, it must be remembered that in cases of injury, the reduction of pain is not an indicator of complete healing, especially in cases of serious injury that may be underestimated or not properly diagnosed.

Functional bandaging provides *non-specific protective* functions: it encourages the quick return of athletes to athletic activities, helps them in the prevention of congenital or acquired functional weakness or instability, and achieves an antalgic and antiphlogistic effect by restricting the wounded structure to a role of functional rest.

Elastic bandages seem to have a significant *trophic vasomotor* action for all chronic and/or degenerative pathologies arising from overexertion; bandaging, in fact, acts as a veritable vascular massage, capable of helping tissues affected by ischemic-degenerative phenomena, improving their functionality, and reducing pain, similar to a pump working on circulation.

Finally, the *psychological* effects of functional bandaging must not be underestimated: athletes, or any subjects who have this type of retention, will experience a beneficial sense of protection and safety accompanied by an increase in the threshold of attention and vigilance.

BASIC TECHNIQUES

On the basis of the need to produce a specific mechanical response, the techniques of application are identified as follows (Table 1):

- *Compressive bandaging for edema or hematoma reabsorption*. Adhesive elastic bandages are used in conjunction with pre-bandaging, done with pre-tape or non-adhesive or cohesive elastic bandages. The reabsorption of hematomas is encouraged by vascularization and the draining effect of the bandaging. The progress of the healing process may be monitored each time the bandaging is changed;
- *Support and retention bandaging*. Elastic (normal or adhesive, with or without pre-tape) or cohesive bandages are used. The aim is to limit movement that causes pain and to guide the healthy parts to a point of controlled mobility;

Table 1 Functional bandaging techniques: objectives, materials, and indications

Techniques	*Objectives*	*Materials*	*Indications*
Compression Bandaging	Reduction of liquids	Normal or adhesive elastic bandage with pre-tape or cohesive bandage 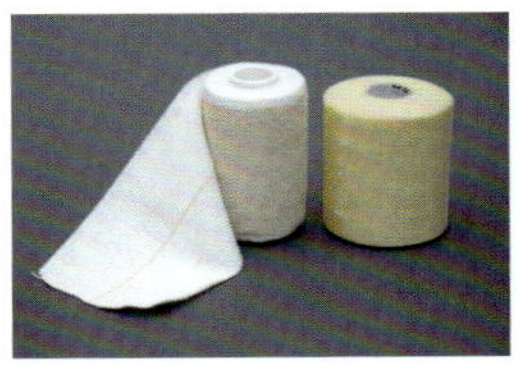 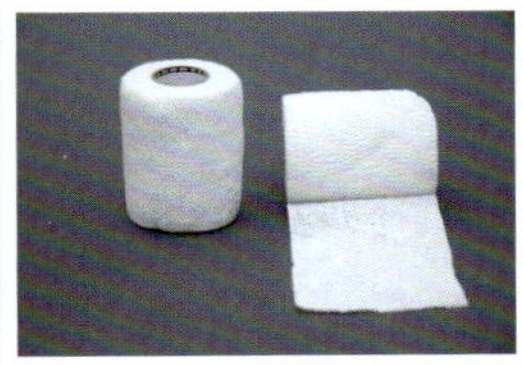	Reabsorption of edema and hematoma Joint effusion
Support and retention bandaging	Limitation and guidance of movement	Normal or adhesive elastic bandage, with or without pre-tape, or cohesive bandage 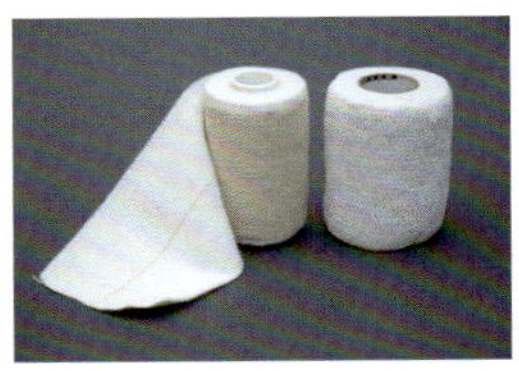	Prevention and rehabilitation
Immobilization bandaging	Inhibition of movement	Adhesive inelastic bandages with or without pre-tape 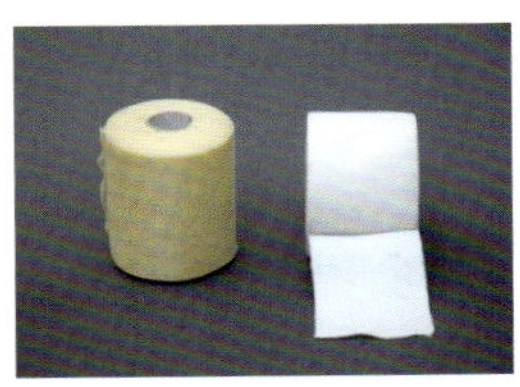	Prevention and rehabilitation in the sports field
Mixed or combined bandaging	Limitation of movement and support on the wounded side; movement guidance	Adhesive elastic bandage, with or without pre-tape, reinforced with adhesive or cohesive inelastic tape 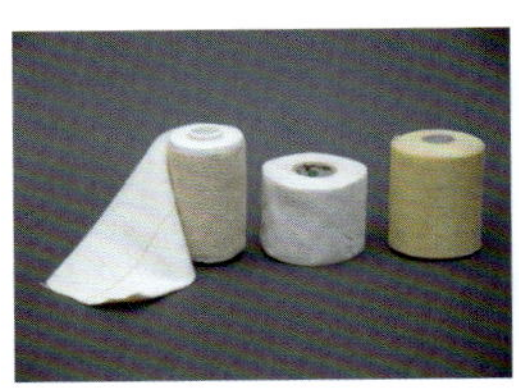 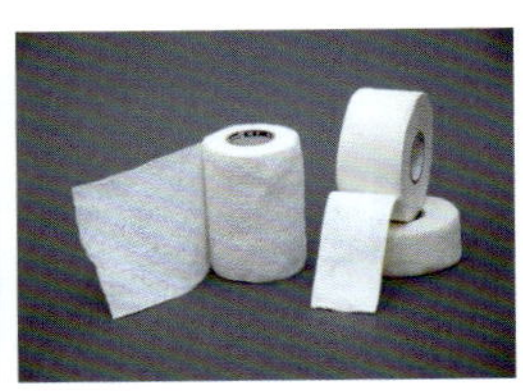	Prevention and rehabilitation

- *Immobilization bandaging*. Inelastic adhesive bandages are used to impede movement that causes pain;
- *Partial immobilization mixed or combined bandaging*. Adhesive or cohesive elastic bandages are used as a base, which are then reinforced by affixing inelastic adhesive tape or inelastic cohesive tape. The aim is to limit movement that causes pain.

Based on the different athletic, therapeutic, or preventative demands, the techniques of application are identified as:

- *Preventative/sports bandaging*. The aim is to prevent joint trauma. This is used in sports disciplines with high rates of trauma linked to specific motions, or for athletes who are predisposed to injury or who may need psychological support. It is useful for subjects with local conditions predisposing them to injury, both constitutional/congenital (ligamentous laxity) and acquired (posttraumatic joint instability);
- *Rehabilitative/therapeutic bandaging*. Various kinesiological treatments and posttraumatic rehabilitations may successfully use functional bandaging, such as in cases of capsuloligamentous and musculotendinous aftereffects following basic orthopedic treatment or surgery. In these cases, the bandaging provides support that protects and guides the functional work of the wounded and incompletely healed structure;
- *Posttraumatic bandaging*. This is used following capsuloligamentous trauma or muscular injuries without significant complications, such as in the presence of large hematomas; it is also useful in cases of injury and fatigue due to myotendinous and aponeurotic functional overload, in synergy with other pharmacological or kinesiotherapeutic treatments.

INDICATIONS, PRECAUTIONS, CONTRAINDICATIONS

Functional bandaging is applied in the field of so-called minor musculoskeletal traumatology, in the areas of prevention, posttraumatic treatment, athletic therapy, and postoperative therapy.

This type of bandaging is used primarily as a system for support, retention, and stabilization in cases of acute or chronic instability and trauma of the ankle, knee, and wrist *joints*, supporting and substituting for the functional underperformance of the capsuloligamentous structures responsible for these instabilities and working against abnormal movements or pathological deviations of the joints.

With regards to the *muscular system*, bandaging plays an important role of therapeutic support and compression, preventing and limiting maximum muscle contraction and/or limiting the excursion of the joint to which the muscle is anchored, thus encouraging the scarring of the wounded muscle tissue.

Primary *indications* and fields of application are:

- First and second degree capsuloligamentous sprains, above all in cases of sprain trauma results (the objective of bandaging is to keep the joint in a physiological position even during movement, encouraging the healing over of the injured tissues);

- Preventative treatment for subjects with ligament laxity or joint instability;
- Preventative sports treatment;
- Indirect muscular traumatology in cases of first- and second-degree injuries (bandaging provides unloading, protecting areas that undergo excessive traction forces, in addition to encouraging proper emptying of any intra-muscular hematoma);
- Insertional myotendinous or pure tendinous pathologies (bandaging relieves the tendon, reducing the forces of traction acting upon it);
- Plantar fasciitis;
- Metatarsalgia;
- Rebalancing of anomalous tendinous tensions that promote static support disorders caused by trauma or postural compromises such as hallux valgus;
- Aftereffects of scapulohumeral subluxation;
- Femur-knee instability;
- Femoral adductor conditions;
- Postural defects from a varus/valgus of the knee;
- Facilitation upon hyperextension of the knee (*recurvatum*);
- Rehabilitative phases after posttraumatic or postoperative immobilization.

Any person implementing functional bandaging must have sufficient knowledge of the anatomy and functional biomechanics of the locomotor apparatus; they must also recognize the mechanisms that did or could cause injury in order to be able to create an ideal retention system with the bandages for countering the detrimental (or potentially detrimental) mechanical stress.

In all cases, certain *precautions* must be observed during the application of bandaging, in order to avoid:
- The formation of folds between the bandage and the skin under the plantar arch;
- The compression of the metatarsal heads, above all at the fifth metatarsus;
- The compression of the Achilles tendon;
- The compression of popliteal fossa;
- The application of an adhesive bandage in direct contact with the popliteal fossa, the underarm, or the inguinal cavity;
- The direct application of adhesive material to the skin without hair removal.

Additionally:
- In cases of acute capsuloligamentous trauma with joint effusion from sprain, it may sometimes be useful to apply a U-shaped foam rubber support under the bandaging in order to encourage the joint's emptying;
- For bandaging of the Achilles tendon, it may be useful to apply a foam rubber

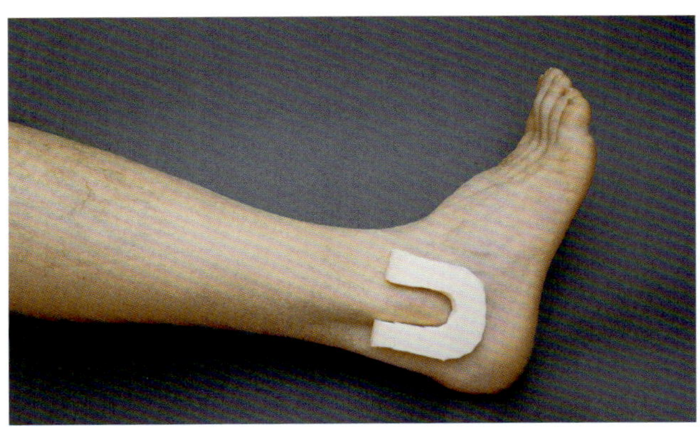

"heel lift" in order to encourage tendinous unloading;
- For the protection of superficial tendinous passages, it may be useful to protect

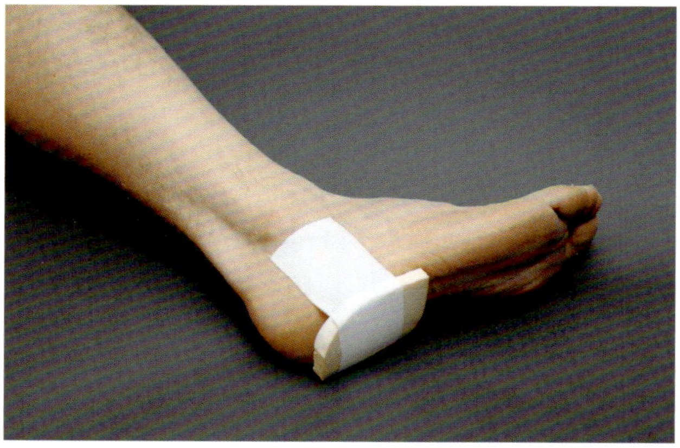

the skin with the application of protective pads before the bandaging of an ankle or knee, either prepackaged or made with pre-tape.

The specific and absolute *contraindications* of functional bandaging, especially in

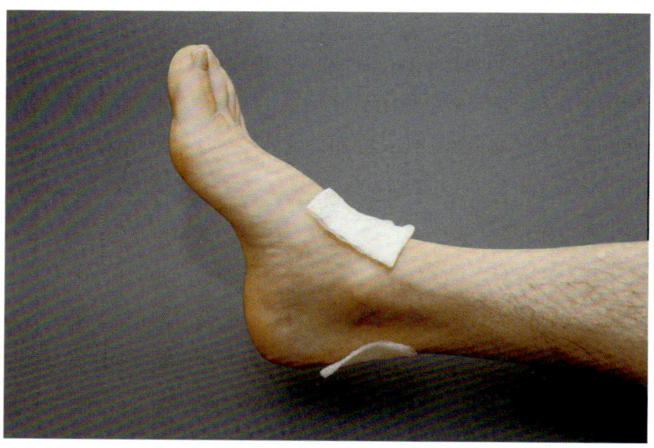

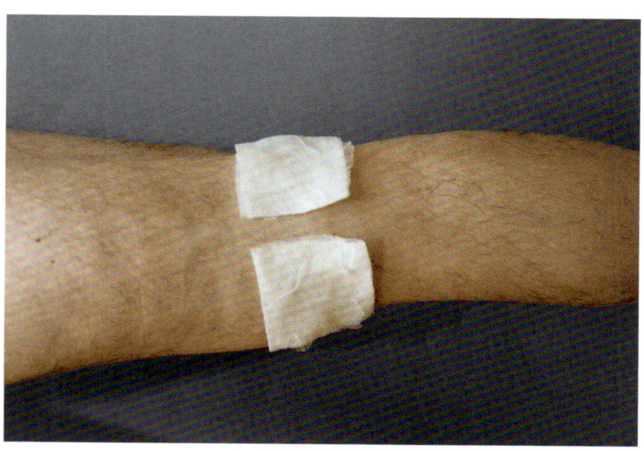

cases of the application of adhesive bandages directly to the skin, are:

- Presence of varicose veins;
- Presence of skin wounds or abrasions, or sores;
- Organized edemas (such as lymphedema);
- Trophic or vascular disturbances;
- Sensitivities or allergies to adhesive products;
- Skin rashes or dermatological conditions of various types;
- Complete ligament breakage with capsular breakage;
- Complete tearing of tendons;
- Muscular tearing;
- Large contusions;
- Non-reduced dislocations;
- Rheumatic conditions;
- Bone fractures;
- Application without precise diagnosis, particularly in the acute phase.

MATERIALS

In recent years, the constant search for new materials and the creation of ever more cutting-edge products have allowed functional bandaging to become more and more efficient and varied. The ability to choose the most suitable material allows for ideal bandaging; the bandaging technique and the material depend on the type of treatment that is chosen for application.

If bandaging is selected wherein the adhesive material is in direct contact with the skin, it must be remembered that the action of the bandaging on the locomotor apparatus is strongly dependent on the conditions of the skin. The skin is normally covered with a film of hydrolipids that render it slightly oily and thus not very suitable for allowing perfect adhesion of the bandage. Even peeling and the presence or loss of hairs impede the adhesion of the bandage, reducing the retention effect; the sweat itself that the skin secretes during particularly intense effort may cause the loss of adhesiveness.

Thus, the skin must be cleaned, dried, and prepared for bandaging, and also protected in order to avoid any irritation problems linked to the adhesive.

The bandage must be chosen on the basis of therapeutic, preventative, or athletic needs, as well as the bandaging techniques to be applied and the area to be covered.

There exist in the market numerous varieties of adhesive and non-adhesive bandages; the choice must fall upon those products that fulfill characteristics of *quality,* such as the ease of unrolling, optimal resistance to functional demands, and acceptable microporosity of the adhesive so as to reduce the retention of sweat and encourage optimal adhesion. Elastic or inelastic bandages must have a continuous action duration throughout the entire time of the bandage's presence and good *tolerability* in relation to the hypoallergenic quality of the adhesive part. If cohesive bandages are used, they must have high resistance in order to optimize the retention of the base bandage.

Pre-tape

This is a thin, highly porous polyurethane foam bandage. It is important to apply pre-tape evenly, ensuring that it adheres well to the skin surface without the formation of wrinkles. Its use is indispensable to protect delicate skin and to facilitate removal of the bandage; it is also used to affix medications or medicated pads, or for the creation of pads to be used under the base bandage, which are useful for the protection of tendinous projections. On the market, there exist cans of spray adhesive that may facilitate the adhesion of the pre-tape.

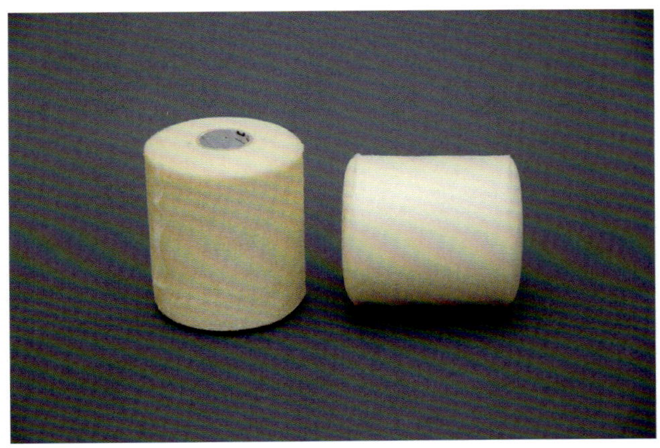

Non-adhesive elastic bandage

This is a bandage that adheres neither to itself nor to the skin: it has no adhesive. It is often used for drainage bandaging with compressive action.

Adhesive elastic bandage

This is an adhesive elastic band made of cotton fabric that is capable of adhering to itself and to the skin; it has a central line of alignment. Hypo-allergenic, it provides a stable base for joint support bandaging.

Cohesive fixation bandage

This is a medium-resistance cohesive bandage that, without adhesive, adheres

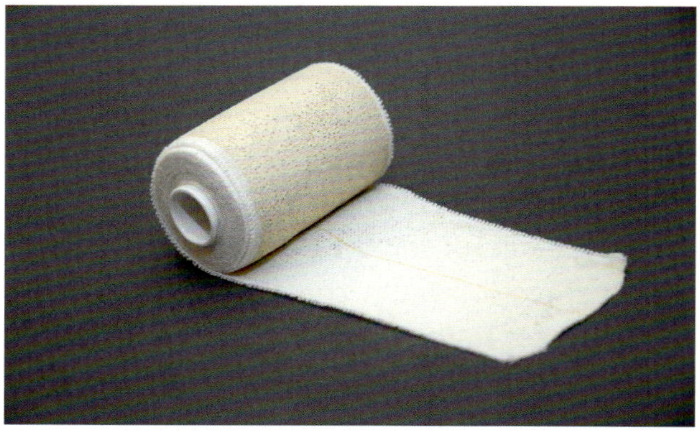

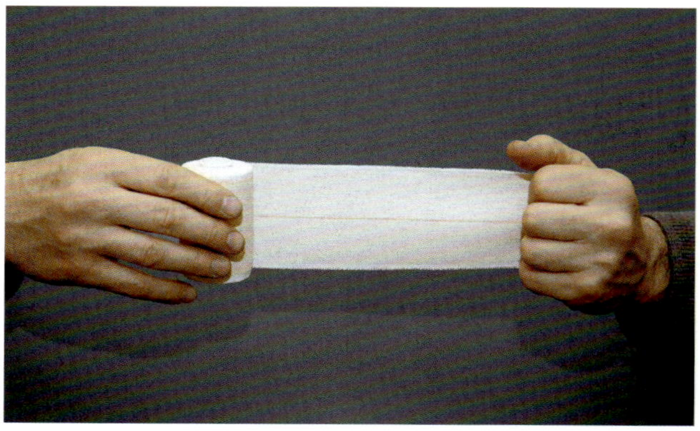

to itself but not to the skin. These are used to refine and finish functional bandaging.

High-resistance cohesive bandage

This is a tearing cohesive bandage, ideal for sports medicine. Light and elastic, it offers optimal holding without obstruction.

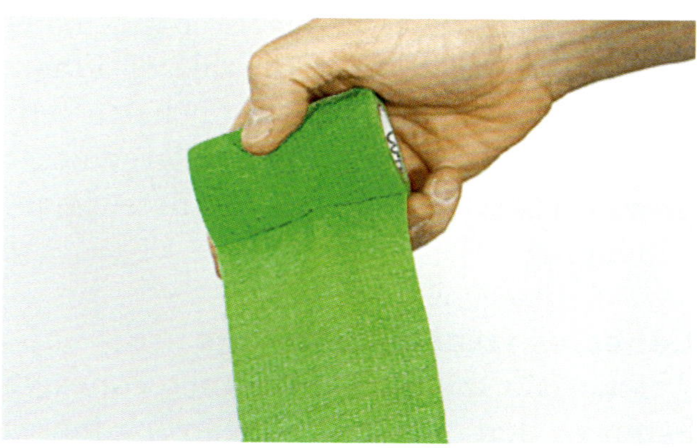

tion. It does not adhere to the skin, only to itself. The application of this bandage is very quick, as it does not require the use of pre-tape and adhesive, and may be used directly on the skin. The compression provided by the bandage ensures the blockage of the tendons and ligaments without impeding mobility or altering sensitivity.

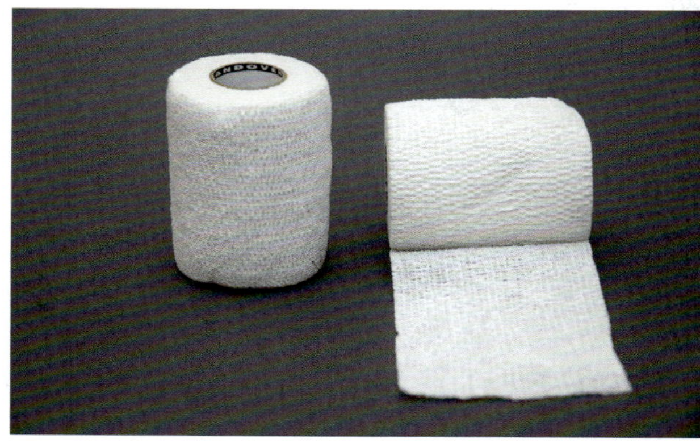

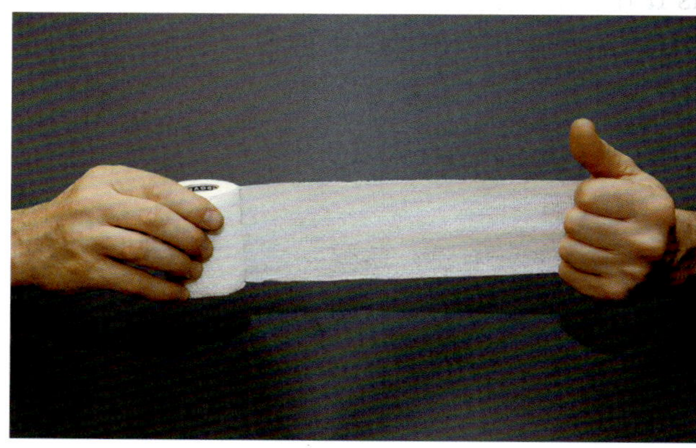

Inelastic adhesive tape

Inelastic bandage with zinc oxide adhesive. This is highly adhesive and adheres securely to the skin. It is useful for immobilization and support bandaging in cases of sprains, dislocations, or joint trauma. It

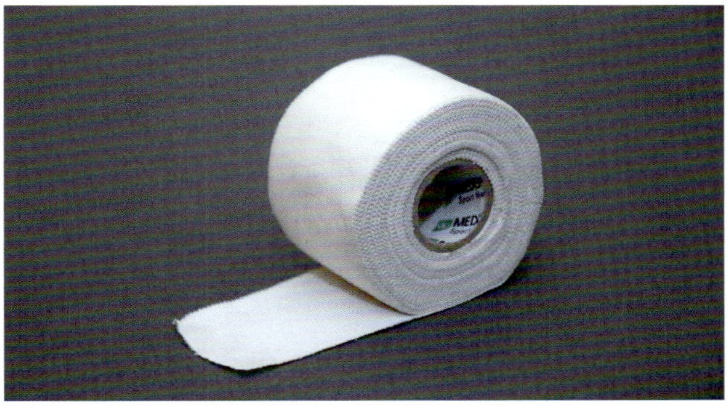

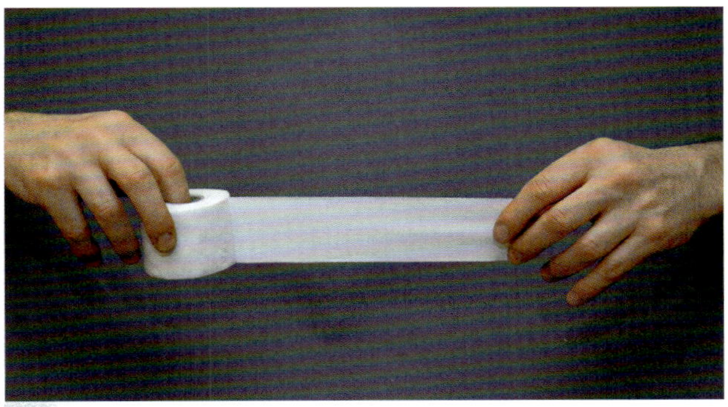

is also suitable for protective joint layering, as it ensures proper blockage and maximum holding strength.

Inelastic cohesive tape

Inelastic cohesive tape is a new and innovative water-repellant and formable material that can substitute for traditional inelastic adhesive tape. It adheres to itself and is made using different synthetic fibers so that it may be used in combination with

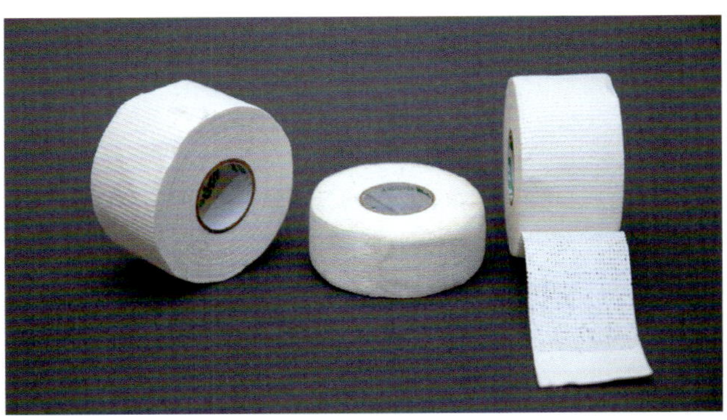

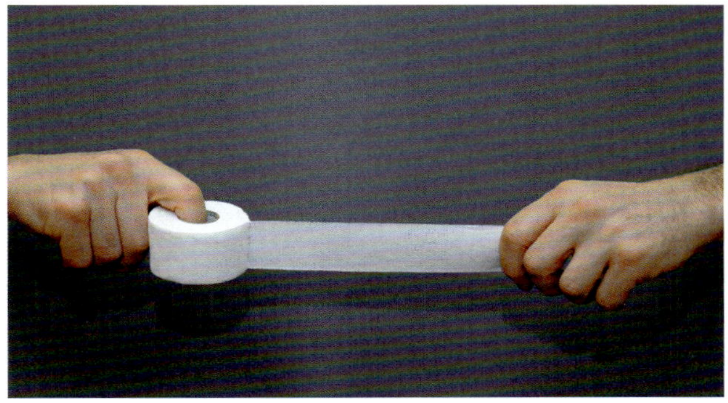

a specific cohesive bandage. It is resistant to water and sweat and is breathable; these characteristics allow the bandaging to remain stable for long periods without losing its support properties. It is easily unwound with the hands, and because it adheres only to itself, renders bandaging simple and fast. Its application, when done with appropriate technique, allows bandaging with strong holding and resistance, guaranteeing optimal containment and freedom of movement.

Foam rubber bandage

This is useful for compressive muscular bandaging; it may be re-cut and shaped according to needs.

Hydrating cream

After the removal of the bandage, it is useful to clean and soften the skin with a hydrating cream.

Razor blade

To encourage the bandage's adhesion, and so that its removal may be less painful, it is recommended that any hair be shaved with a razor several hours before the application of the bandage.

Lister scissors

These are specific scissors for cutting and removing bandages. Their blunt tip allows the safe and easy removal of adhesive bandages from the skin.

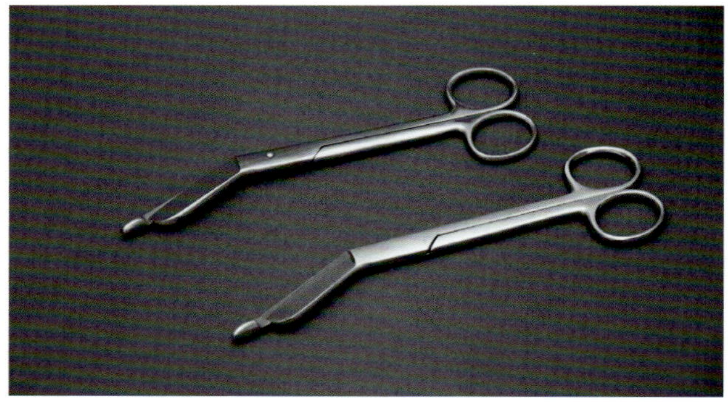

Upper limb

- **Acromioclavicular joint**
- **Glenohumeral joint**
- **Elbow joint**
- **Supinator muscle**
- **Radiocarpal joint**
- **Metacarpophalangeal joints**
- **Proximal interphalangeal joints**

ACROMIOCLAVICULAR JOINT

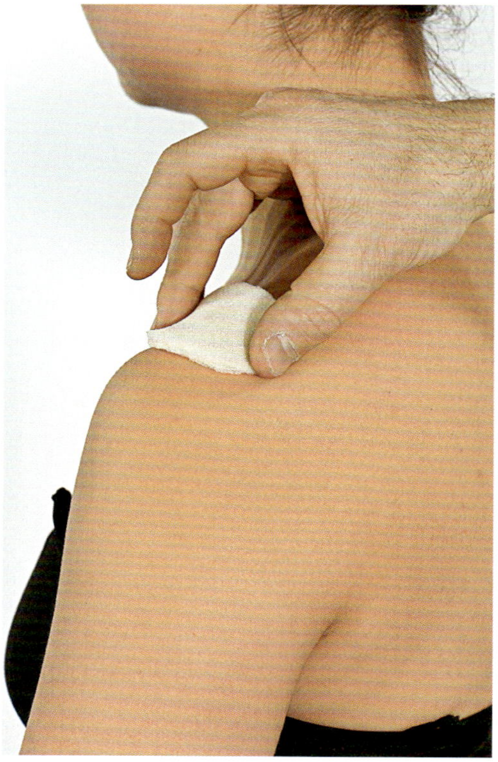

1

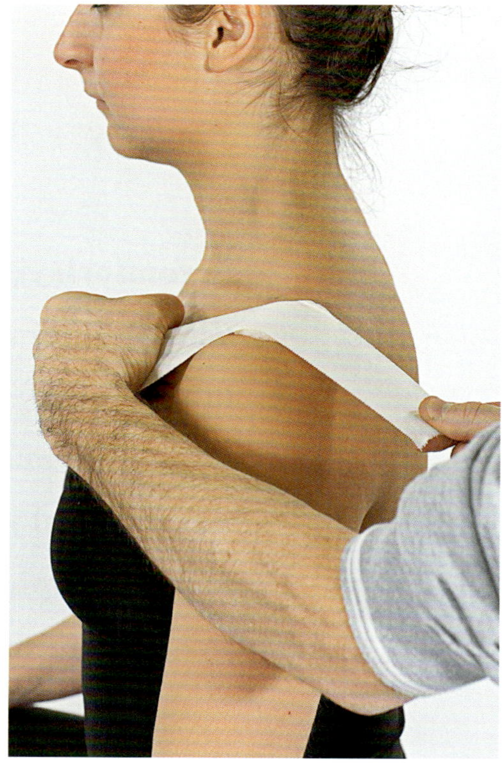

2

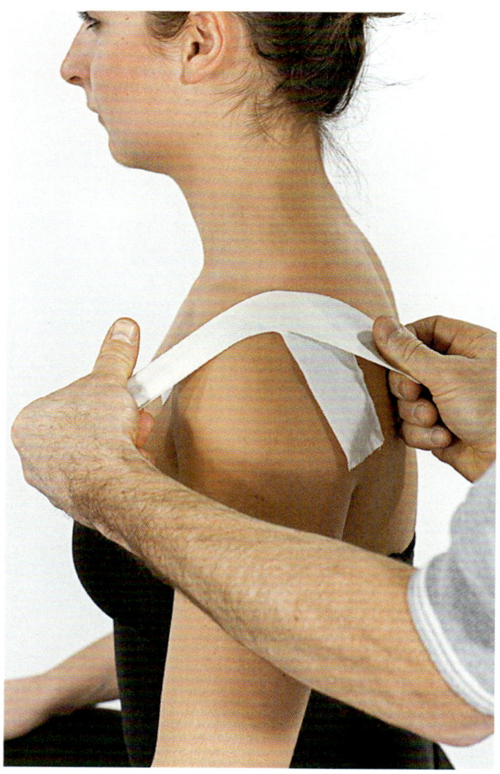

3

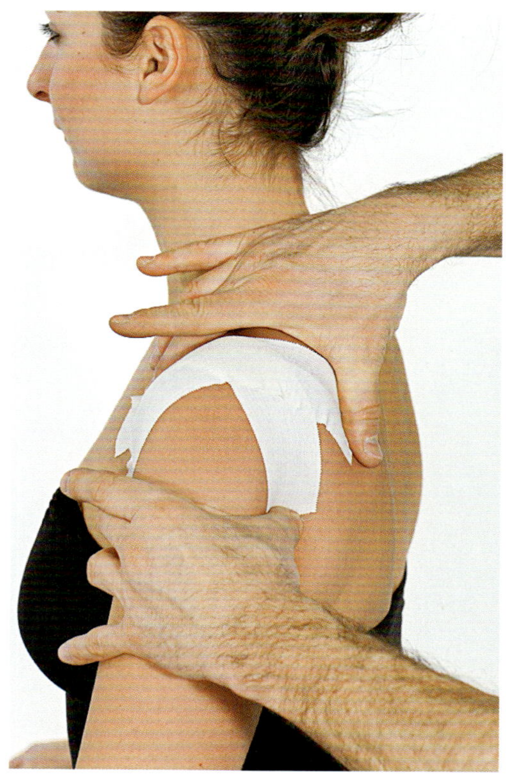

4

Stabilization for "piano key" injury

MATERIAL

✓ Foam rubber or pre-tape compress for creating a compressive pad
✓ Inelastic adhesive tape

APPLICATION

1 The subject is seated; a latex foam or polyurethane compress is placed on the skin projection of the acromion in order to compress the area.

2 The compress is fixed in place with a strip of inelastic adhesive tape.

3 A second strip of inelastic material is then crossed over the first.

4 Bandaging is complete.

When applying the inelastic adhesive tape, the pad must be compressed downward and the strip adhered well to the skin, keeping it under tension.

INDICATIONS

✓ *Pain symptoms in the acromioclavicular joint for results of direct trauma with subluxation of the acromion*

GLENOHUMERAL JOINT

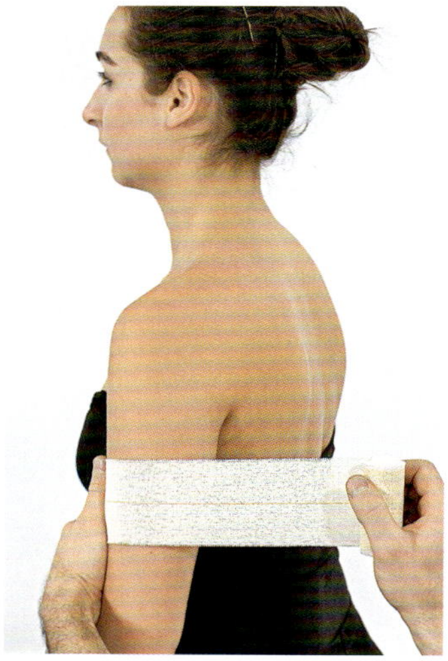

1

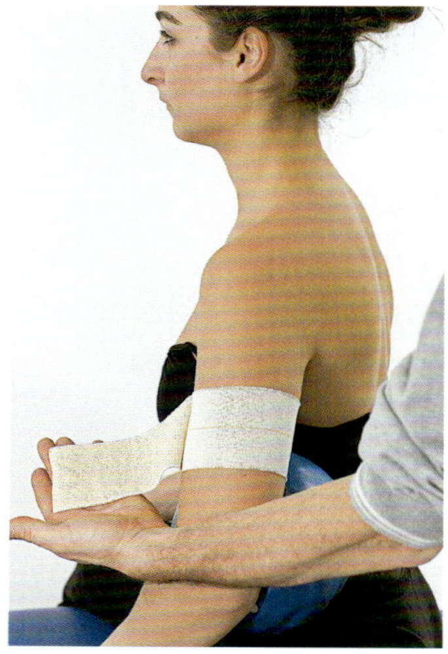

2

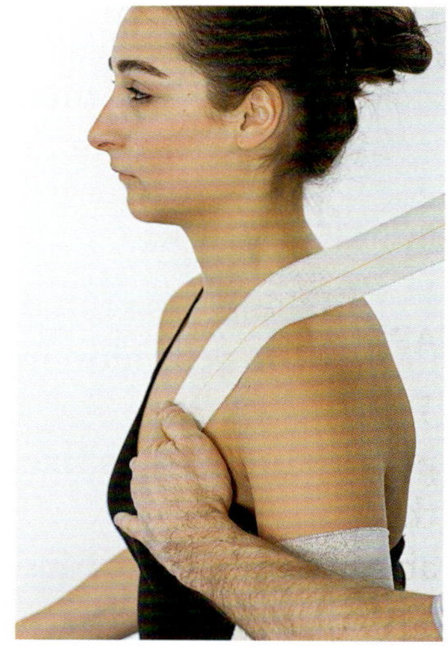

3

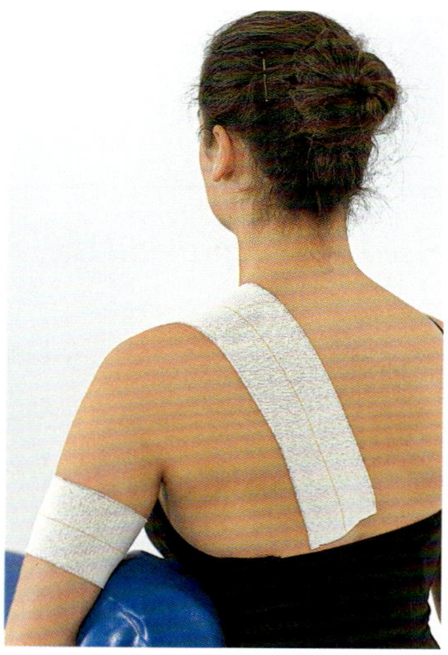

4

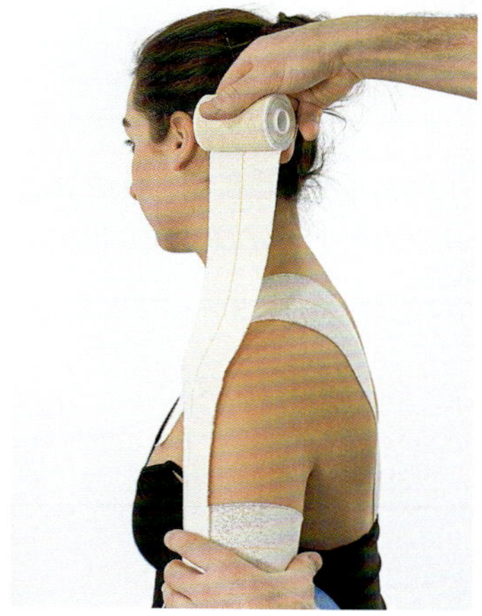

5

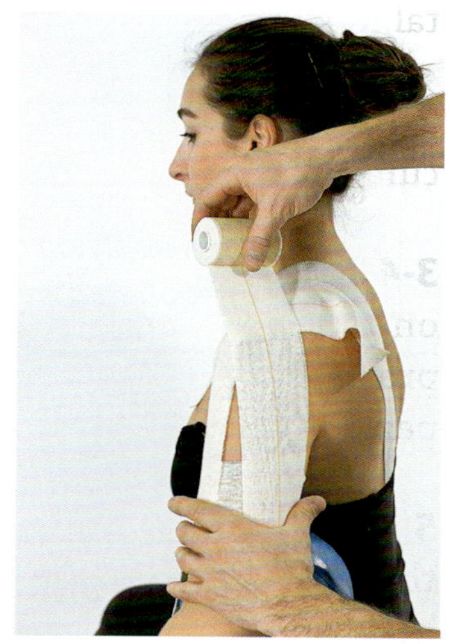

6

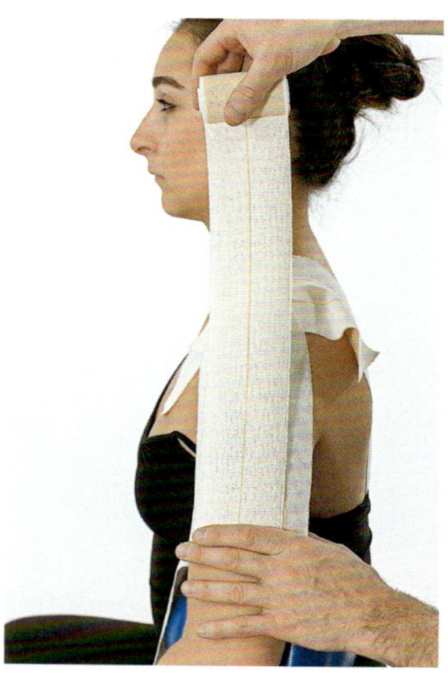

7

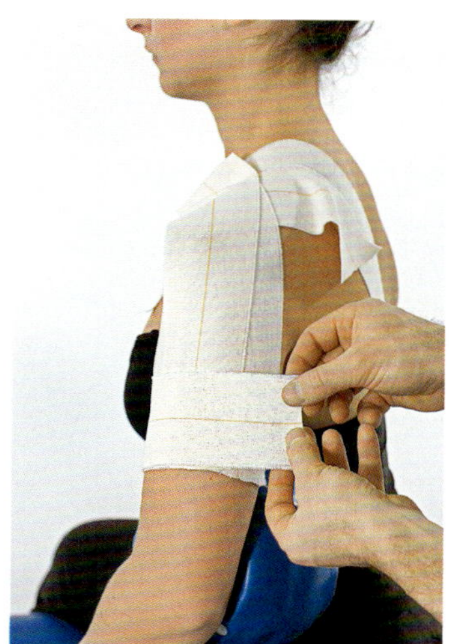

8

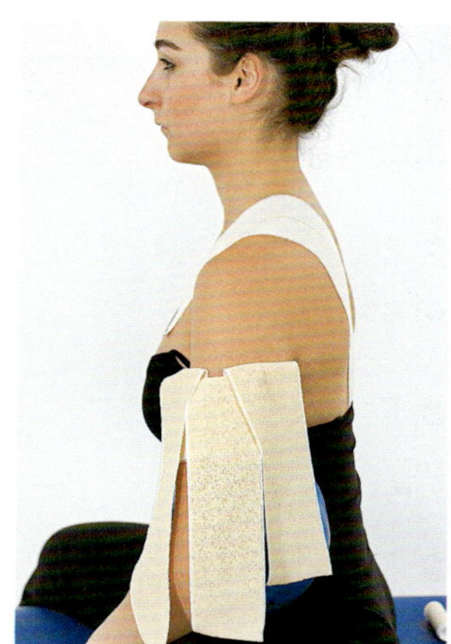

9

Base bandaging with elastic adhesive bandage

MATERIAL

- ✓ Cotton fabric porous elastic adhesive bandage that can be stretched lengthwise, 7.5 cm in width
- ✓ Pre-tape or foam rubber compress for making a protective pad
- ✓ Inelastic adhesive tape for affixing the bandage

APPLICATION

1 The subject is seated, preferably with a pad between the upper limb and the side of the thorax in order to keep the arm in light abduction. Make a distal anchoring point by wrapping the mono-extensible elastic adhesive bandage around the arm under the distal insertion of the deltoid.

Before bandaging, it is recommended that a compress of a soft material be applied in order to protect the skin projection of the acromion.

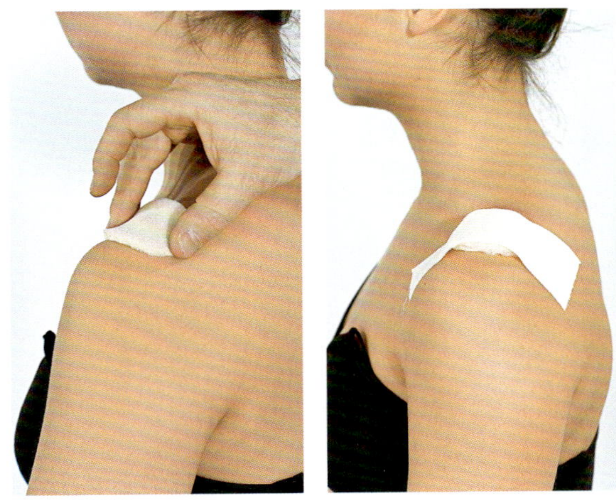

2 A strip of bandage is left free so as to secure it later.

3-4 The proximal anchoring point is made on the shoulder, perpendicular to the skin projection of the superior bundle of the trapezius.

5 Several strips of bandage are applied to the distal anchoring point without being adhered to the skin. The first, positioned anteriorly, is supported on the skin projection of the anterior bundle of the deltoid.

6 The second, positioned posteriorly, is supported on the skin projection of the posterior bundle of the deltoid.

7 The third, positioned laterally, is supported on the skin projection of the medial bundle of the deltoid.

8 The three strips of bandage are affixed with the strip left free on the distal anchoring point.

9 The three strips are left to fall backward.

GLENOHUMERAL JOINT

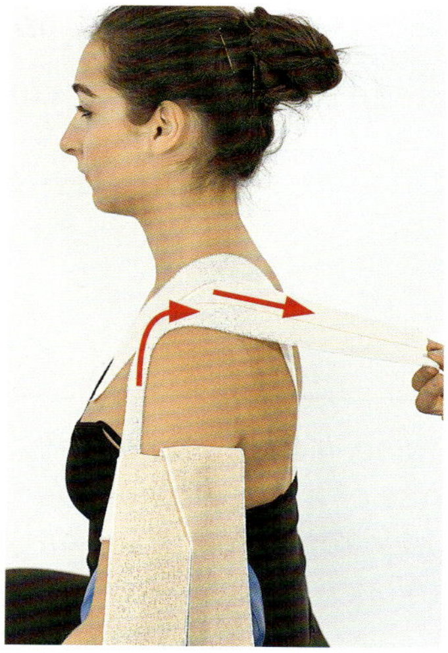
10

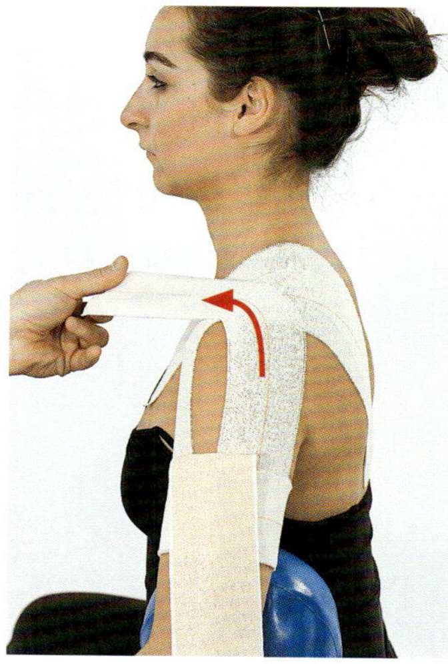
11

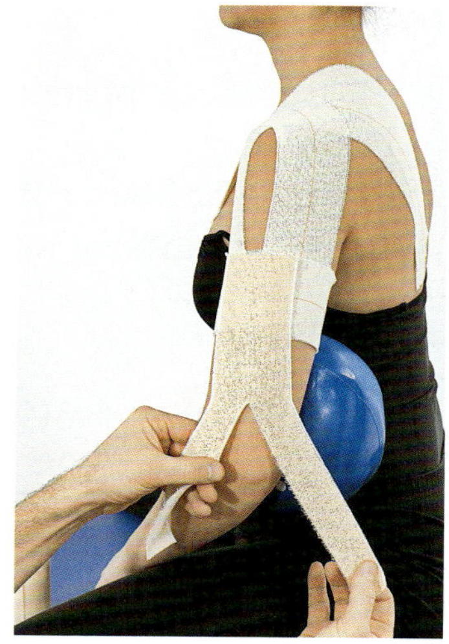
12

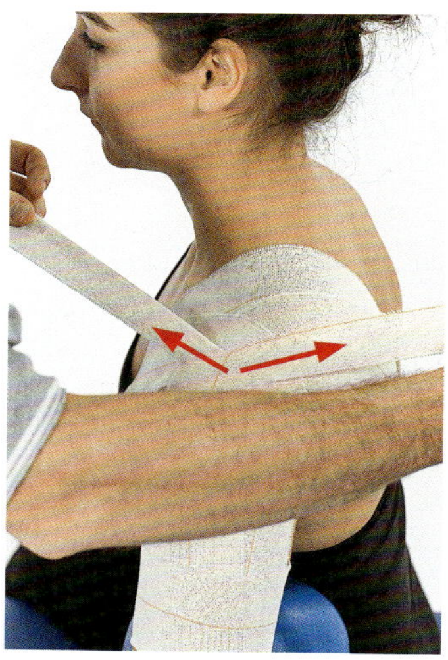
13

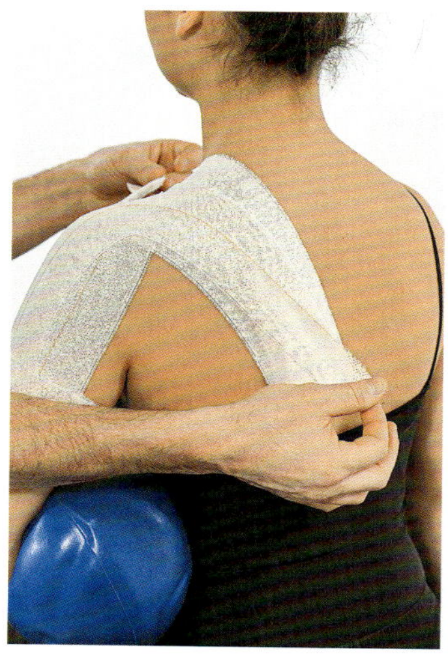
14

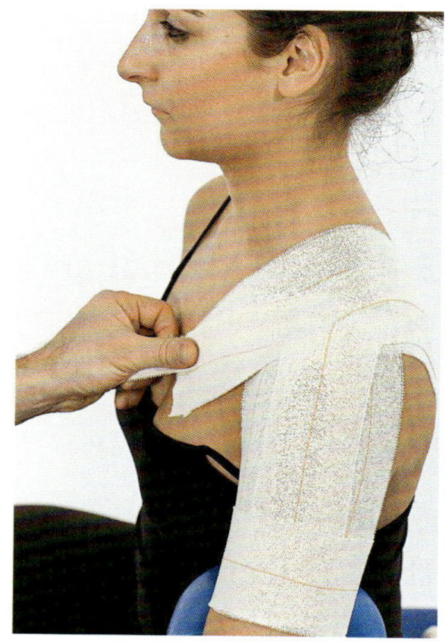
15

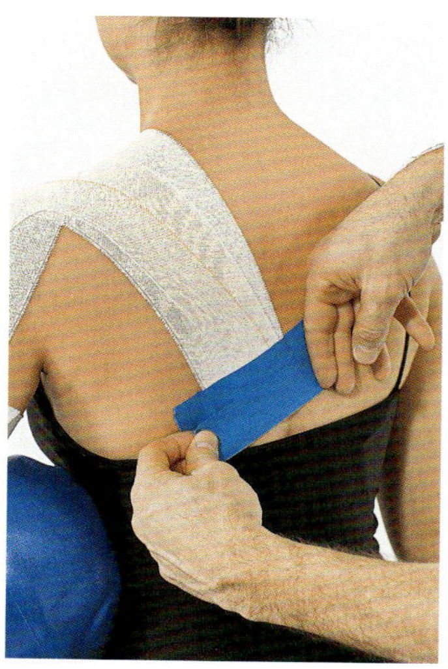
16

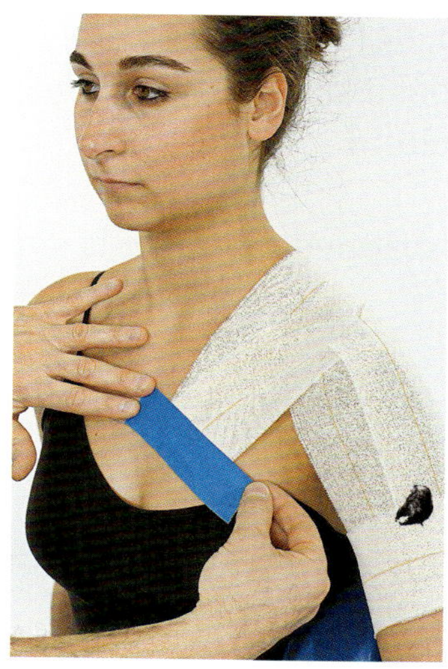
17

Base bandaging with elastic adhesive bandage

10 The bandage affixed anteriorly is put under tension and passed over the skin projection of the acromion to adhere posteriorly to the proximal anchoring point.

11 After the posteriorly affixed bandage has been put under tension, it is crossed over itself at the acromion, on the first stretch of bandage, and is affixed anteriorly at the proximal anchoring point.

12-13 The third strip of bandage is cut longitudinally so that the two pieces separate at the level of the skin projection of the acromion.

14-15 Once put under tension, the two pieces are applied at the proximal anchoring point, one anteriorly and the other posteriorly.

16-17 The bandage is affixed, applying two strips of inelastic adhesive tape posteriorly and anteriorly on the proximal anchoring point.

The adhesive elastic bandaging may be completed with the application of a cohesive bandage to secure the retention and improve its holding strength, or adhesive elastic bandages may be applied to the cohesive base bandage. For the application of this technique, see the bandaging described on page 36.

INDICATIONS

- ✓ *Pain symptoms upon movement of the glenohumeral joint*
- ✓ *Aftereffects of traumatic dislocation of the glenohumeral joint*
- ✓ *Chronic instability of the shoulder*

GLENOHUMERAL JOINT

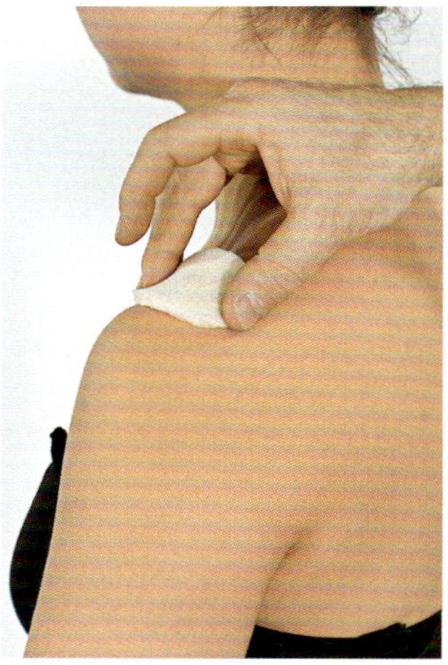
1

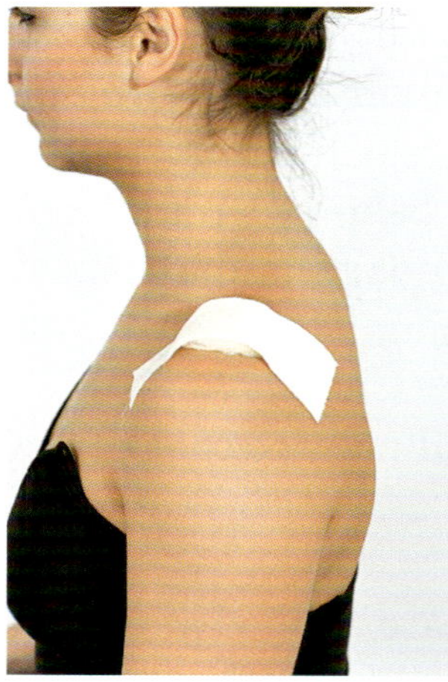
2

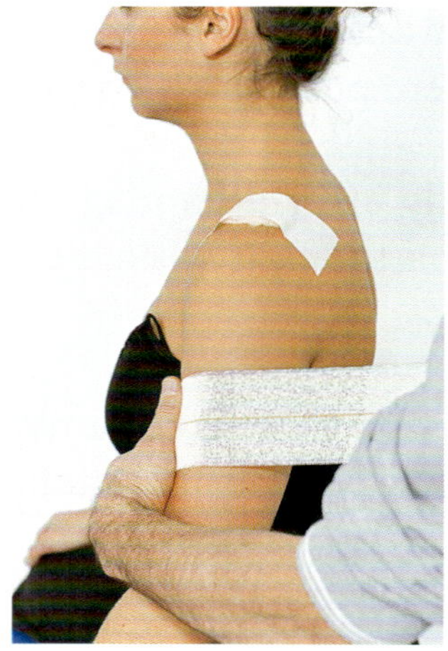
3

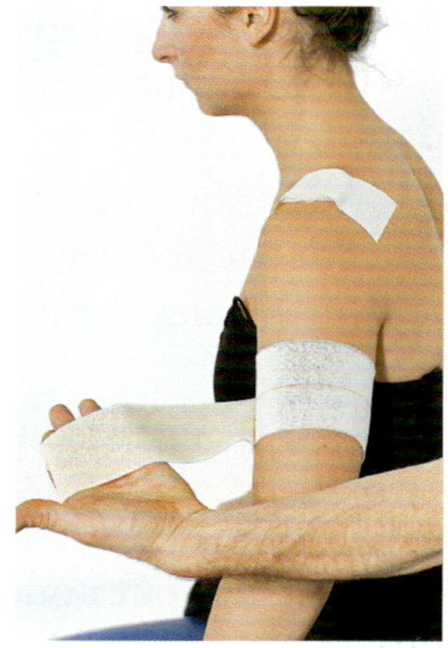
4

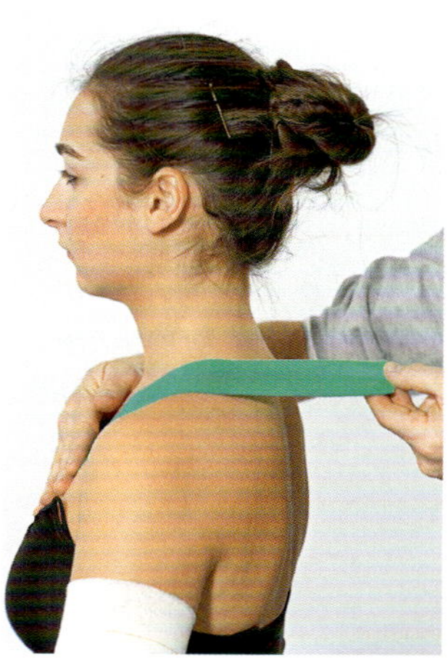
5

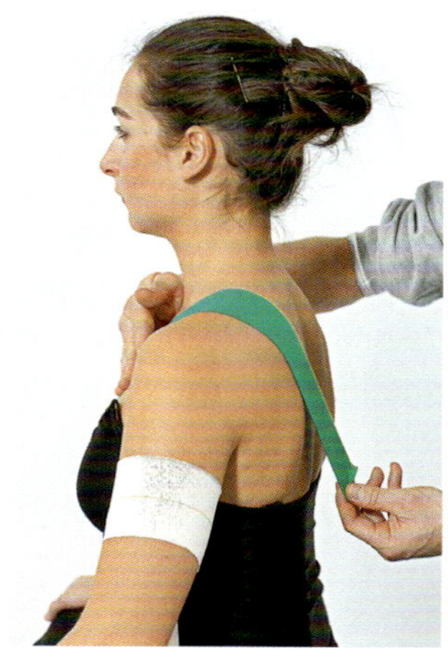
6

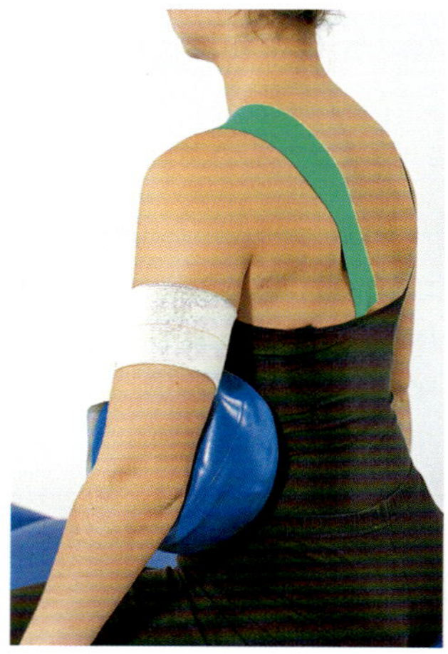
7

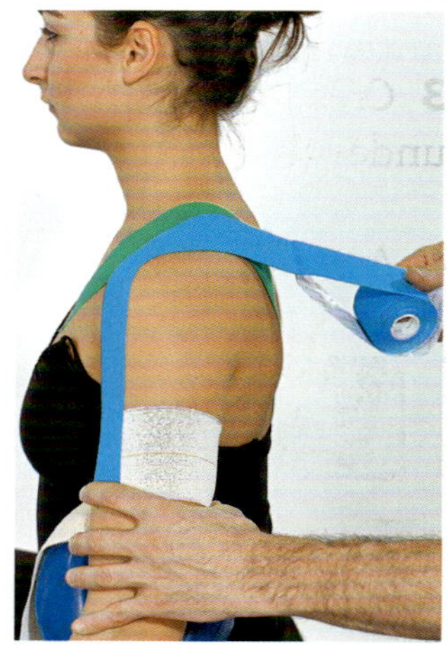
8

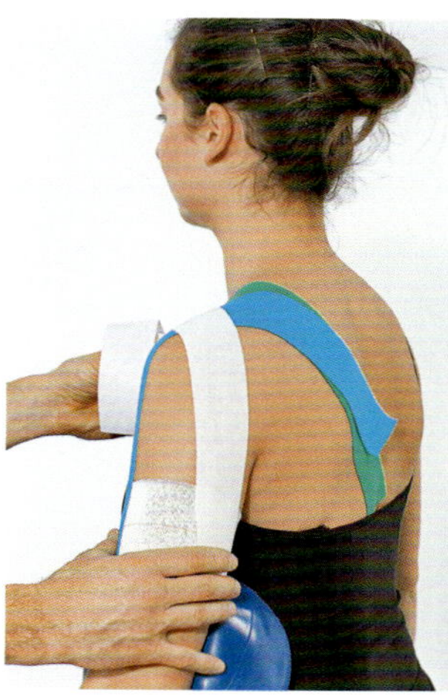
9

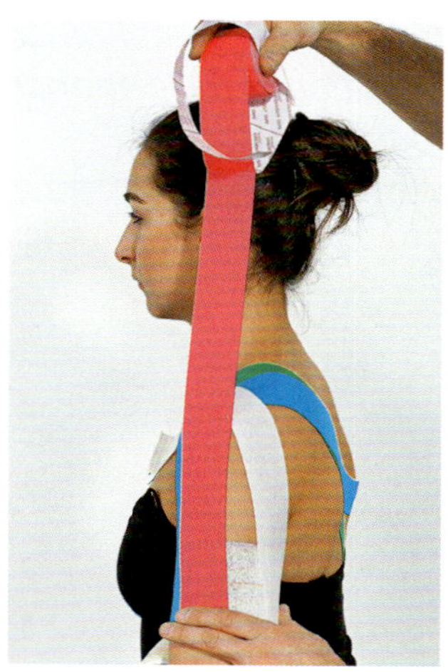
10

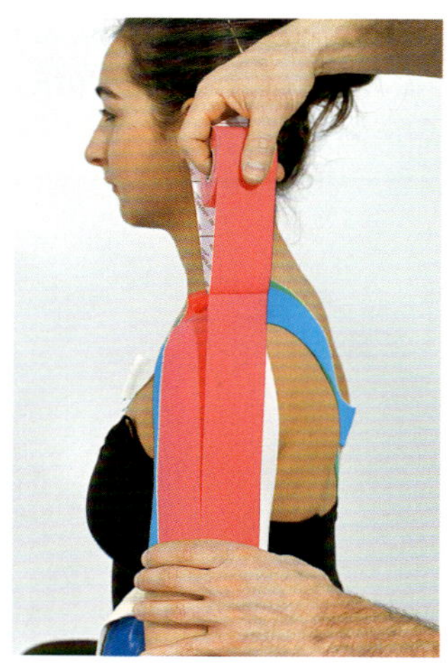
11

Base bandaging with elastic adhesive tape

MATERIAL

- ✓ Elastic adhesive tape, extensible lengthwise, 5 cm in width
- ✓ Cotton fabric porous elastic adhesive bandage that can be stretched lengthwise, 10 cm in width
- ✓ Pre-tape or foam rubber compress for making a protective pad
- ✓ Inelastic adhesive tape for affixing the compress and the bandaging

APPLICATION

1 The subject is seated with a cushion or ball between the arm and the thorax so as to keep the limb slightly abducted. A compress, made of a soft material, is positioned on the skin projection of the acromion.

2 The compress is fixed in place with a strip of inelastic adhesive tape.

3 Create a distal anchoring point by wrapping the elastic adhesive bandage around the arm under the distal insertion of the deltoid.

4 A strip of bandage is left free to later secure the bandage.

> *Although the compress is no longer seen in the following images, in actual bandaging it is kept. In this case, it was removed in order to allow better visualization of the subsequent steps.*

5-6-7 A strip of elastic adhesive tape is needed for the proximal anchoring point. The anchoring point is applied from the sternocostal skin projection, in line with the nipple, then coming out to cover the pectoralis muscle, passing perpendicularly over the skin projection of the trapezius, and covering the scapula before affixing beyond its lower border.

8 Bandaging proceeds by applying several pieces of elastic adhesive tape to the distal anchoring point; the strips are tightened without being adhered to the skin. The first tape leaves from the anterior surface of the distal anchoring point and is brought over the skin projection of the anterior bundle of the deltoid.

9 The second tape leaves from the posterior surface of the distal anchoring point and is brought over the skin projection of the posterior bundle of the deltoid.

10-11 The third and fourth pieces of bandage leave from the lateral surface of the distal anchoring point and are brought over the skin projection of the medial bundle of the deltoid.

GLENOHUMERAL JOINT

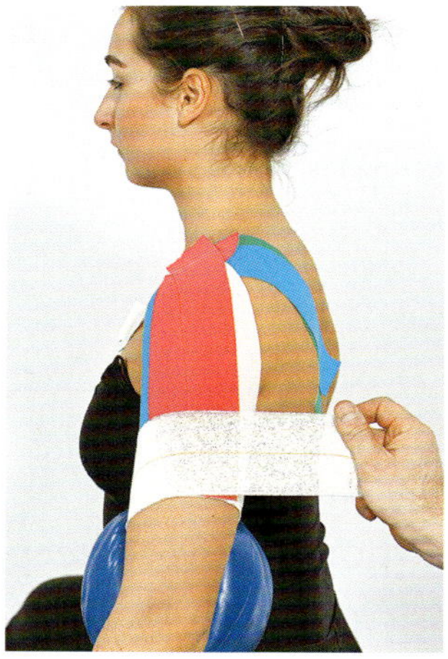
12

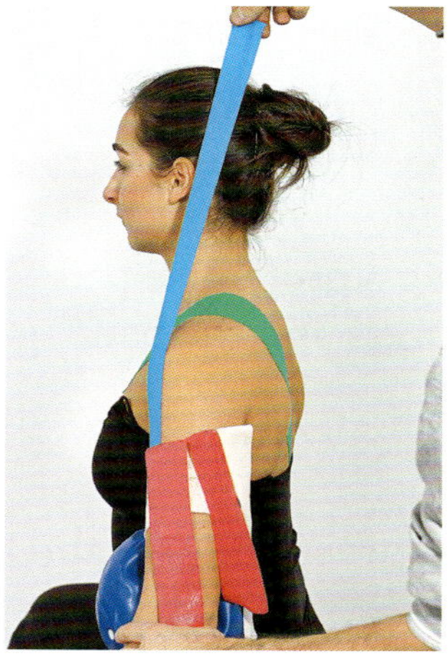
13

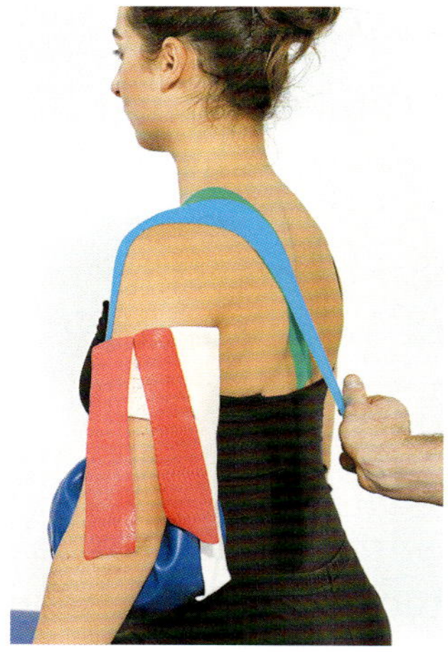
14

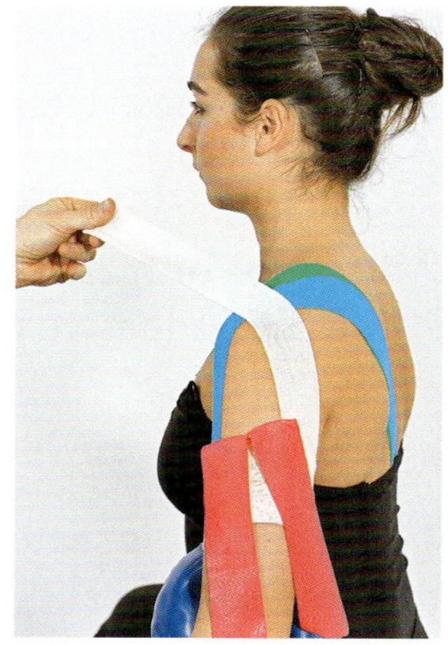
15

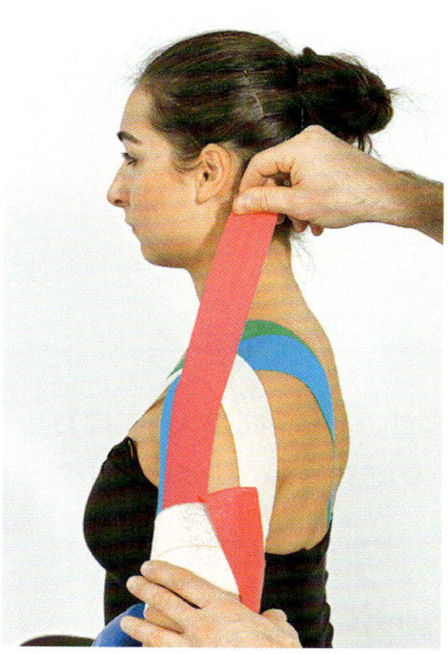
16

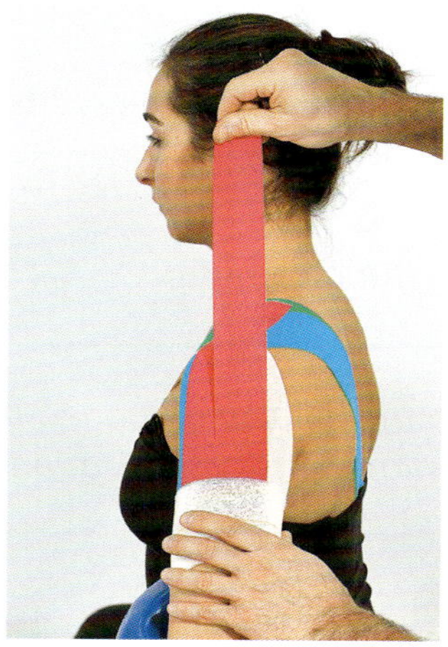
17

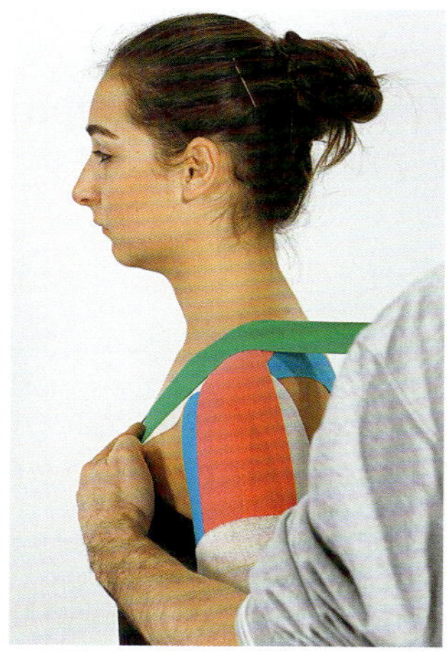
18

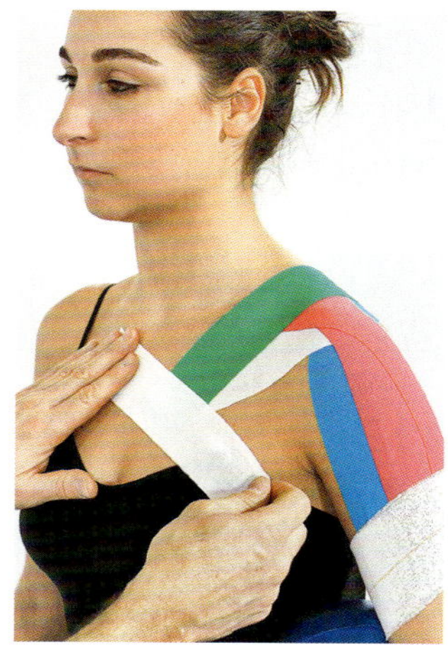
19

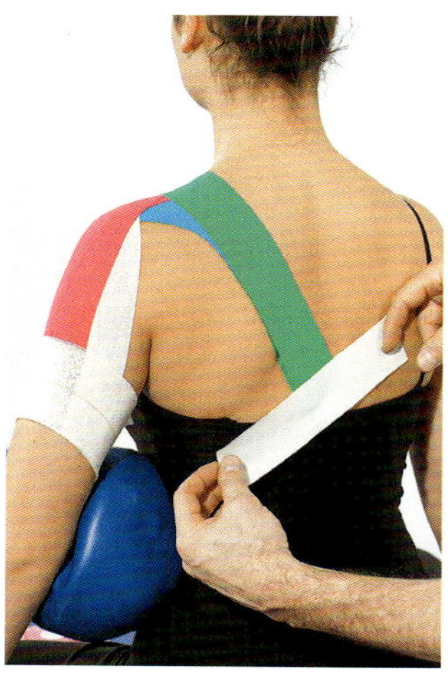
20

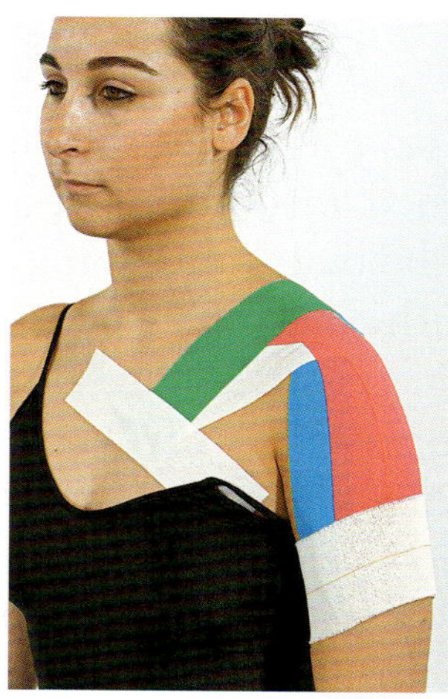
21

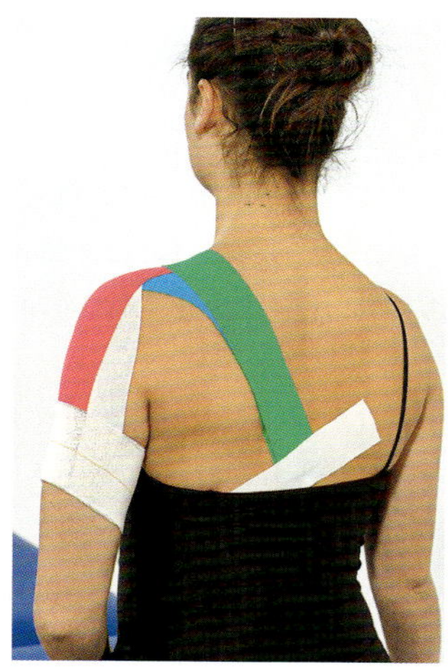
22

Base bandaging with elastic adhesive tape

12 With the piece of bandage at the distal anchorage point that had been left free for this purpose, the pieces of tape applied in the previous steps are affixed.

13-14 With the pieces of bandage allowed to fall backward, bandaging proceeds by stretching the first with 70% tension and bringing it over the skin projection of the acromion (the site of the compress), adhering it posteriorly on the proximal anchoring point.

When applying the pieces of elastic adhesive bandage, the compress must be turned downward in order to create an area of compression.

15 The piece of bandage applied posteriorly on the distal anchoring point is now brought to 70% tension before crossing the first piece of tape at the acromion, and is then affixed anteriorly on the proximal anchoring point.

16-17 Next, the third and fourth pieces of bandage are pulled into 70% tension and are affixed centrally on the proximal anchoring point after crossing over the acromial projection.

18 The pieces of bandage applied in the previous steps are fixed in place with another piece of elastic adhesive tape at the proximal anchoring point.

19-20 Two pieces of inelastic adhesive tape are used to affix the proximal anchoring point anteriorly and posteriorly.

21-22 Bandaging is complete.

INDICATIONS

- ✓ *Chronic instability of the shoulder*
- ✓ *Effects of glenohumeral dislocation or subluxation*
- ✓ *Pain upon movement*

GLENOHUMERAL JOINT

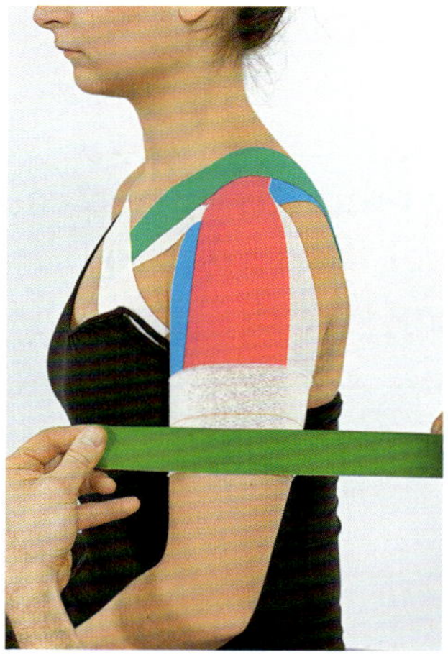

1

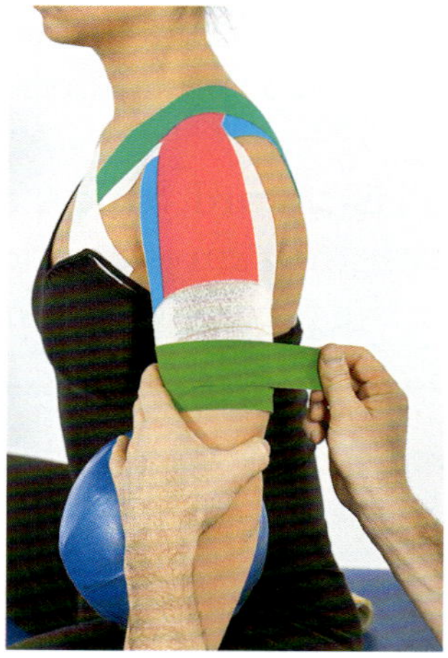

2

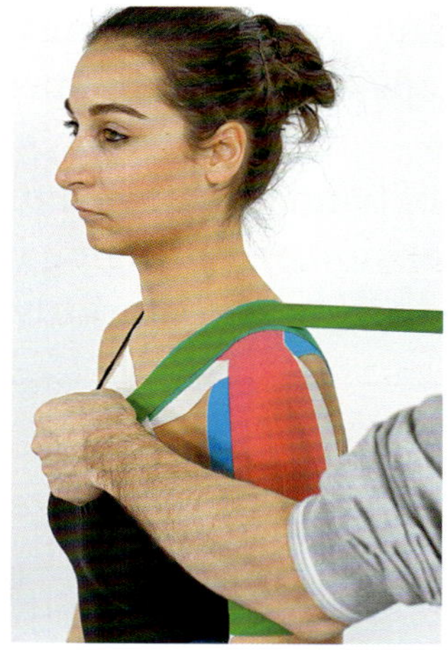

3

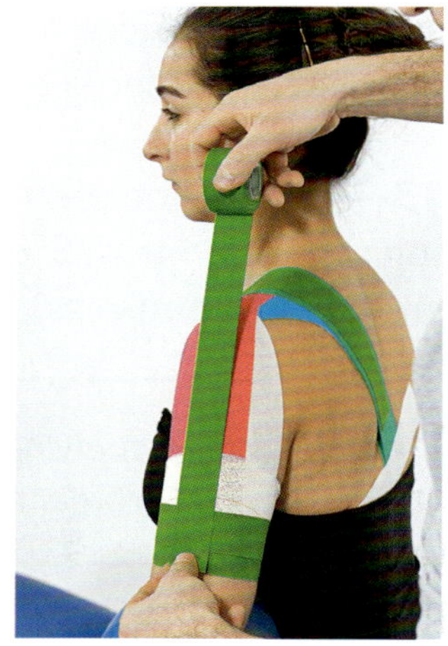

4

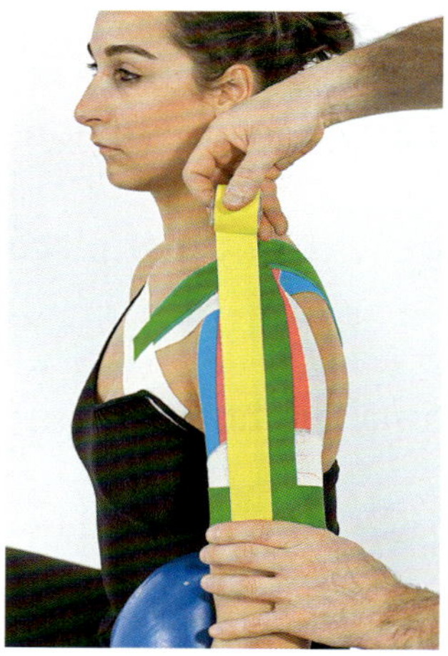

5

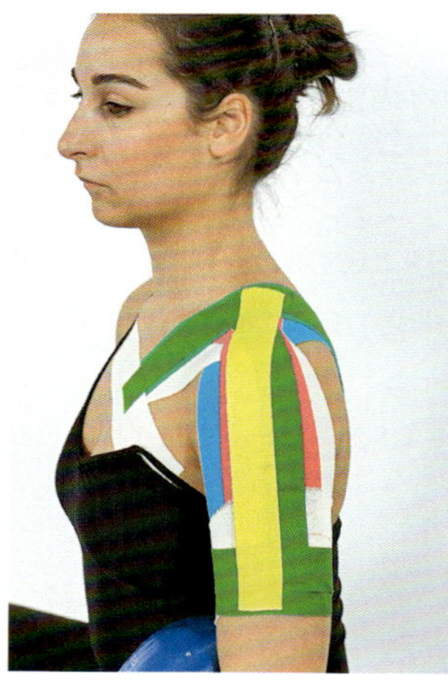

6

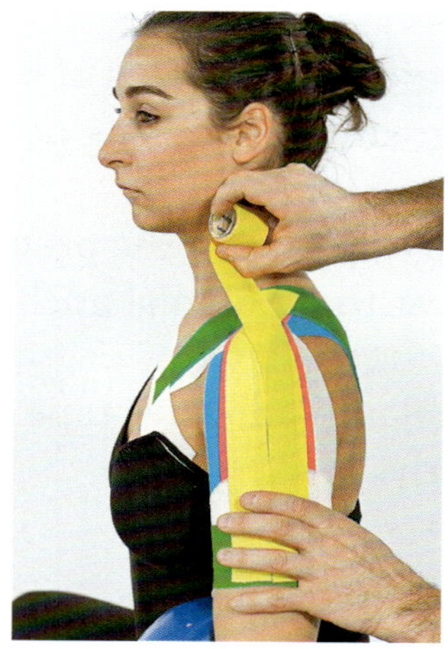

7

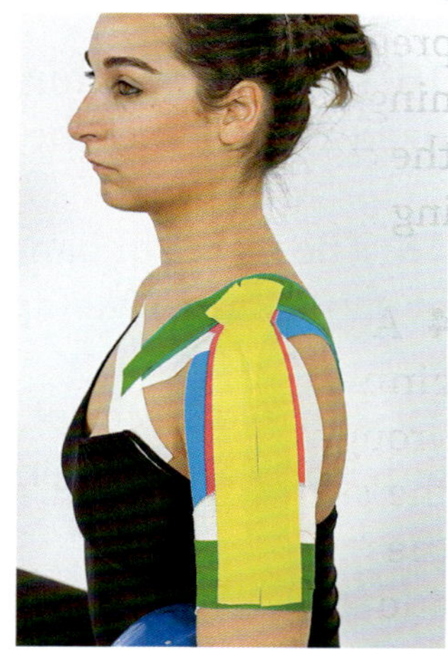

8

Tape-based stabilization and reinforcement of base bandaging

MATERIAL

- ✓ Inelastic adhesive tape
- ✓ 5 cm wide elastic adhesive tape and 10 cm wide porous elastic adhesive bandage for base bandaging
- ✓ Foam rubber or pre-tape compress for creating a compressive pad

APPLICATION

The base bandaging can also be done by using only a cotton fabric porous elastic adhesive bandage of 7.5 cm width.

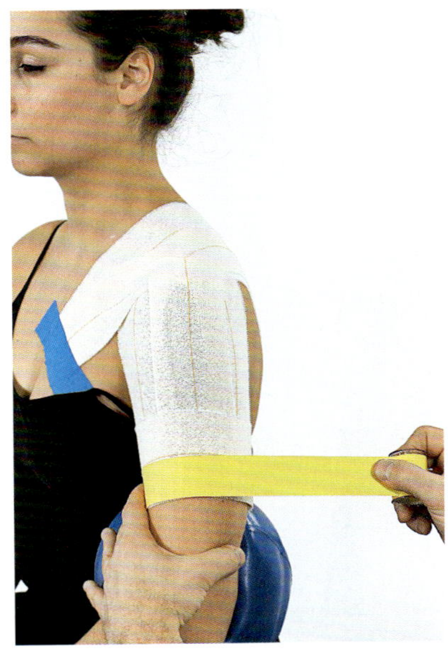

1-2 A distal anchoring point is prepared on the base bandaging with elastic adhesive tape and bandage (see pages 18-21) by applying two strips of inelastic adhesive tape in a semicircle.

3 Another strip of tape is applied in order to prepare a proximal anchoring point, beginning perpendicular to the skin projection of the clavicle at the base of the neck and arriving at the medial bundles of the trapezius.

4 An inelastic adhesive tape is applied beginning at the distal anchoring point and brought in a distal-proximal direction over the skin projection of the medial bundle of the deltoid, then over the acromial process, and finally over the proximal anchoring point.

5-6 Another piece of inelastic adhesive tape is applied to the anterior bundle of the deltoid, going on to cover 25-50% of the previous application.

7-8 A third strip of inelastic adhesive tape proceeds over the posterior bundle of the deltoid, covering 25-50% of the first application.

GLENOHUMERAL JOINT

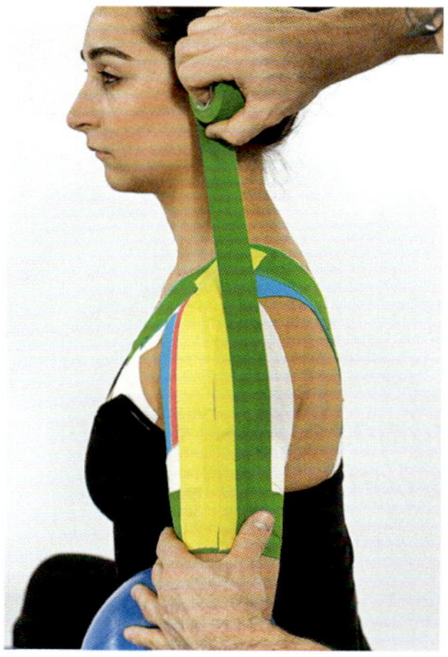
9

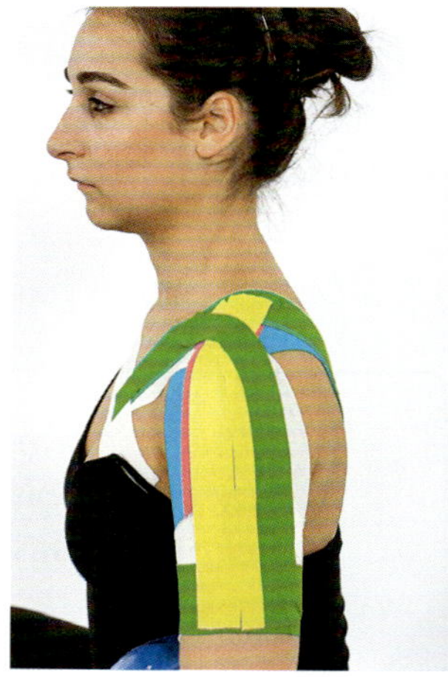
10

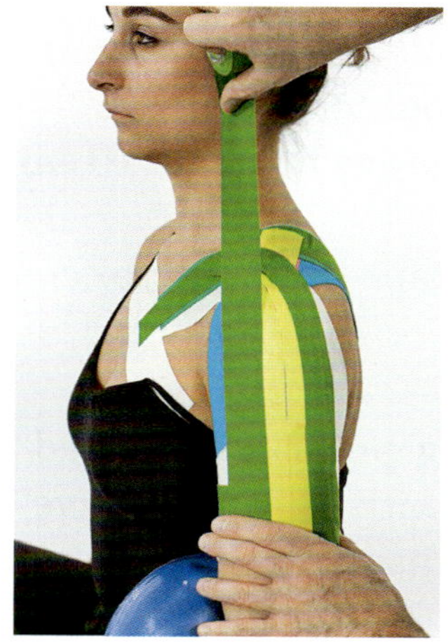
11

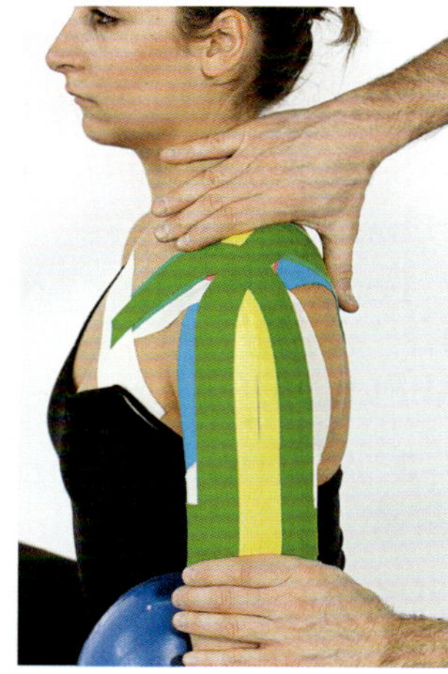
12

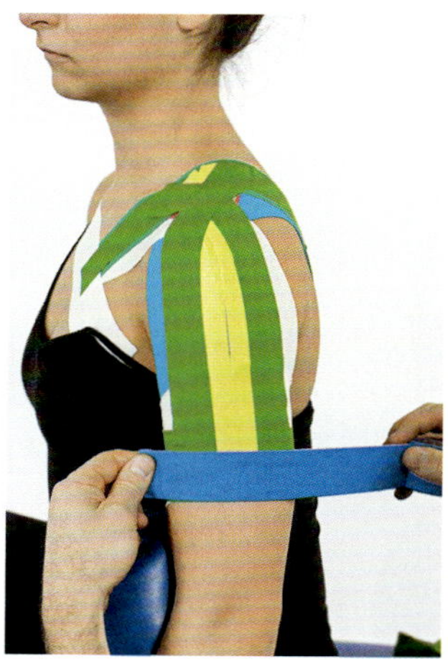
13

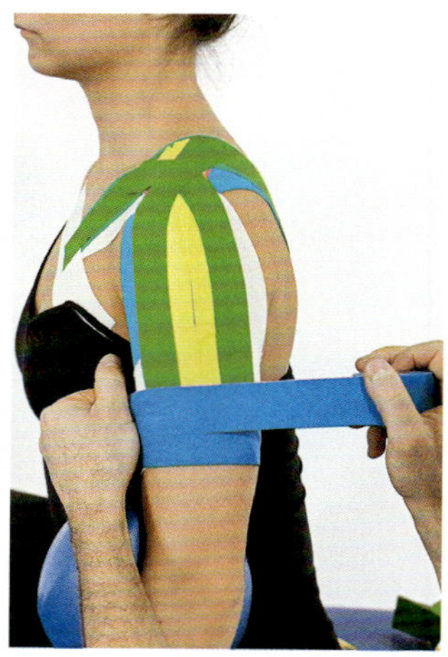
14

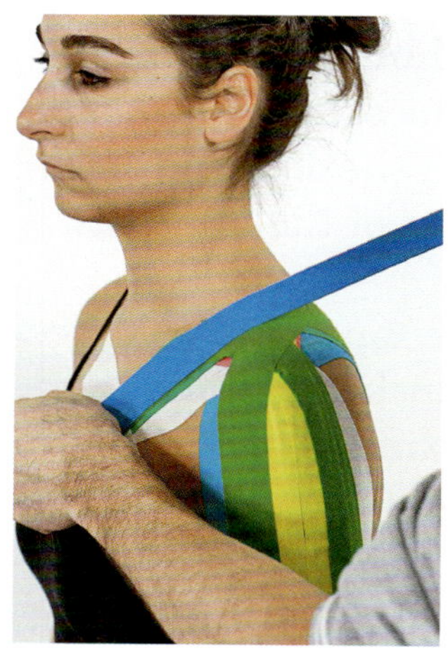
15

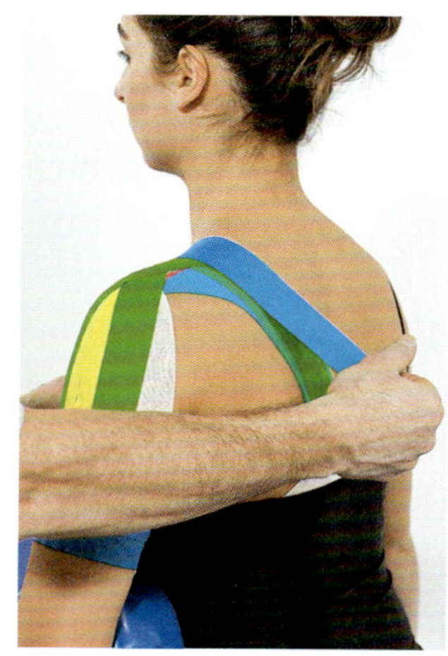
16

Tape-based stabilization and reinforcement of base bandaging

9-10-11-12 Bandaging proceeds by applying two more pieces of tape, placed posteriorly and anteriorly to the previous ones, in such a way as to cover them by 25-50%. The two pieces of tape cross over at the skin projection of the acromion and end on the proximal anchoring point.

13-14-15-16 Bandaging ends with the application of affixing tape on the distal and proximal anchoring points.

INDICATIONS

✓ *Chronic instability of the shoulder*
✓ *Effects of glenohumeral dislocation or subluxation*
✓ *Pain upon movement*

GLENOHUMERAL JOINT

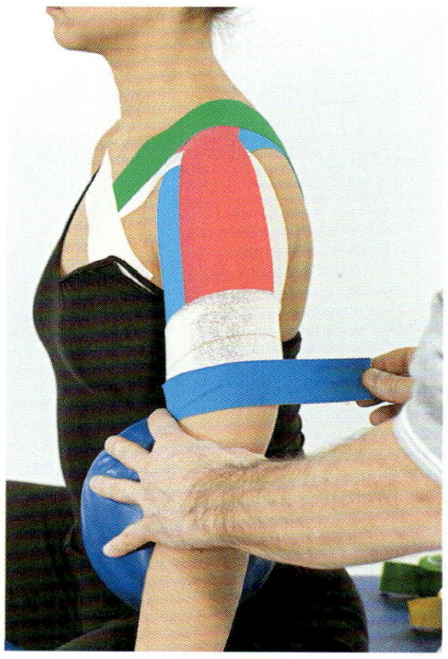

1

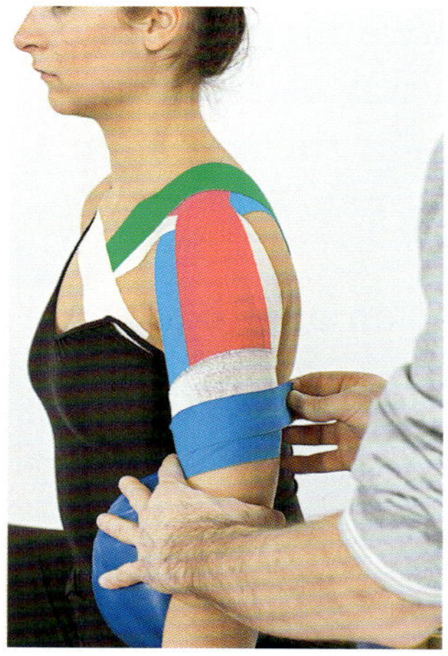

2

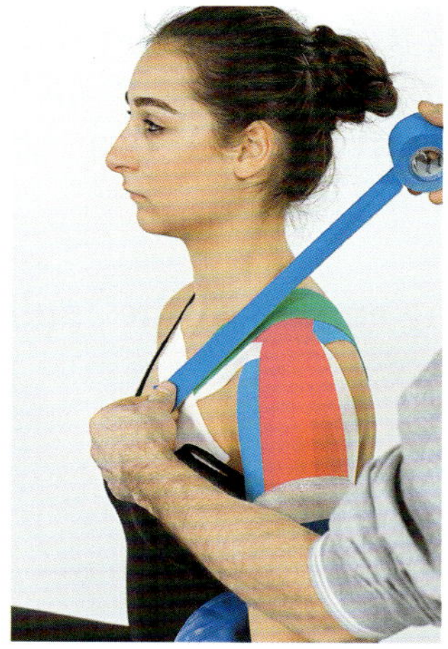

3

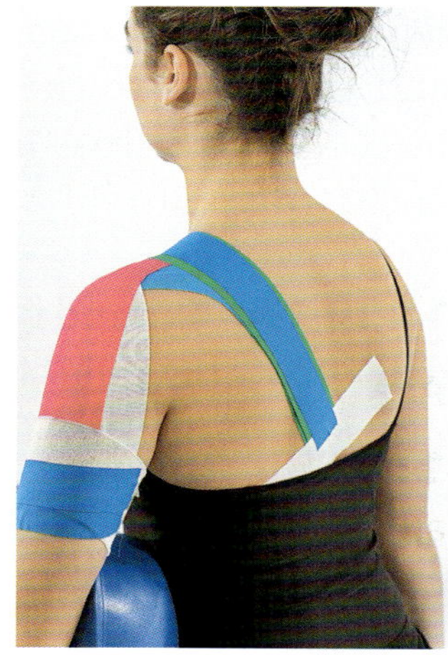

4

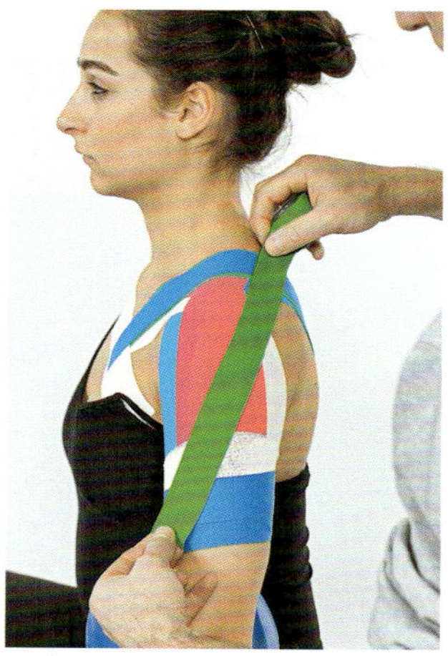

5

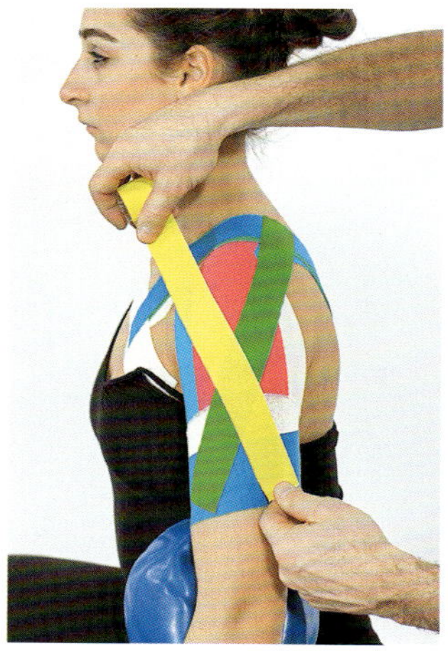

6

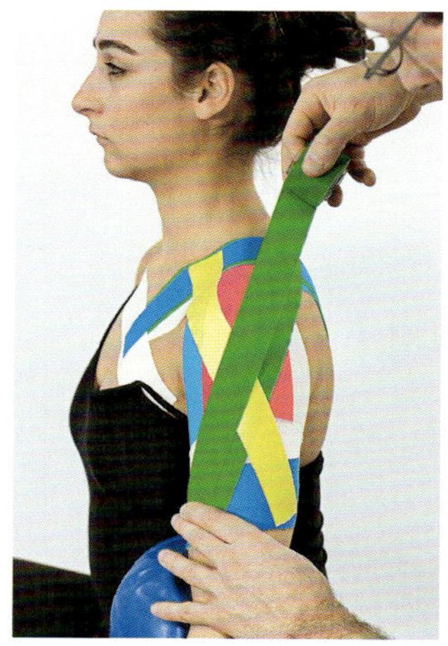

7

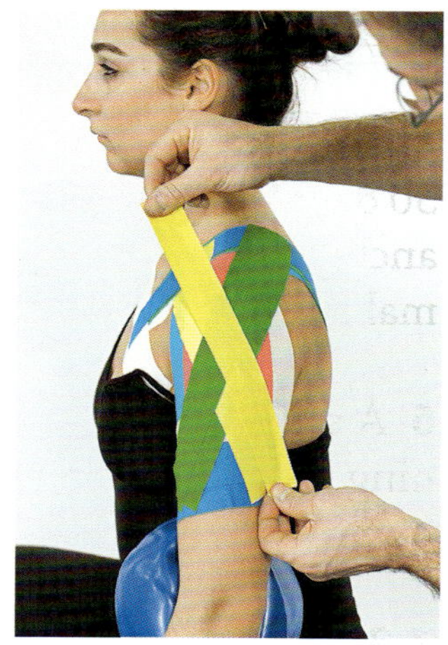

8

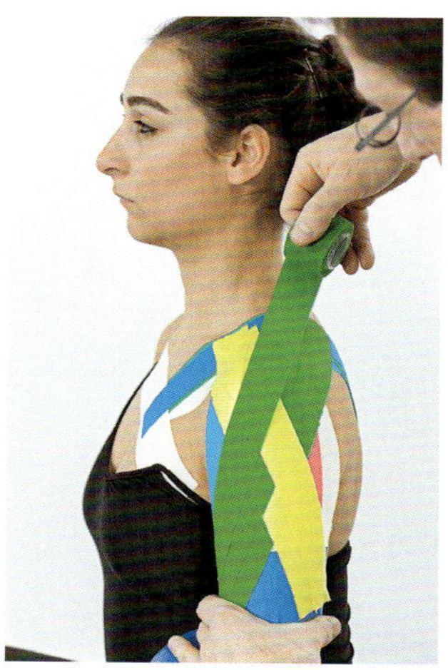

9

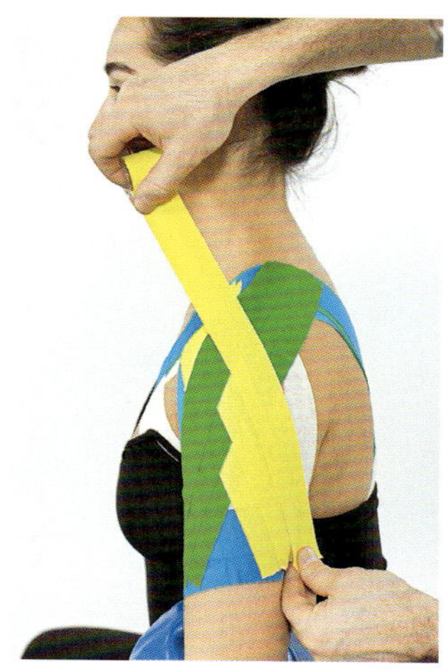

10

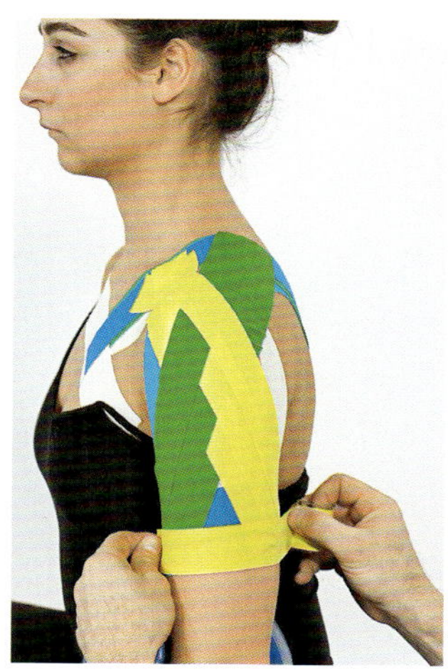

11

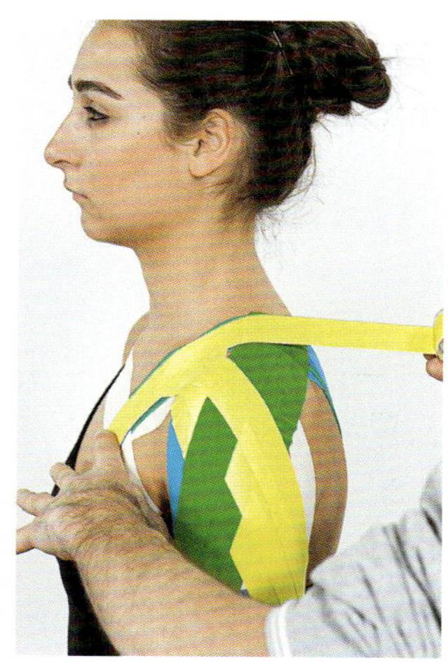

12

Crossing stabilization and reinforcement of base bandaging

MATERIAL

- ✓ Inelastic adhesive tape
- ✓ 5 cm wide elastic adhesive tape and 10 cm wide porous elastic adhesive bandage for base bandaging
- ✓ Pre-tape or foam rubber compress for making a protective pad

APPLICATION

1-2 A distal anchorage point is prepared on the base bandaging with elastic adhesive tape and bandage (see pages 18-21) by applying two strips of inelastic adhesive tape in a semicircle.

3-4 Another strip of tape is applied in order to prepare a proximal anchoring point, beginning perpendicular to the skin projection of the clavicle at the base of the neck and arriving at the medial bundles of the trapezius.

5 The first piece of inelastic adhesive tape is applied with an inclination between 15 and 30 degrees (depending on muscle volume), beginning from the anterior surface of the distal anchoring point, passing over the posterior bundle of the deltoid, and affixing to the proximal anchoring point.

6 A second strip of tape is applied with an inclination between 15 and 30 degrees, beginning from the posterior surface of the distal anchoring point, passing over the anterior bundle of the deltoid, and affixing to the proximal anchoring point.

7-8-9-10 Bandaging proceeds, covering the entire deltoid with strips of inelastic adhesive material, positioned parallel to the previous ones and overlapping them by 25-50%.

11-12 Bandaging ends with the application of affixing tape on the distal and proximal anchoring points.

INDICATIONS

- ✓ *Chronic instability of the shoulder*
- ✓ *Effects of glenohumeral dislocation or subluxation*
- ✓ *Pain upon movement*

GLENOHUMERAL JOINT

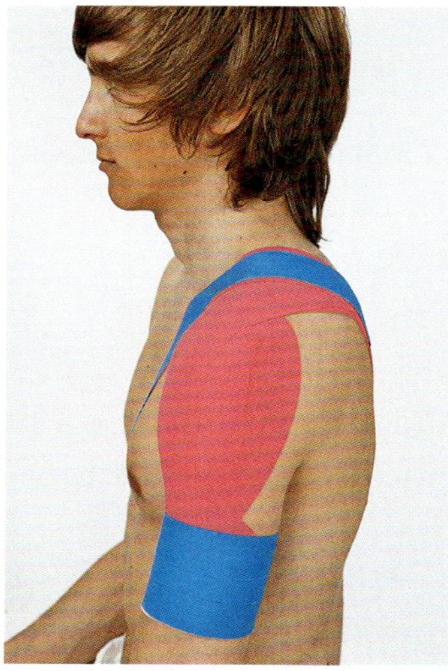
1

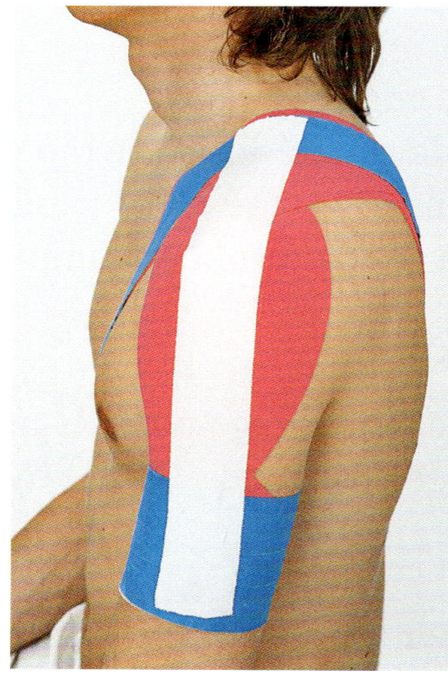
2

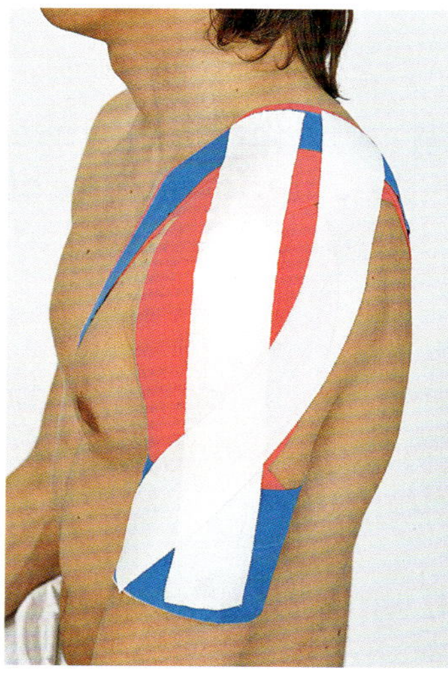
3

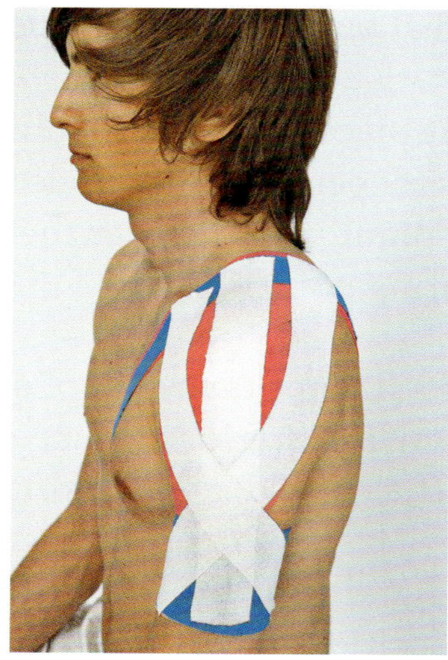
4

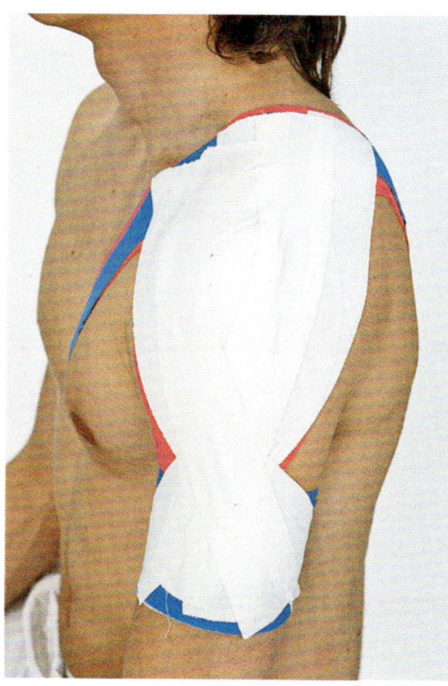
5

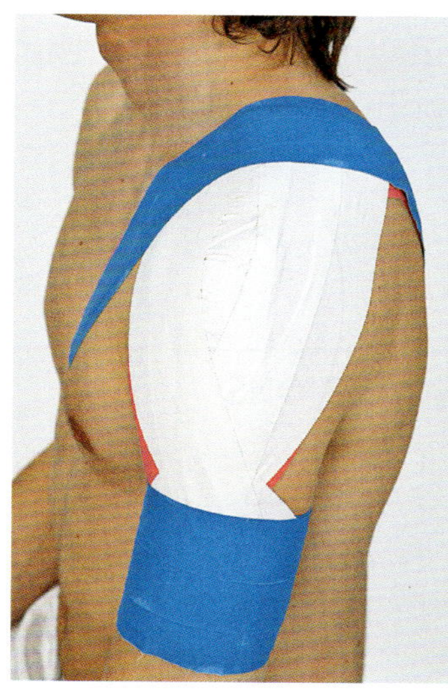
6

Stabilization and reinforcement of tape base bandaging

MATERIAL

- ✓ Inelastic adhesive tape, 5 cm in width
- ✓ 5 cm wide elastic adhesive tape for base bandaging
- ✓ Pre-tape or foam rubber compress for making a protective pad

APPLICATION

1 To begin, base bandaging is prepared (see pages 18-21) using only elastic adhesive tape strips, also to establish anchoring points and affix the tape.

2 A strip of inelastic adhesive tape is applied following the longitudinal direction of the arm, beginning from the distal anchoring point and proceeding to the proximal one, passing over the skin projection of the acromion.

3 A second strip of inelastic adhesive tape is applied, following the skin projection of the anterior bundle of the deltoid.

4 A third strip of inelastic adhesive tape is applied, following the skin projection of the posterior bundle of the deltoid.

5 Bandaging proceeds by applying some strips of inelastic adhesive tape running parallel to the previous ones until all open spaces are covered.

6 Bandaging is refined and set in place by applying strips of elastic or inelastic adhesive tape.

INDICATIONS

- ✓ *Chronic instability of the shoulder*
- ✓ *Effects of glenohumeral dislocation or subluxation*
- ✓ *Pain upon movement*

GLENOHUMERAL JOINT

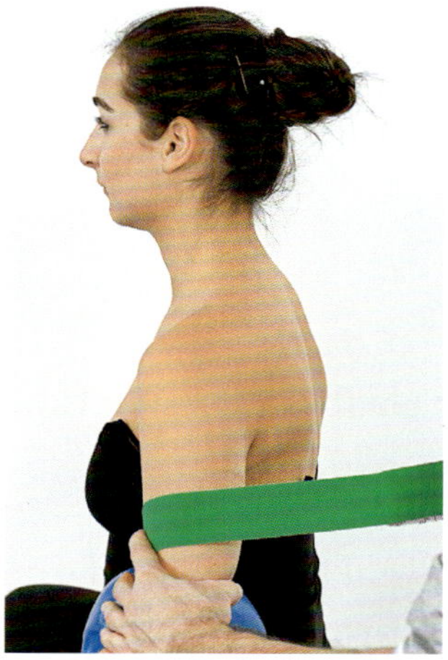

1

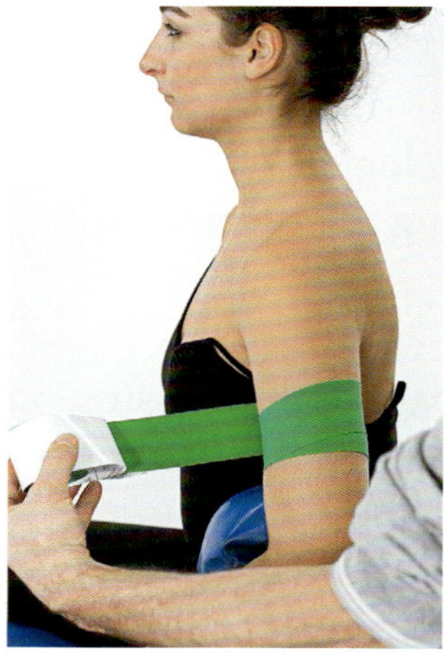

2

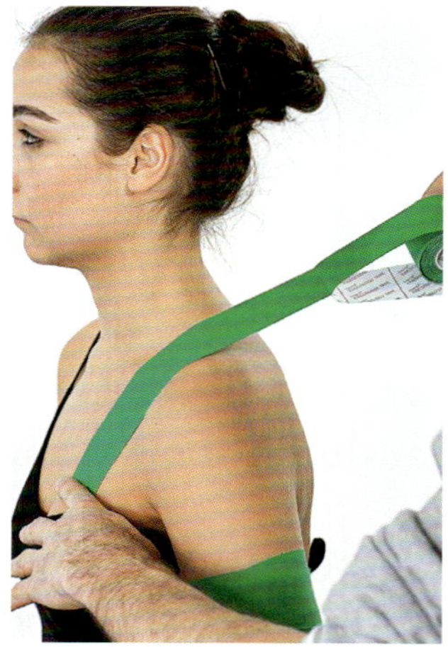

3

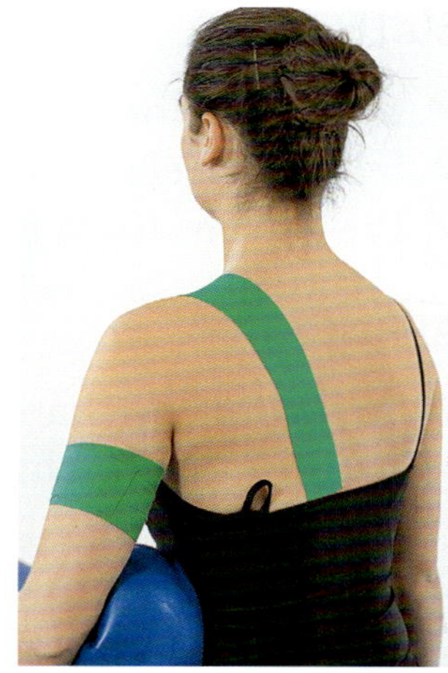

4

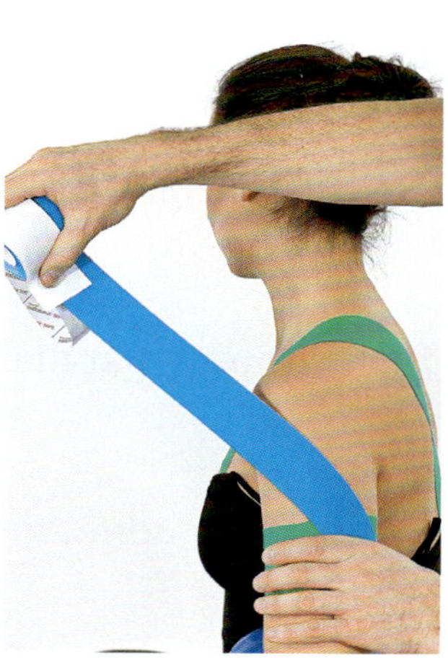

5

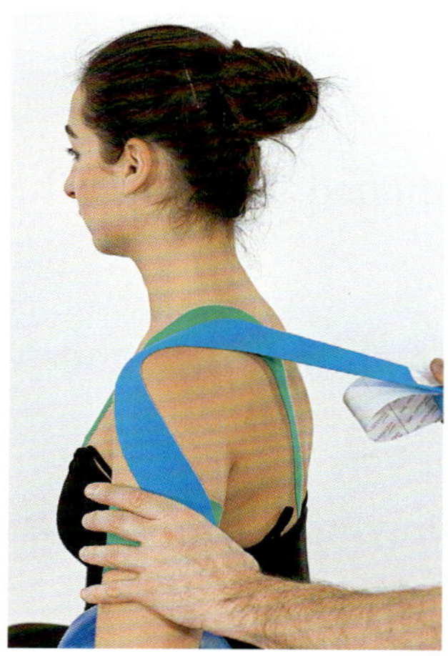

6

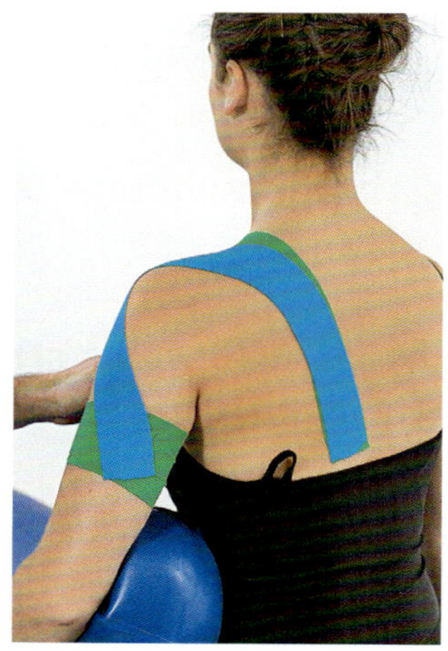

7

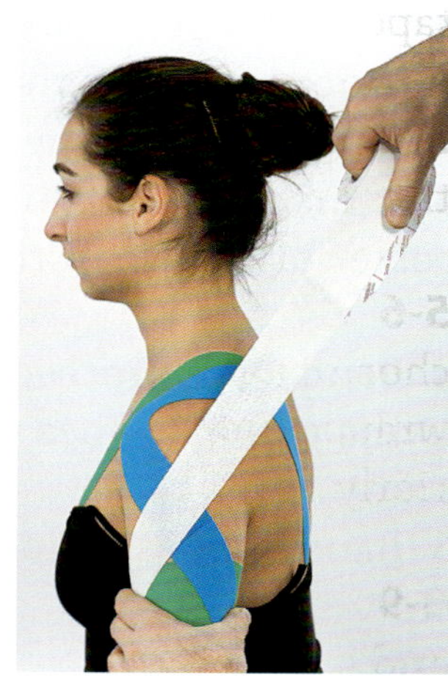

8

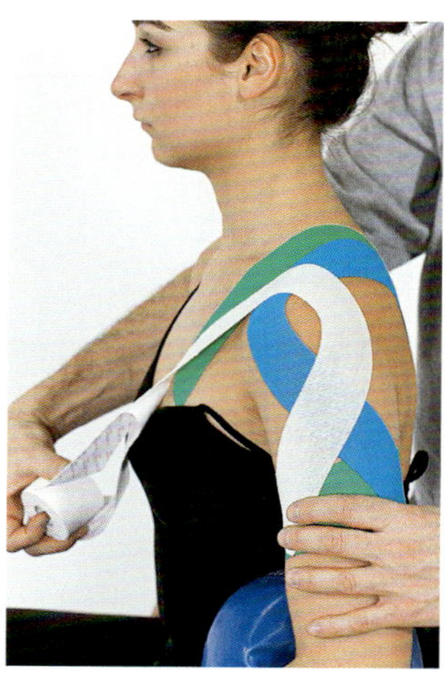

9

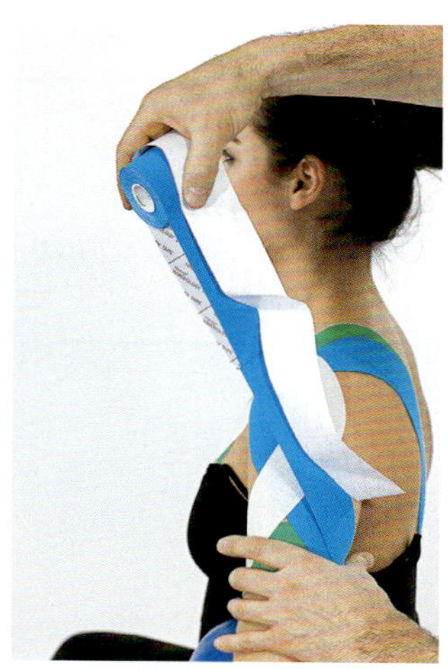

10

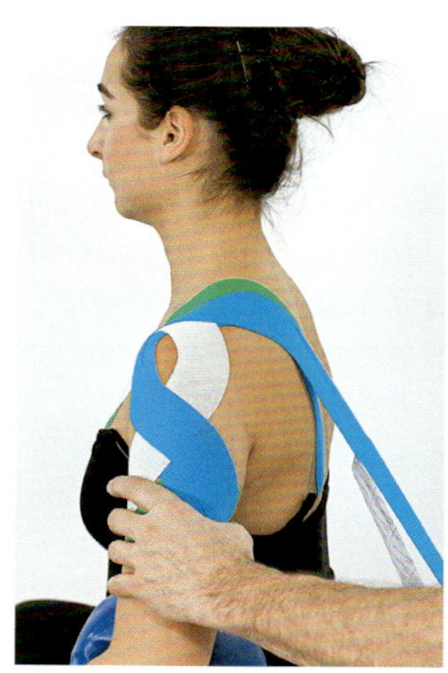

11

Unloading, retention, and guidance of movement

MATERIAL

✓ Elastic adhesive tape, extensible lengthwise, 5 cm in width
✓ 5 cm wide inelastic adhesive tape to affix bandaging

The use of elastic adhesive tape is particularly recommended when dealing with sensitive skin, and above all if it is necessary to maintain bandaging for several days.

APPLICATION

1-2 The subject is seated with a cushion or ball between the arm and the thorax so as to keep the limb slightly abducted. A distal anchoring point is prepared with a full wrap of the tape around the arm at the tendinous insertion of the deltoid.

3-4 The proximal anchoring point is made with a strip of tape applied from the clavicle to the medial bundle of the trapezius.

5-6-7 A piece of elastic adhesive tape is adhered to the posterior surface of the distal anchoring point and is put under tension, guiding it in an anterior direction. The tape is wrapped around the anterior skin projection of the humeral head, then is directed posteriorly and is affixed to the back above the posterior part of the proximal anchoring point.

8-9 Another strip of tape is applied to the anterior surface of the distal anchoring point and put under tension, then directed posteriorly to wrap around the humeral head; the tape is pulled anteriorly and affixed at the anterior part of the proximal anchoring point.

10-11 At this point, another piece of tape is applied over the first, covering it by 50%. The same course is repeated, beginning from the posterior surface of the distal anchoring point, wrapping around the humeral head, and arriving over the posterior part of the proximal anchoring point.

GLENOHUMERAL JOINT

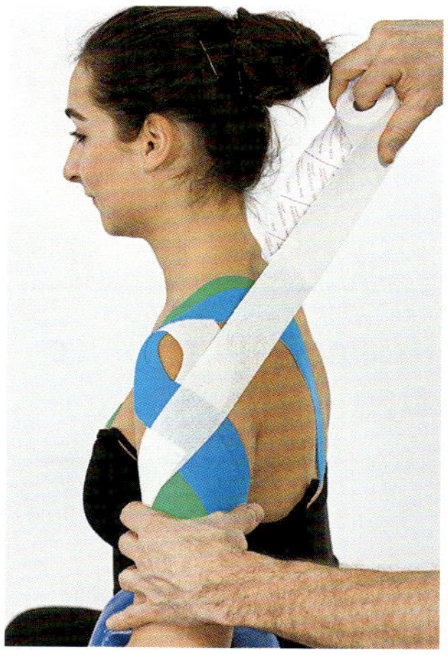

12

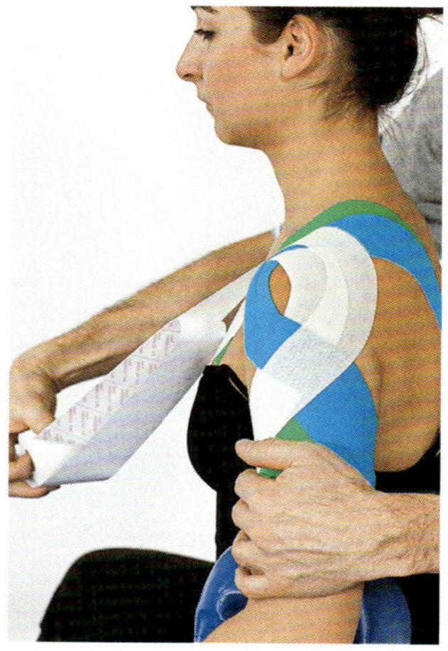

13

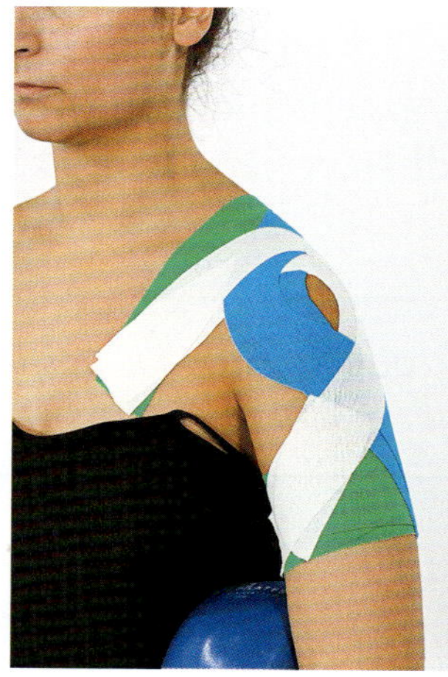

14

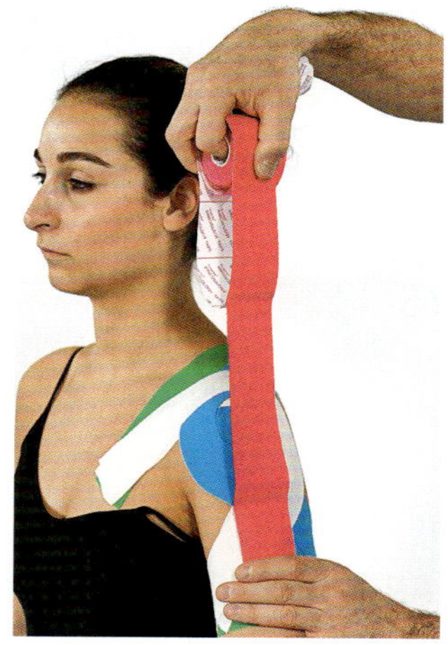

15

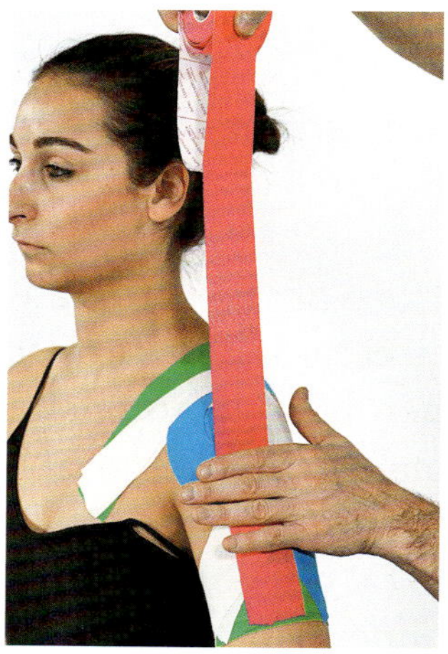

16

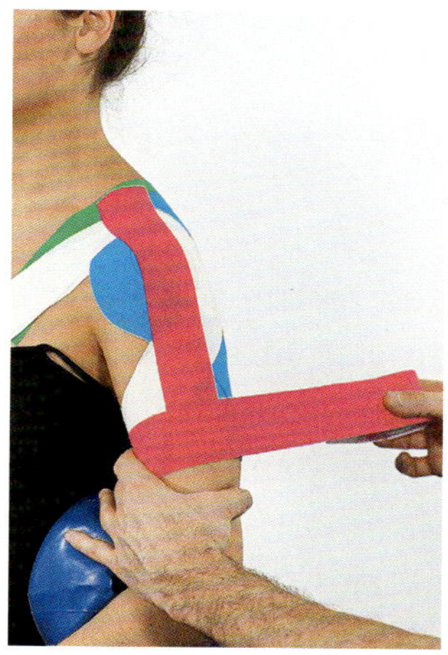

17

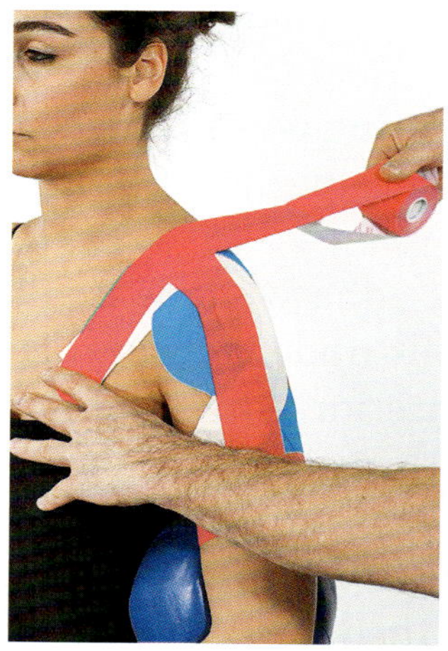

18

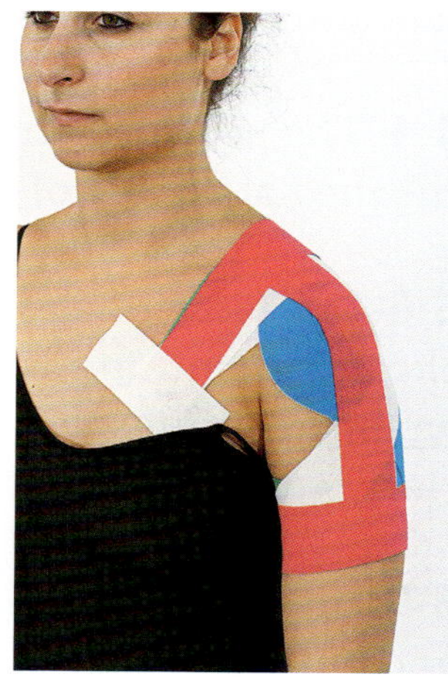

19

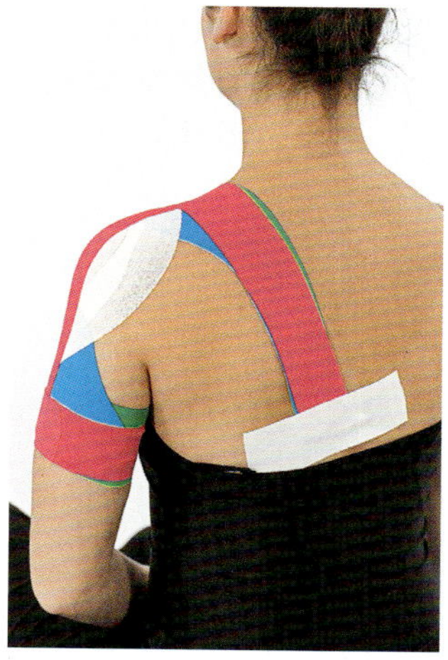

20

Unloading, retention, and guidance of movement

12-13-14 At this point, a fourth piece of tape is applied over the second, covering it by 50%. The same course is repeated, beginning from the anterior surface of the distal anchoring point, wrapping around the humeral head, and arriving over the anterior part of the proximal anchoring point.

15-16 Finally, a piece of tape is applied to cover the skin projection of the medial bundle of the deltoid, from the distal anchoring point to the proximal one.

17-18 Bandaging finishes with the application of affixing tape on the distal and proximal anchoring points.

19-20 The proximal anchoring point is affixed anteriorly and posteriorly with two pieces of inelastic adhesive tape.

Bandaging is completed with the application of elastic retention using a cohesive bandage to hold everything in place, following the base bandaging described on page 36.

INDICATIONS

- ✓ *Chronic instability of the shoulder*
- ✓ *Posttraumatic functional recovery*
- ✓ *Guide to technical motion*
- ✓ *Retention for aftereffects of glenohumeral dislocation and subluxation*

GLENOHUMERAL JOINT

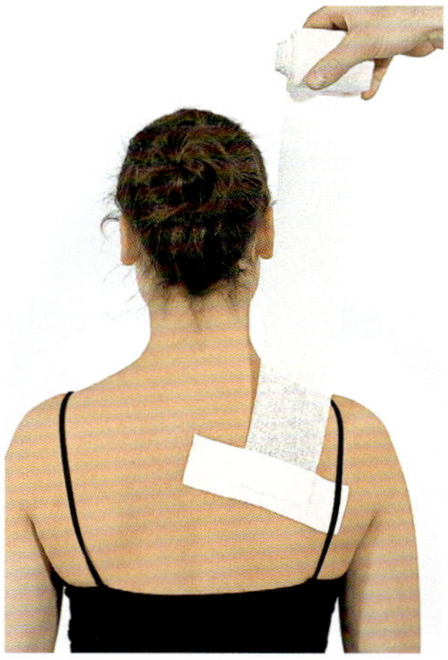

1

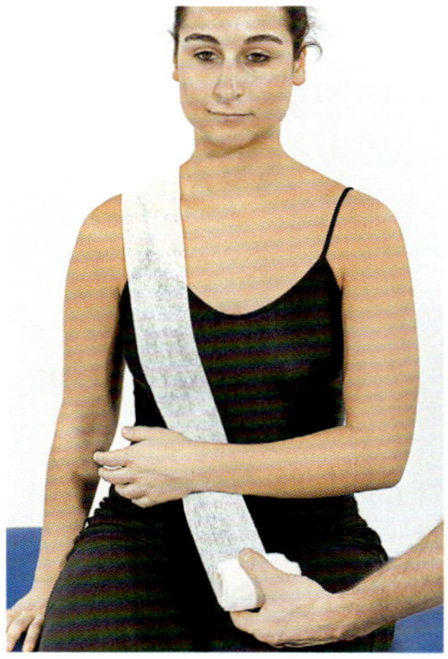

2

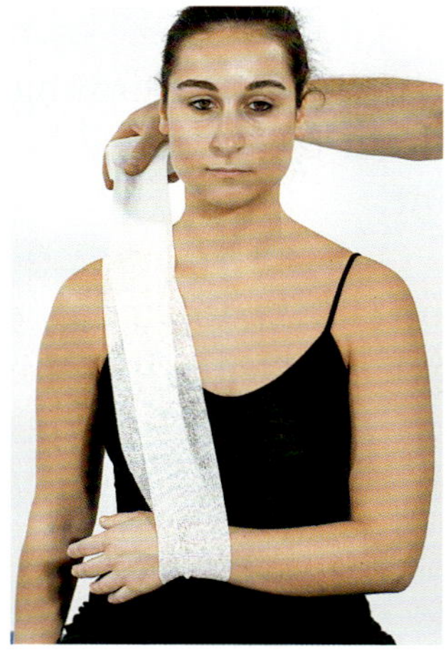

3

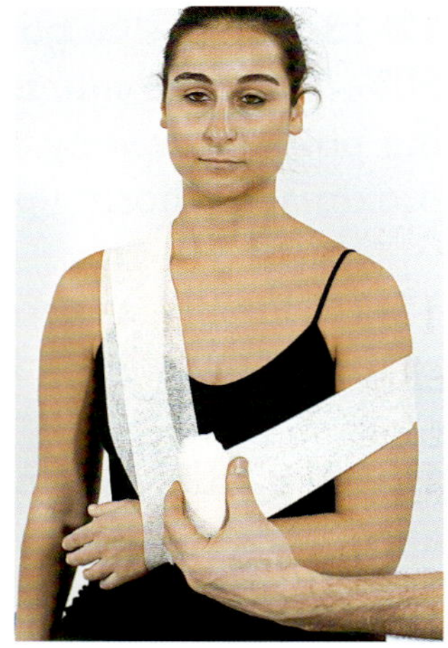

4

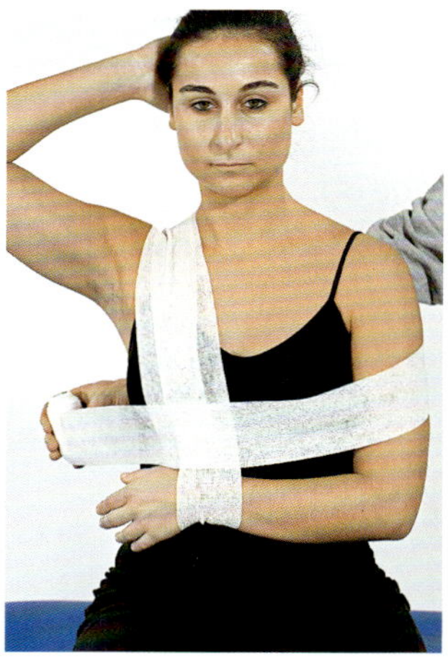

5

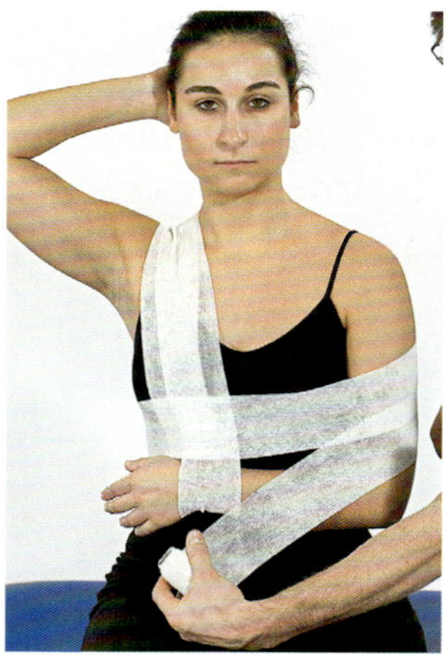

6

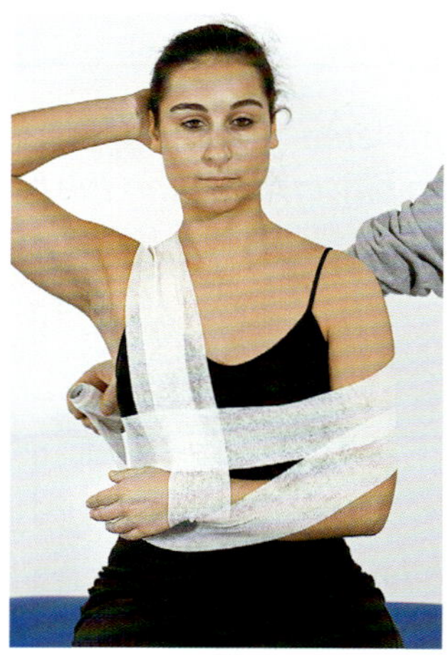

7

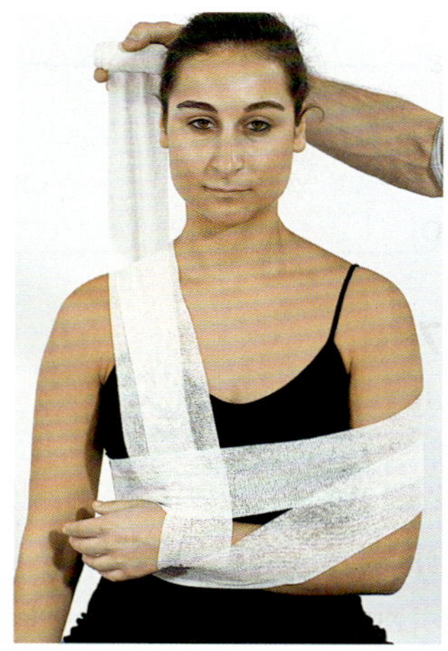

8

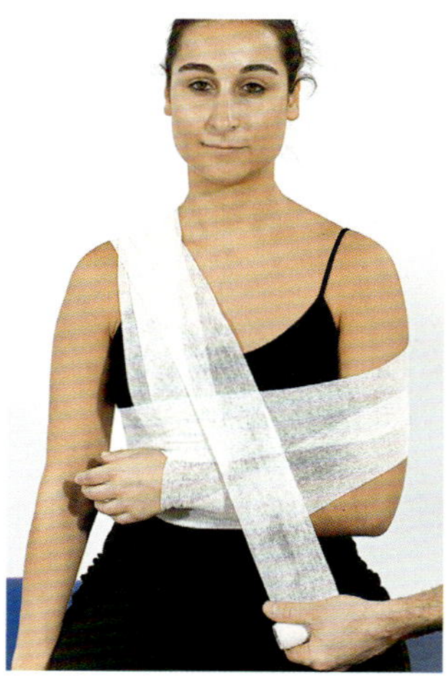

9

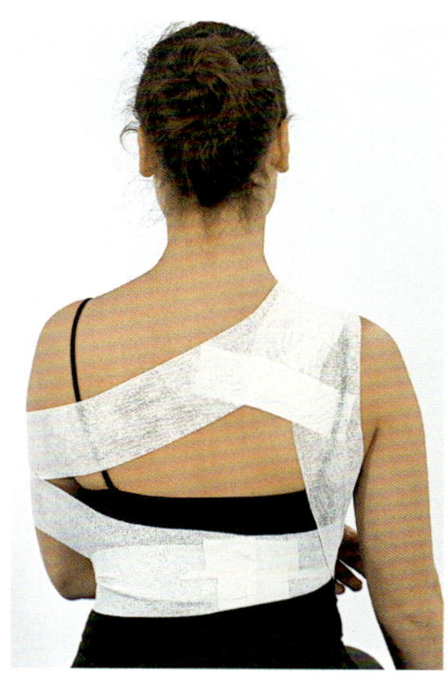

10

Limitation of outward rotation and abduction

MATERIAL

✓ Elastic bandaging, extensible lengthwise, 8-10 cm in width
✓ Inelastic adhesive tape for affixing the bandage

APPLICATION

1 The subject is seated with the upper limb adducted and rotated inwardly, and with the elbow flexed. The elastic bandage is affixed posteriorly with a strip of inelastic adhesive tape applied on the back at the skin projection of the posterior surface of the scapula. The elastic bandage is put under tension by pulling it upward.

2-3 The bandage is brought over the shoulder, then anteriorly downward, bringing it between the abdomen and the wrist, to then return upward toward the same shoulder.

4 The bandage then crosses the back and goes on to wrap around the arm, reappearing anteriorly.

5-6 Crossing the vertical path of the bandage acting as support for the forearm, one wrap of the bandage is made around the chest.

7-8 At this point, the bandage is brought diagonally over the forearm so as to reinforce the support, passes posteriorly, and is then directed upward to the shoulder.

9-10 After passing the shoulder, the bandage crosses the chest diagonally, passes under the elbow, and reaches the back, where it is affixed to the previous wrap of bandage using a strip of inelastic adhesive tape.

INDICATIONS

✓ *Posttraumatic support*

GLENOHUMERAL JOINT

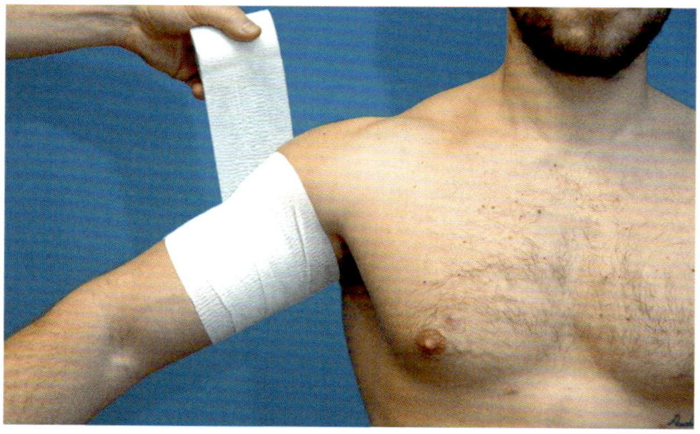

1

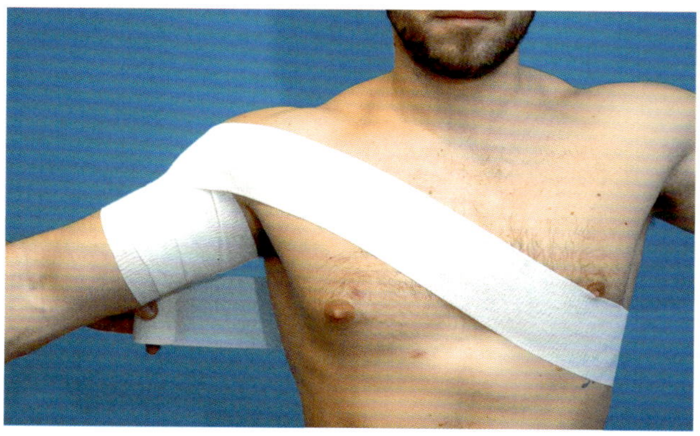

2

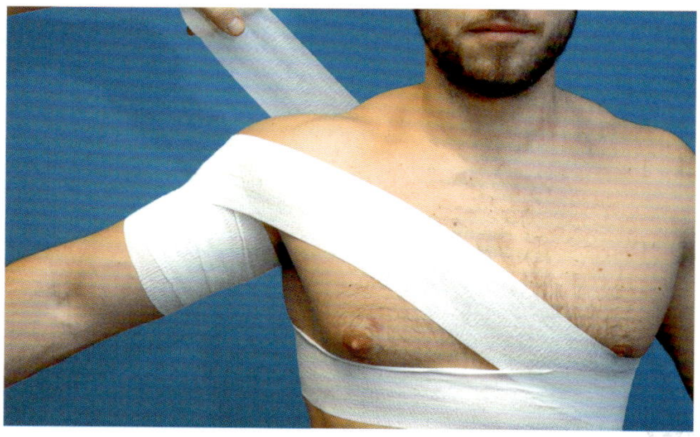

3

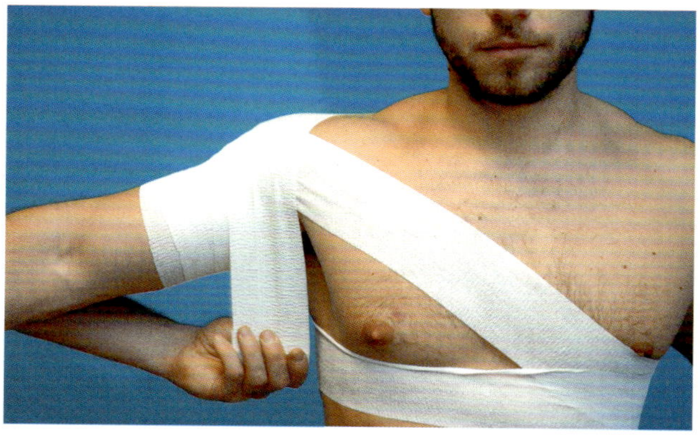

4

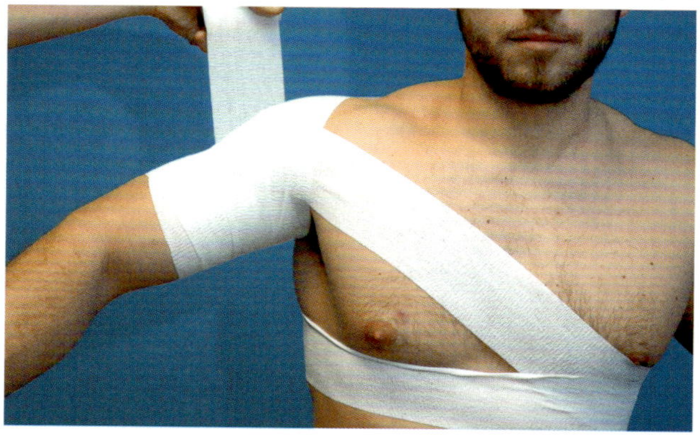

5

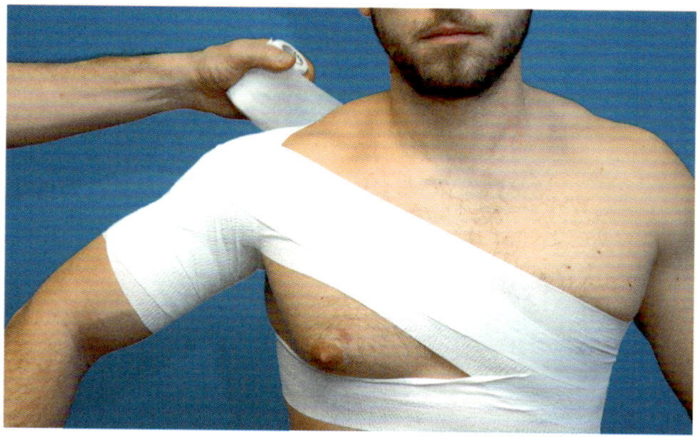

6

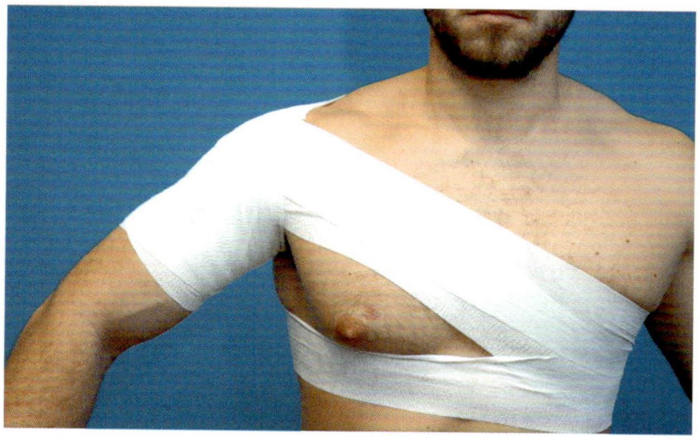

7

Stabilization and limitation of outward rotation

MATERIAL

- ✓ Elastic cohesive bandage
- ✓ Cotton fabric porous elastic adhesive bandage that can be stretched lengthwise, 7.5 cm in width

APPLICATION

1 The subject positions their arm in abduction and internal rotation. With the cohesive bandage, some wrappings are made to cover the axis of the humerus in a distal-proximal direction, from the distal third of the arm to the proximal third. The bandage wrappings follow the direction of inward rotation of the arm.

2 The bandage is brought diagonally across to wrap around the thorax.

3 The bandage is wrapped around the thorax.

4 The bandage goes toward the shoulder in order to cover the acromioclavicular joint.

5 A complete wrapping of the bandage is made proximally around the arm.

6-7 The bandage is brought in a diagonal direction to wrap around the thorax and then return posteriorly toward the shoulder, where it is affixed.

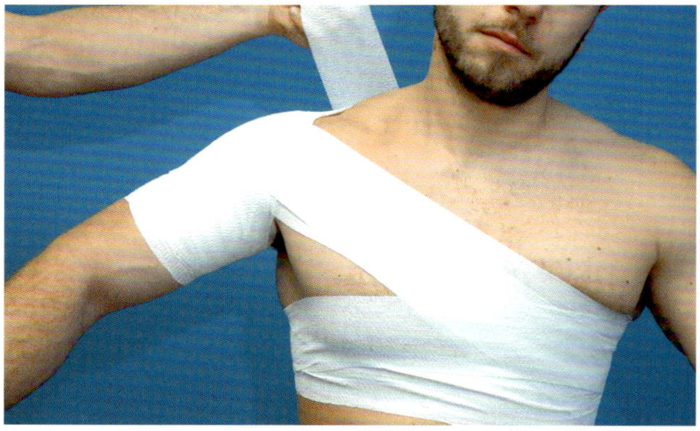
8

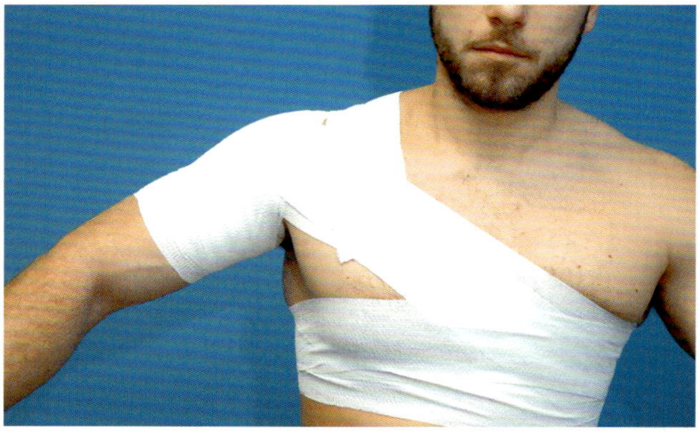
9

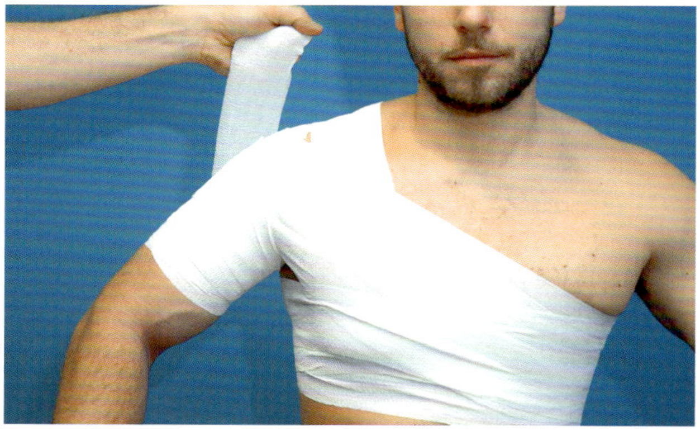
10

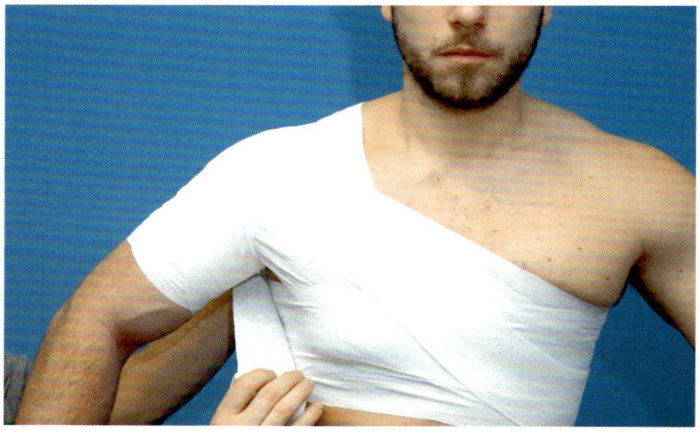
11

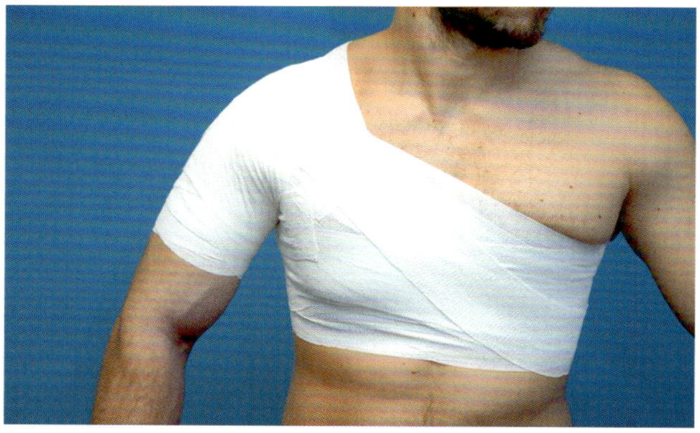
12

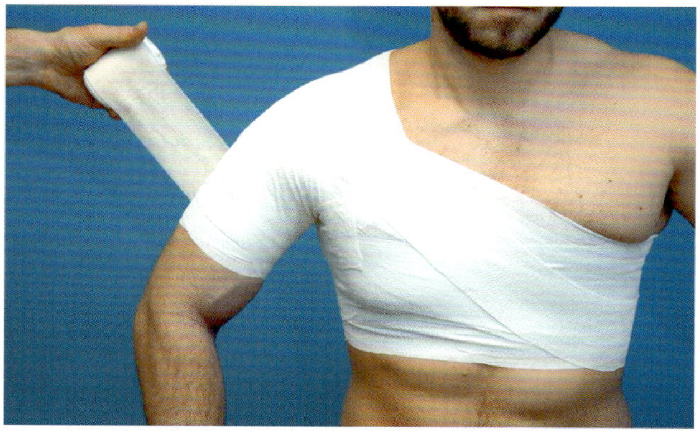
13

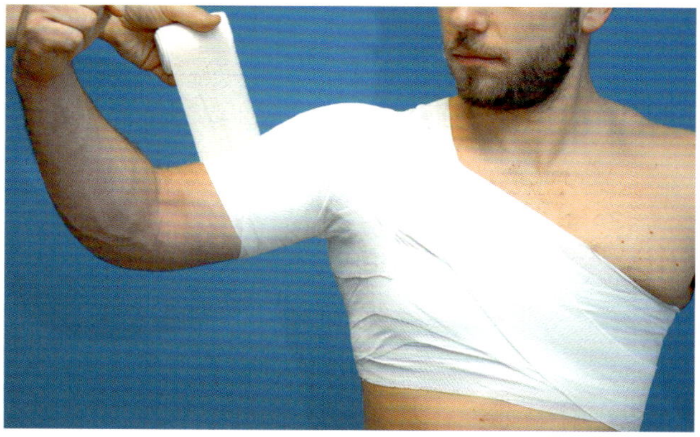
14

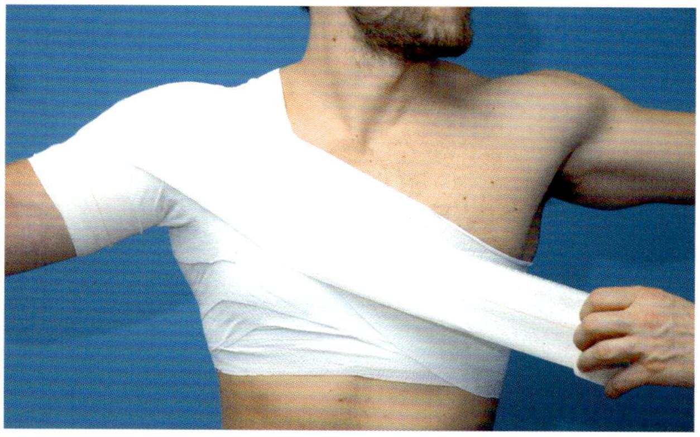
15

Stabilization and limitation of outward rotation

8-9 Several strips of cohesive bandage are applied over the open spaces in order to cover the skin projection of the trapezius. The strips are applied transversely to the direction of the muscle fibers of the scapula in the direction of the pectoralis muscle.

10-11-12 Final bandaging begins from the proximal third of the arm, directed toward the shoulder, then diagonally over the chest to again wrap around the thorax before turning to the opposite side to cover the open spaces over the axillary cavity. Base bandaging is thus completed.

13-14 A complete wrapping is done with the mono-extensible elastic adhesive bandage, distally wrapping around the axis of the humerus. The bandage is directed so as to favor inward rotation and limit outward. The subject's arm is still in abduction, but is now slightly rotated outward.

15 The bandage is brought diagonally until it wraps around the thorax.

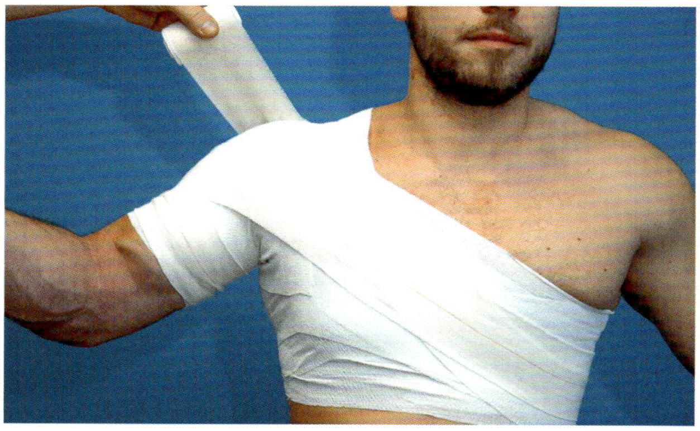

16

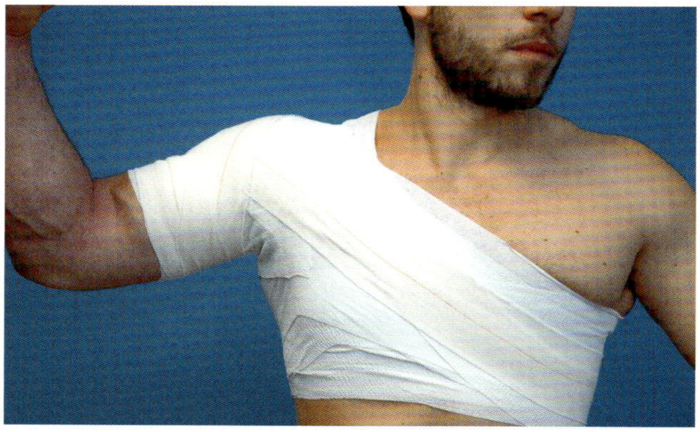

17

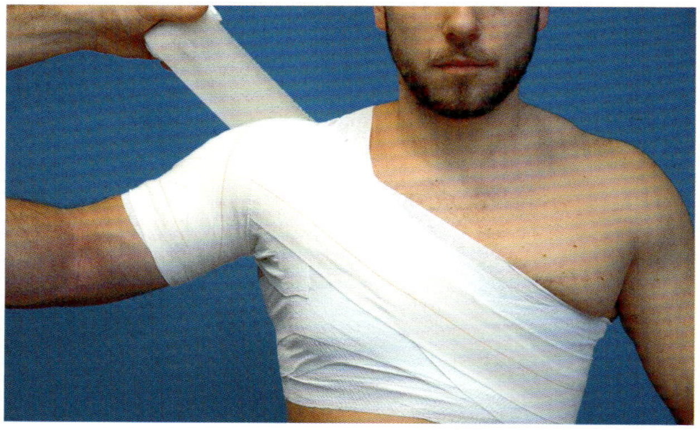

18

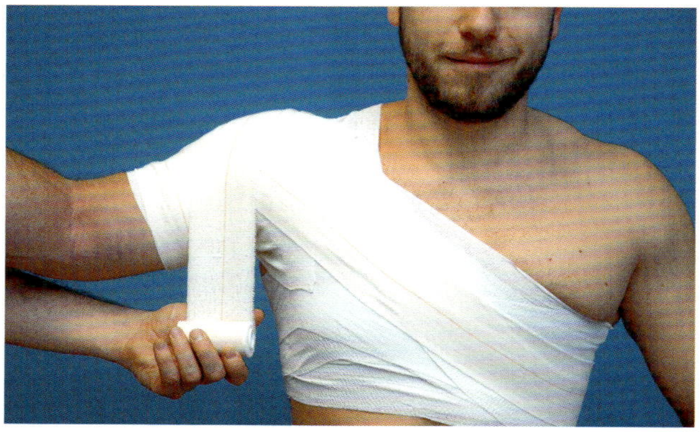

19

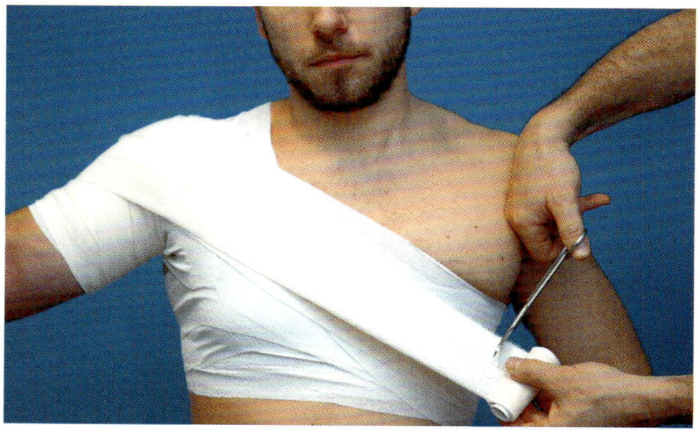

20

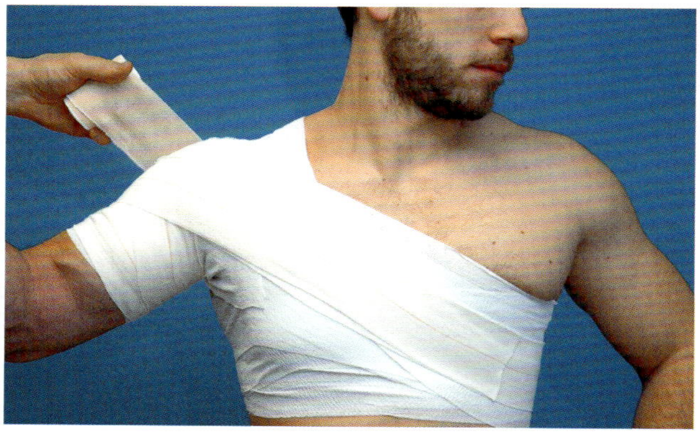

21

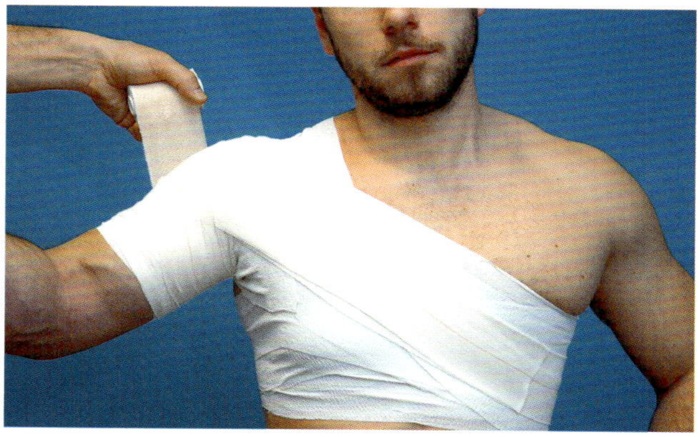

22

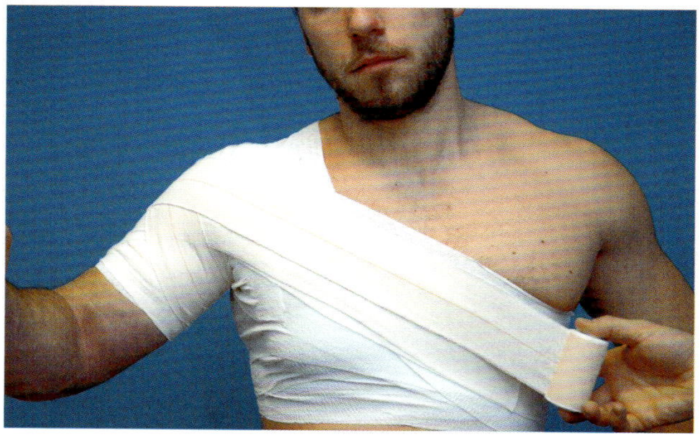

23

Stabilization and limitation of outward rotation

16-17 The bandage is brought toward the shoulder in order to cover the acromion and the glenohumeral joint. Another complete wrap is made around the arm, after crossing the path of the previous bandage.

18-19 Two mono-extensible adhesive elastic bandages are applied in a figure eight in order to stabilize the glenohumeral joint. First, the first strip of bandage is affixed posteriorly on the scapular projection, and is directed to cover the glenohumeral joint. Next, a complete wrapping is done around the axis of the humerus.

20 The bandage is directed anteriorly over the thorax and is cut once the contralateral half of the thorax is reached.

21-22-23 Bandaging proceeds with the application of the second strip of bandage parallel to the first: the bandage begins from the scapular projection, wraps around the glenohumeral joint, does a complete turn around the arm, is brought anteriorly, and is cut once it reaches the contralateral half of the thorax.

GLENOHUMERAL JOINT

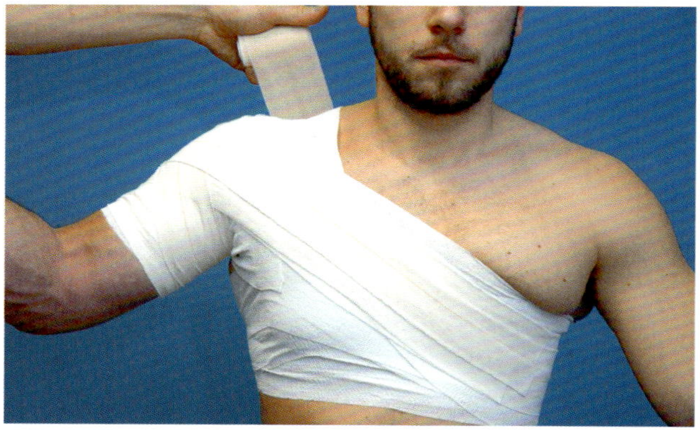
24

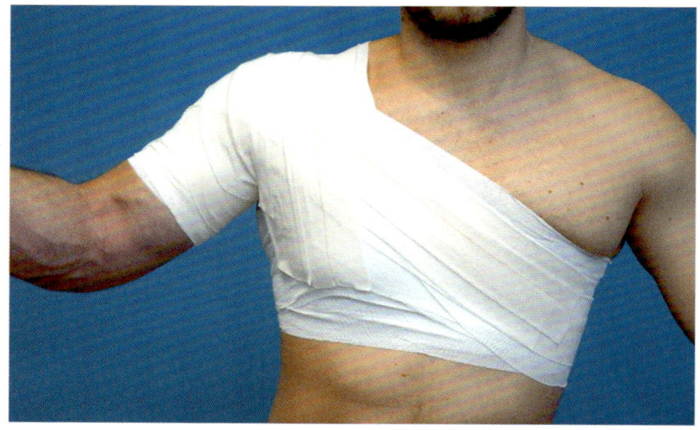
25

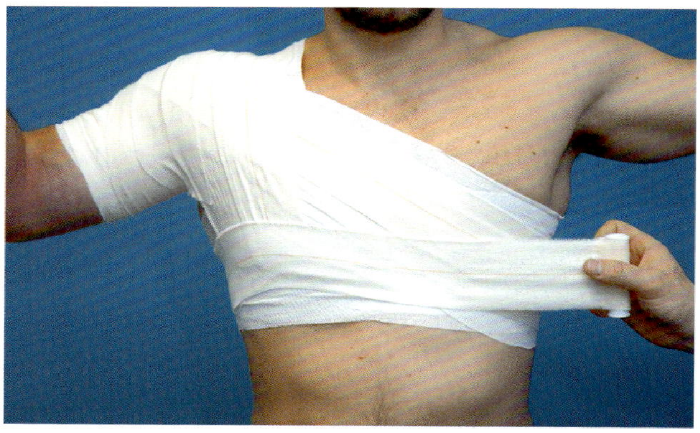
26

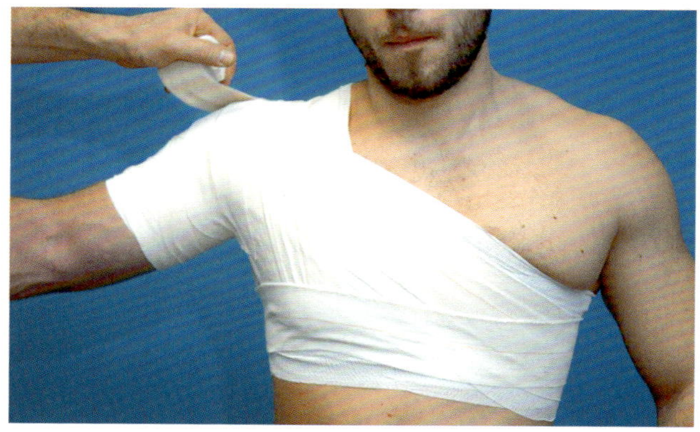
27

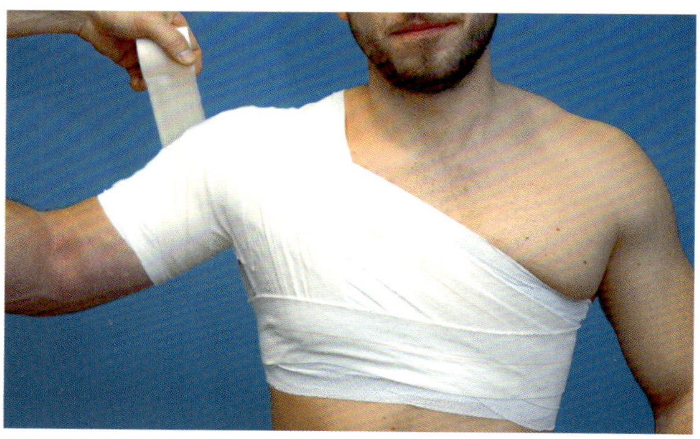
28

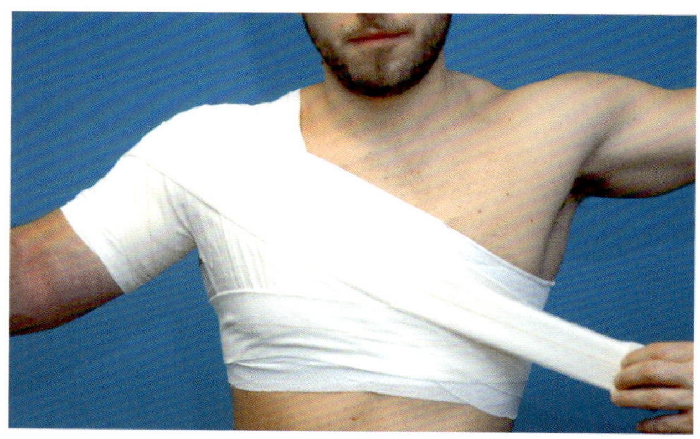
29

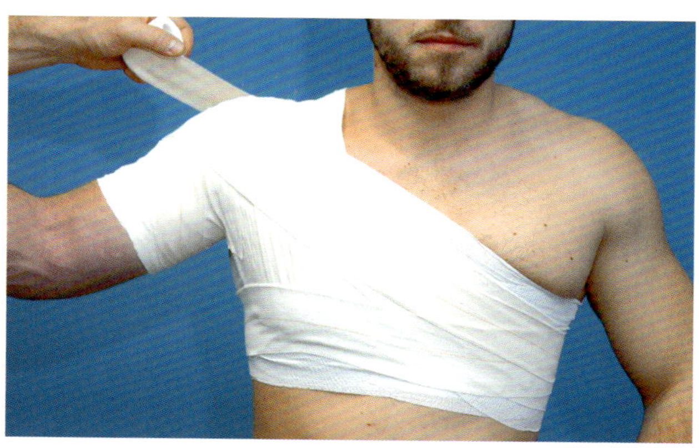
30

Stabilization and limitation of outward rotation

24-25 The bandage is affixed with some strips of mono-extensible adhesive elastic bandage applied transversally, beginning from the scapula and going to the pectoralis muscle.

26 A complete wrap of adhesive elastic bandage is made around the thorax in order to affix the bandage.

27 In order to increase congruency and the stabilization of the glenohumeral joint, the bandage is reinforced with additional strips of bandage applied in a figure eight. The bandage must begin posteriorly from the scapular projection.

28 The bandage is brought anteriorly to wrap around the glenohumeral joint, and then a full wrap is done around the axis of the humerus.

29 The bandage is brought diagonally until it wraps around the thorax.

30 The bandage is brought toward the shoulder.

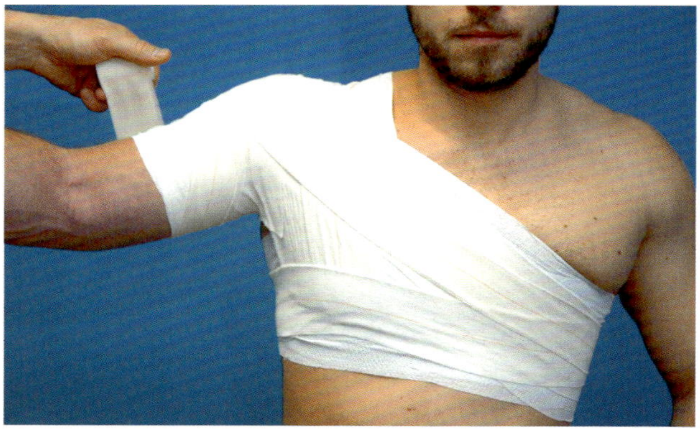
31

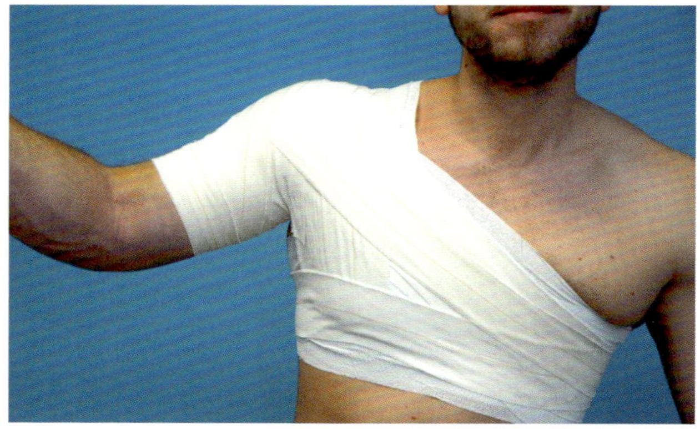
32

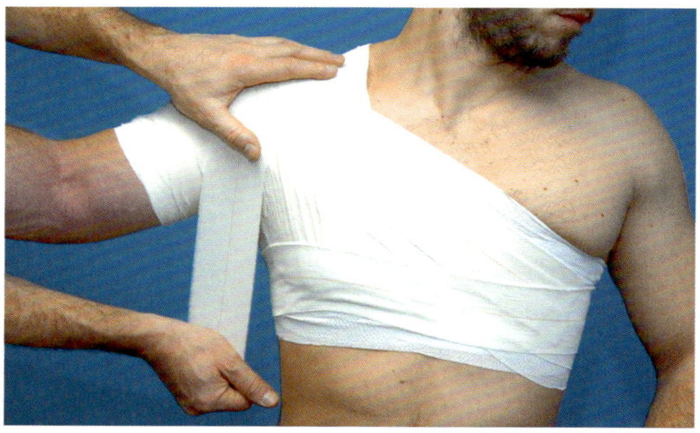
33

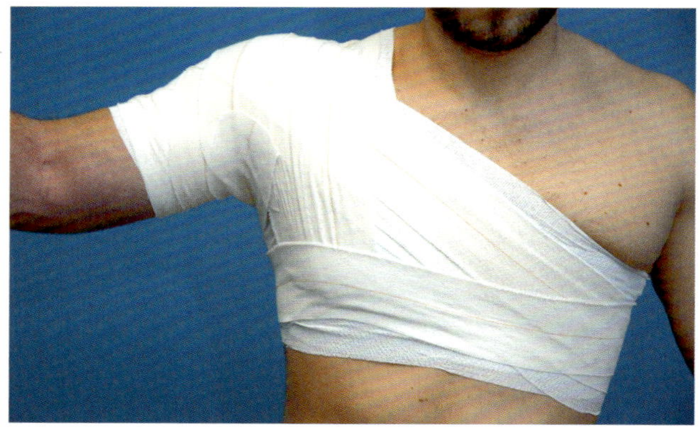
34

Stabilization and limitation of outward rotation

31-32 The glenohumeral joint is covered, crossing paths with the previous bandage, and is then affixed to the arm.

33 A reinforcing strip is applied at the underarm.

34 Bandaging is complete.

INDICACIONES

- ✓ *Aftereffects of subluxation of the glenohumeral joint*
- ✓ *Aftereffects of surgery of the glenohumeral joint*
- ✓ *High-impact athletic activity for athletes to return to the field (rugby, American football)*

ELBOW JOINT

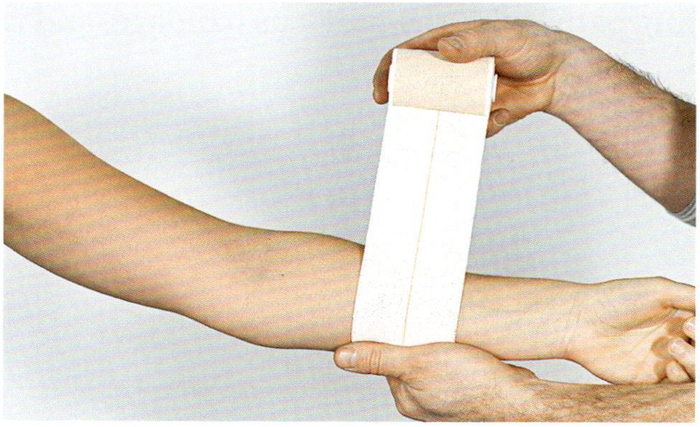
1

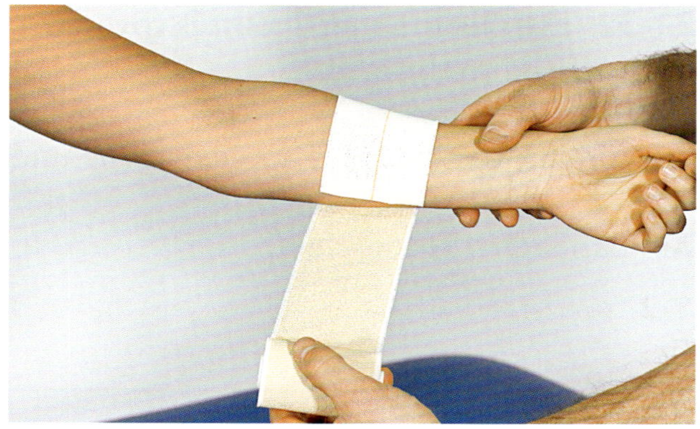
2

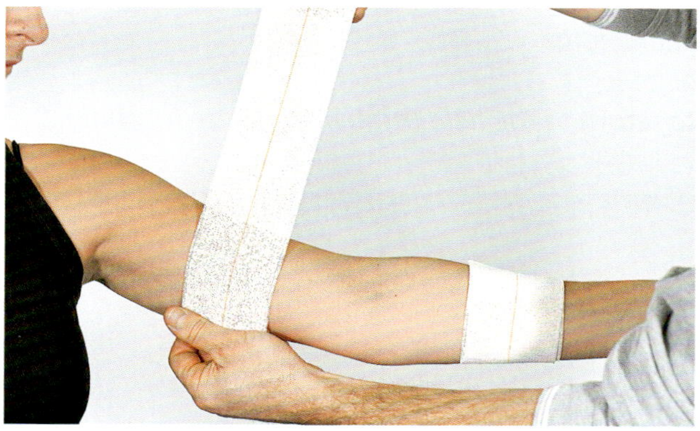
3

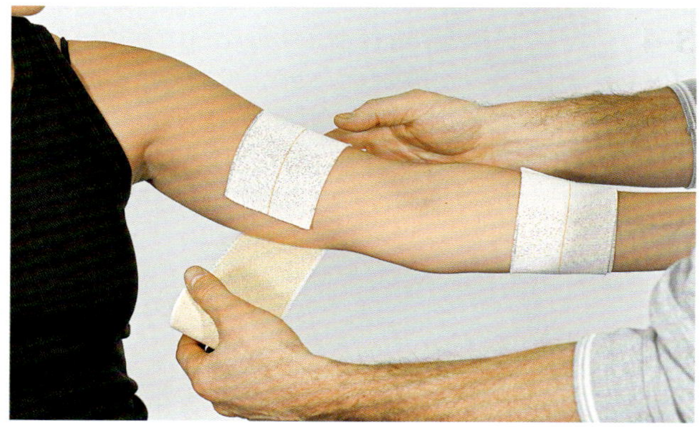
4

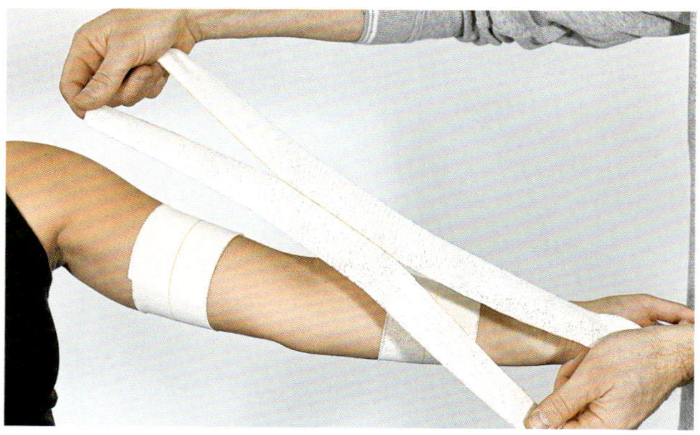
5

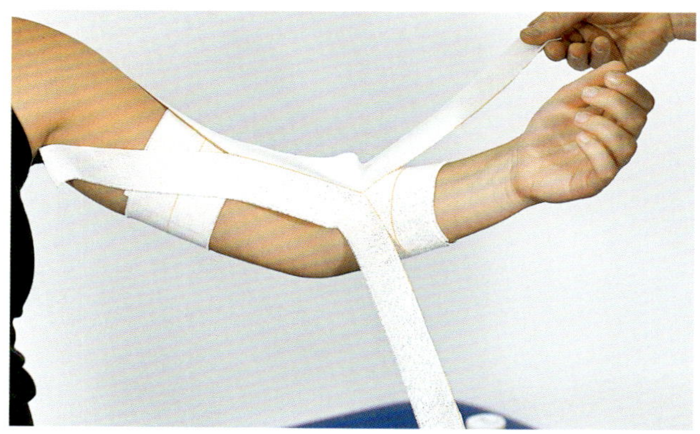
6

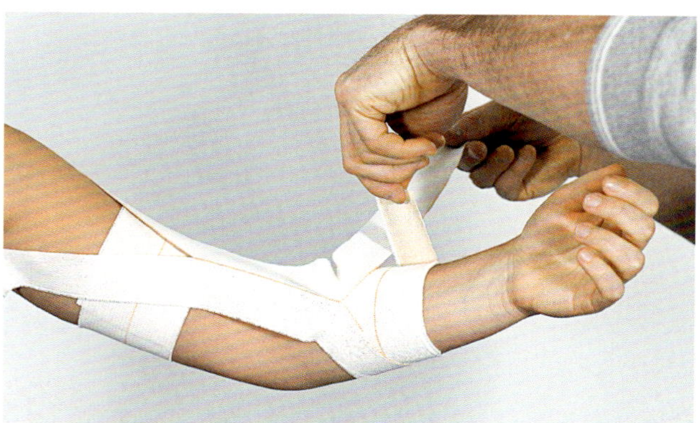
7

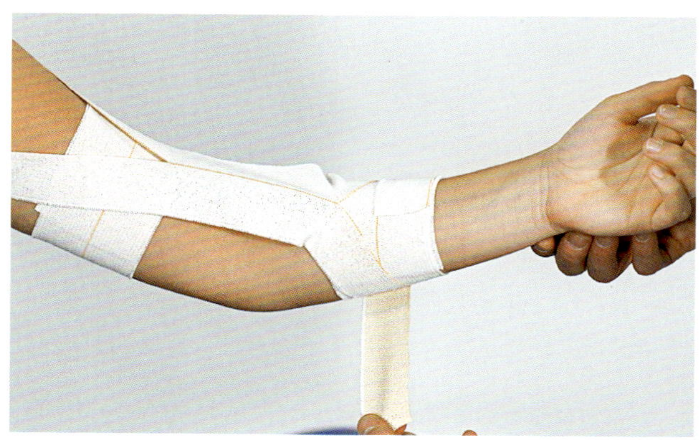
8

Unloading and limitation of extension

MATERIAL

- ✓ Cotton fabric porous elastic adhesive bandage that can be stretched lengthwise, 7.5 cm in width
- ✓ Elastic cohesive bandage

APPLICATION

1-2 The subject is seated with the upper limb in neutral position and the elbow slightly flexed. The distal anchoring point is prepared with the application of a full wrap of elastic adhesive bandage at the middle third of the forearm.

3-4 The proximal anchoring point is applied with a full wrap of elastic adhesive bandage at the middle third of the arm.

5 An X-shaped bandage is made by cutting a strip of elastic adhesive bandage, of the ideal length for bandaging, longitudinally and beginning from the extremity. The uncut portion of bandage should be approximately 10 cm long.

6-7-8 Two pieces of bandage are applied and affixed at the distal anchoring point.

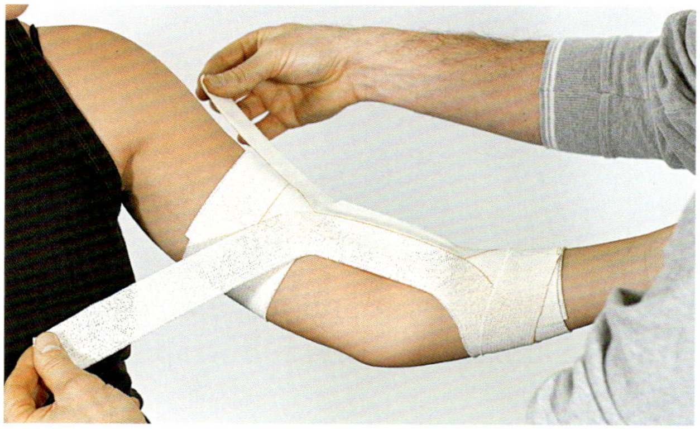

9

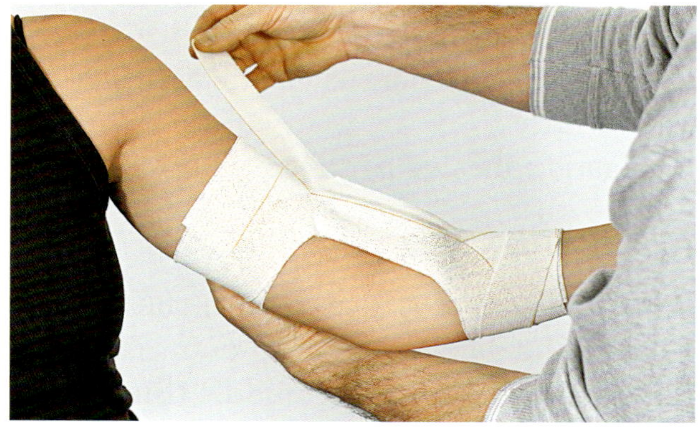

10

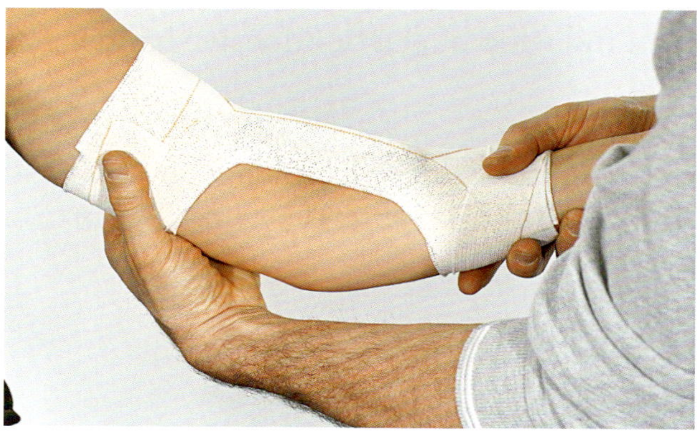

11

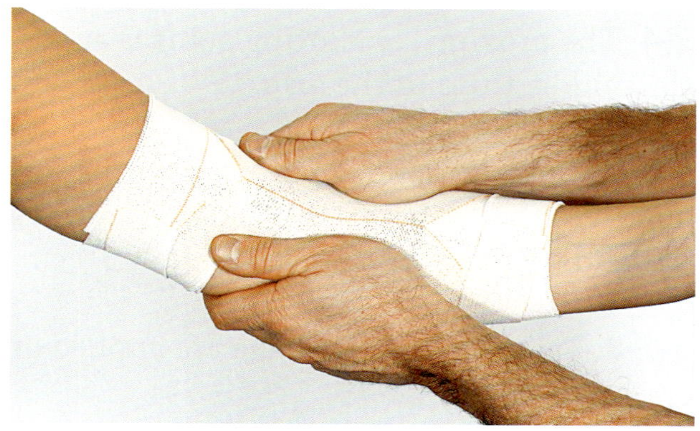

12

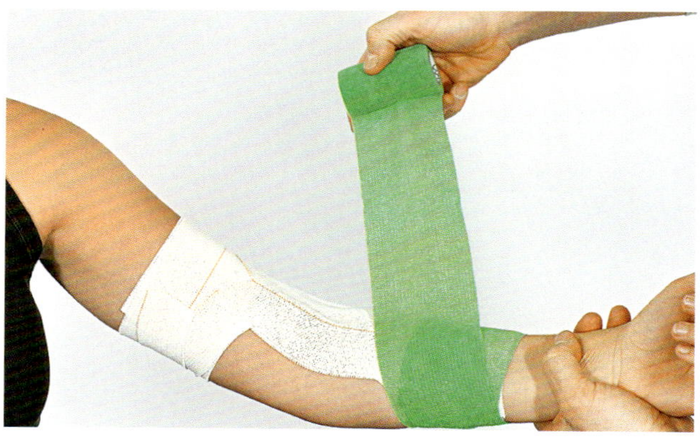

13

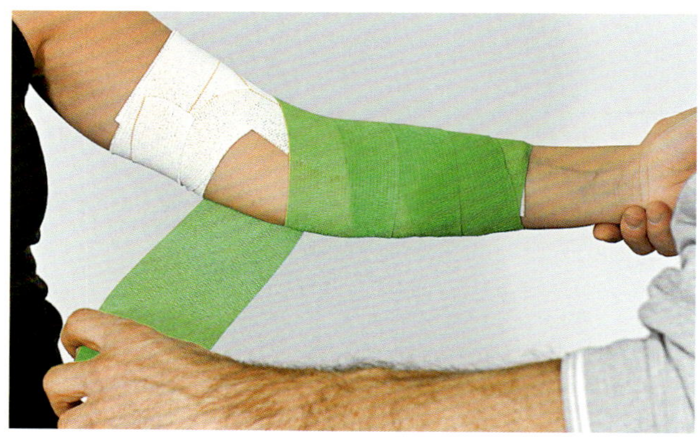

14

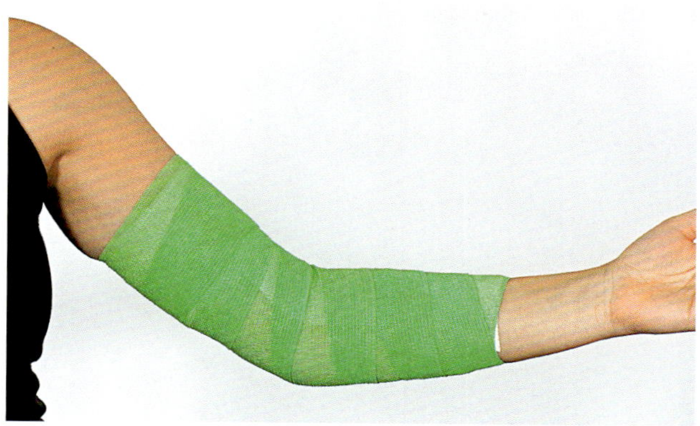

15

Unloading and limitation of extension

9-10-11 With the elbow in slight flexion, the free pieces of bandage are pulled and applied to the proximal anchoring point.

12 The bandage is carefully made to adhere to the skin of the inner surface of the elbow.

13-14 The bandaging is finished by applying a cohesive bandage with spiral wrappings in the distal-proximal direction.

15 Bandaging is complete.

The objective of cohesive bandaging is to increase the efficacy of the base adhesive bandaging and to keep the bandage adhered to the arm.
The adhesive elastic bandaging can also be done on a base covering made with cohesive bandages.

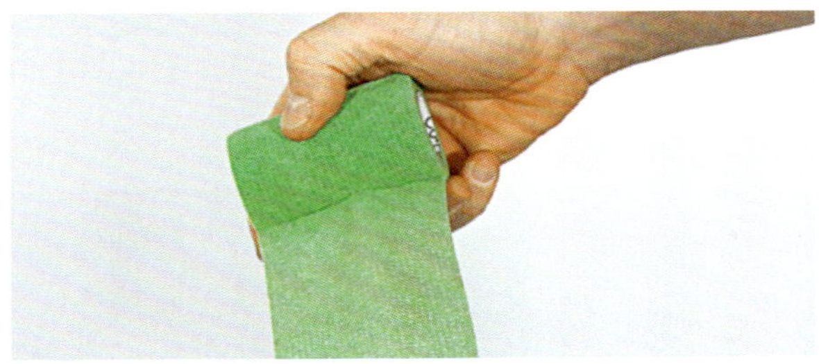

INDICATIONS

✓ *Olecranon pain upon hyperextension of the elbow*

ELBOW JOINT

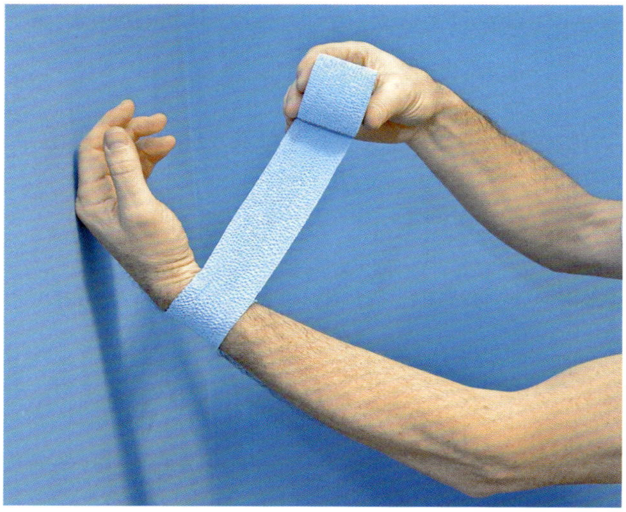

1

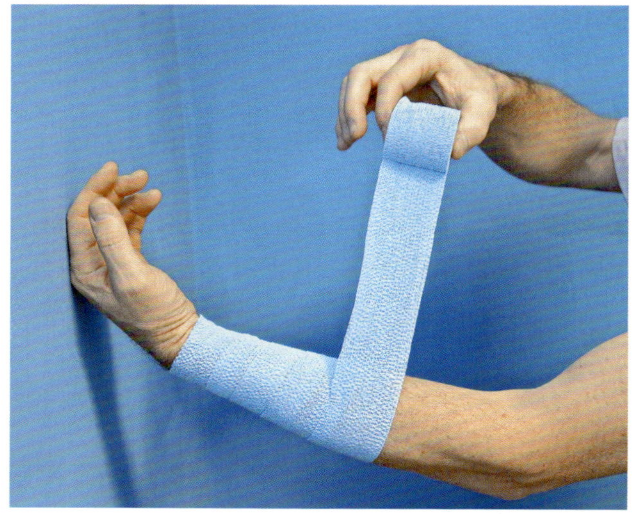

2

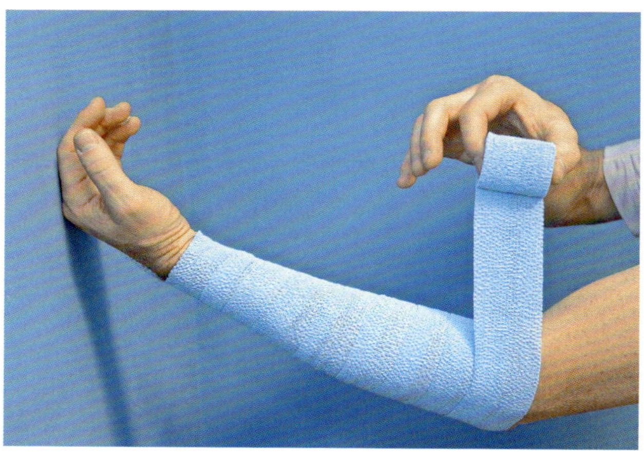

3

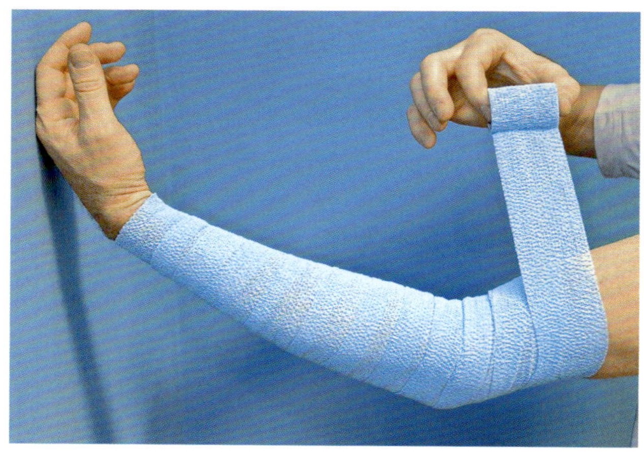

4

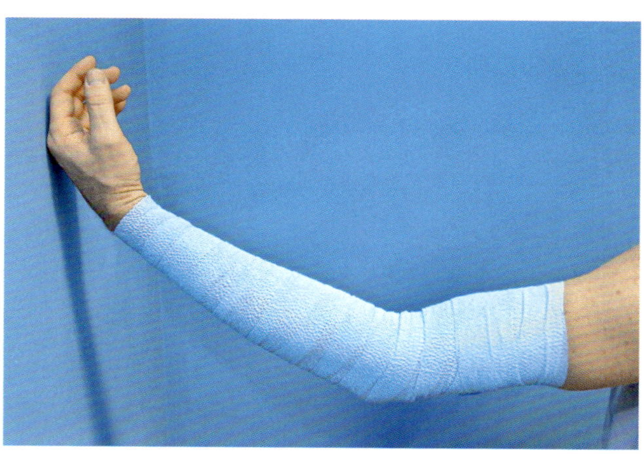

5

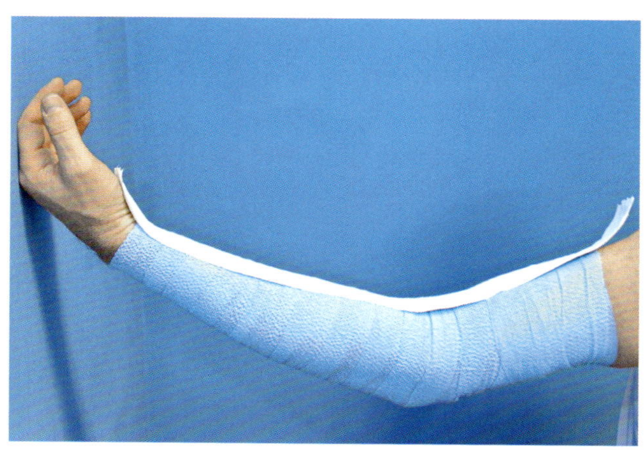

6

Stabilization and limitation of extension

MATERIAL

- ✓ 5 or 7.5 cm wide elastic cohesive bandage
- ✓ Inelastic cohesive tape, 5 or 7.5 cm in width

APPLICATION

1-2-3-4-5 Base bandaging is done with the cohesive elastic bandage, wrapping the forearm and the arm with several spiral wraps in the distal-proximal direction. The elbow must be kept in a semi-flexed position, at an angle of about 20 degrees.

6 A reinforced inelastic tape is prepared by overlapping five strips on top of one another, then all of these over the base bandaging, keeping the elbow's angle of flexion at around 20 degrees at all times.

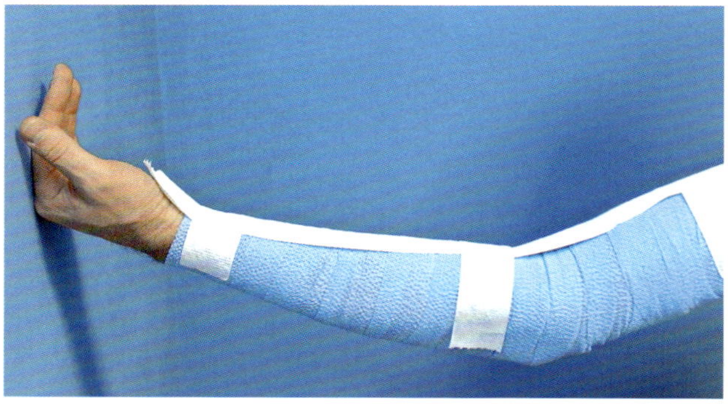
7

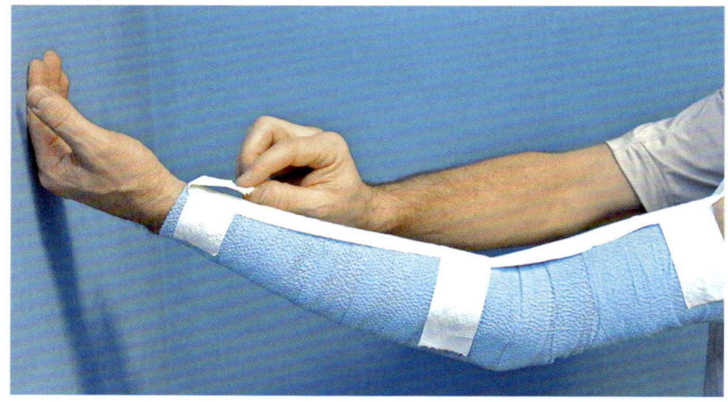
8

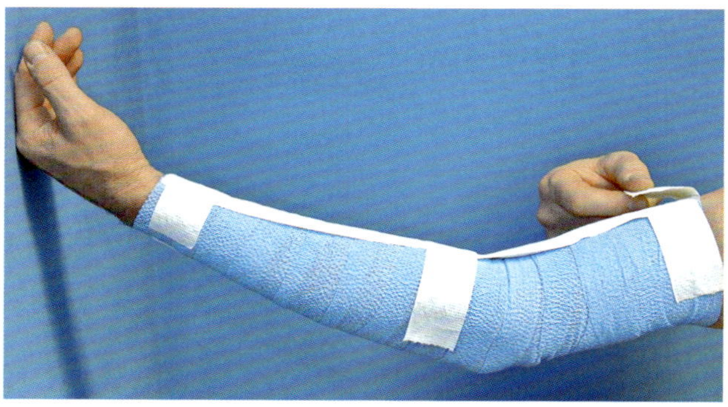
9

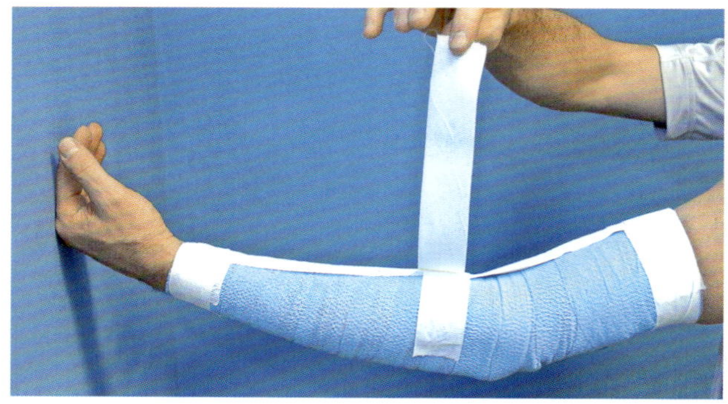
10

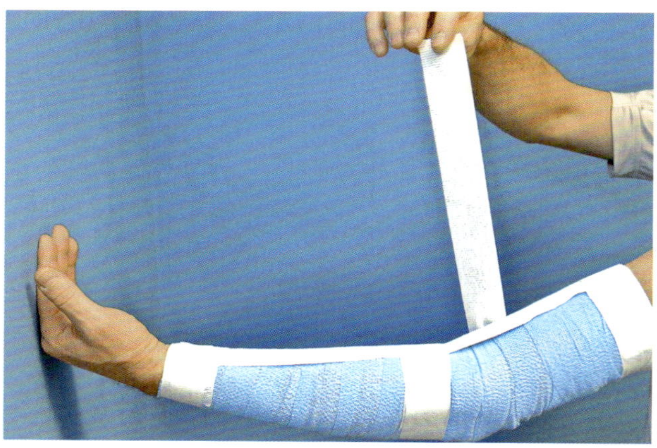
11

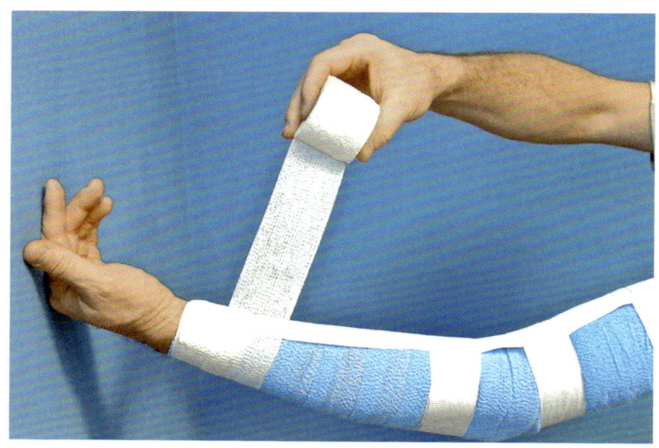
12

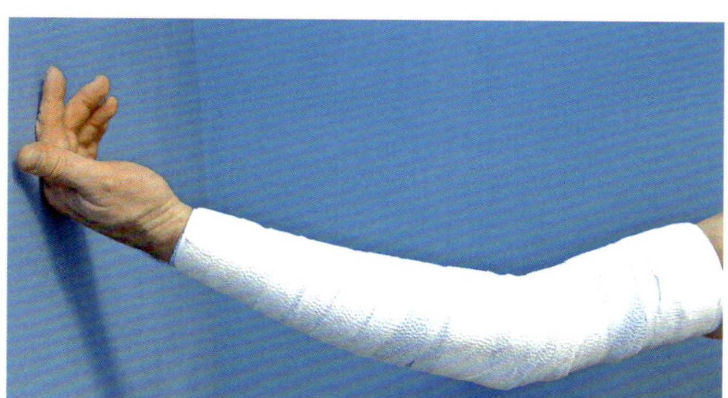
13

Stabilization and limitation of extension

7 The reinforced tape is affixed with several fastening pieces, always made from inelastic material, applied in a semicircle.

8-9 The excess edges of the tape are folded and affixed over the distal and proximal anchoring points.

10-11 Several complete wrappings of inelastic tape are made around the arm in order to set the bandaging in place.

12 Now using the cohesive bandage, the bandaging is set in place by covering the arm with spiral wrappings applied in a distal-proximal direction.

13 Bandaging is complete.

INDICATIONS

- ✓ *Posttraumatic conditions*
- ✓ *Preventative sports treatment*

ELBOW JOINT

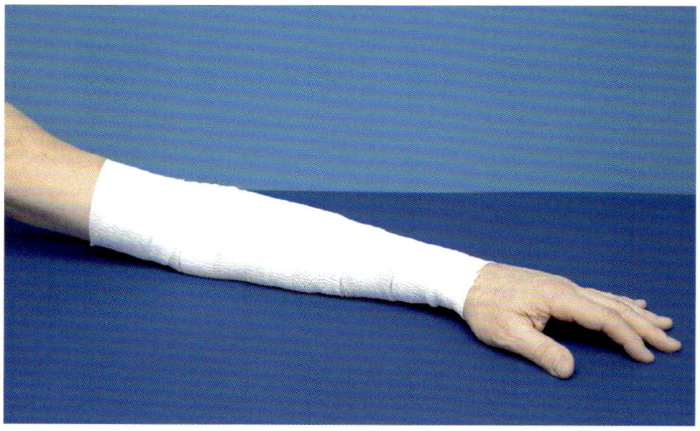
1

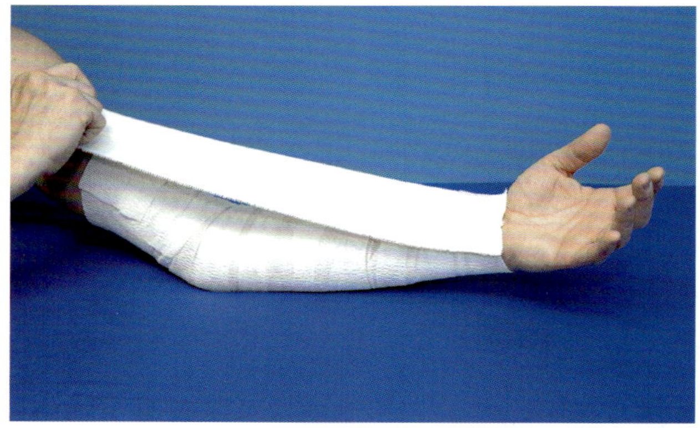
2

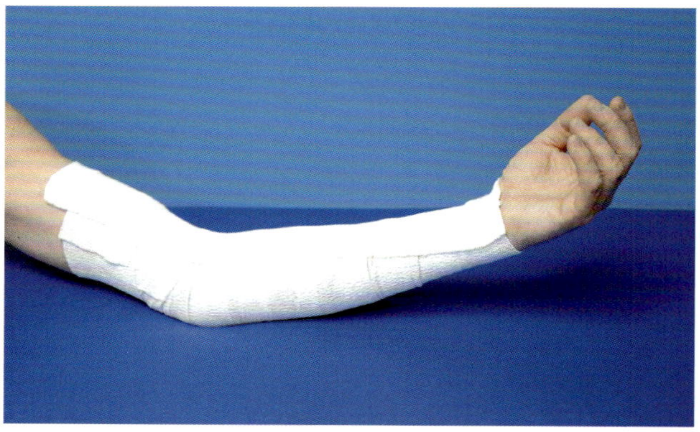
3

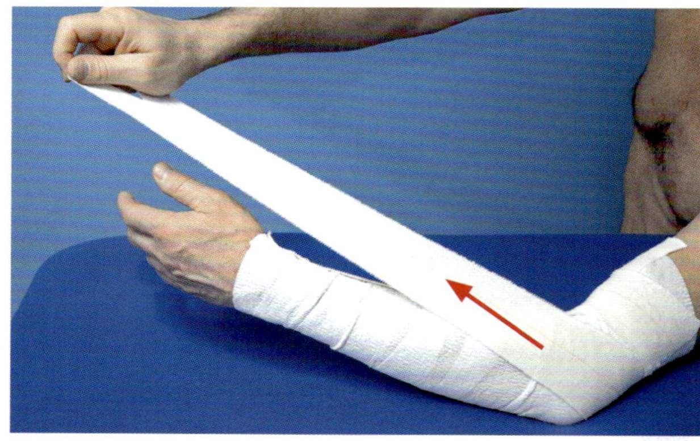
4

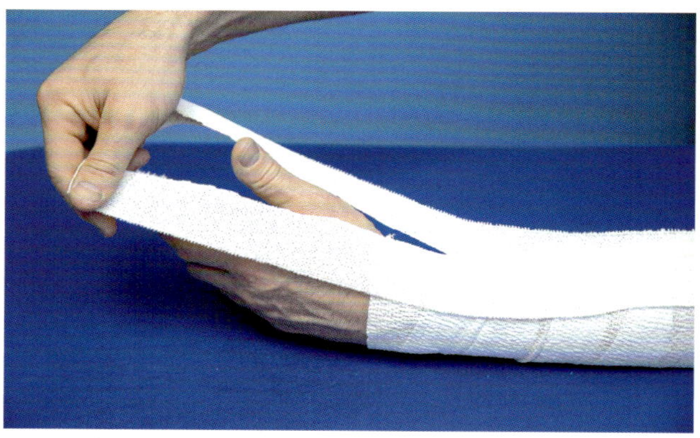
5

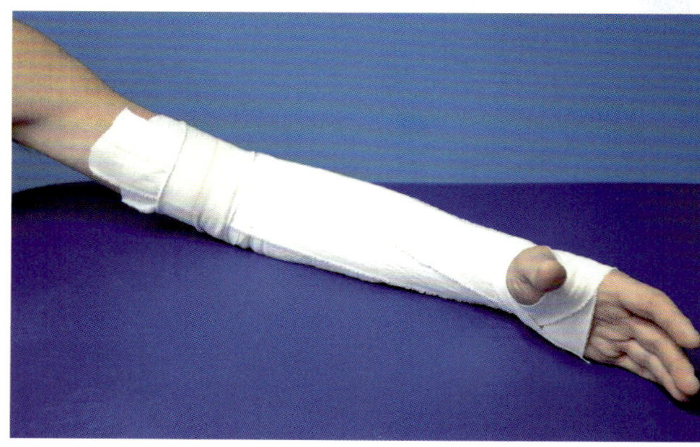
6

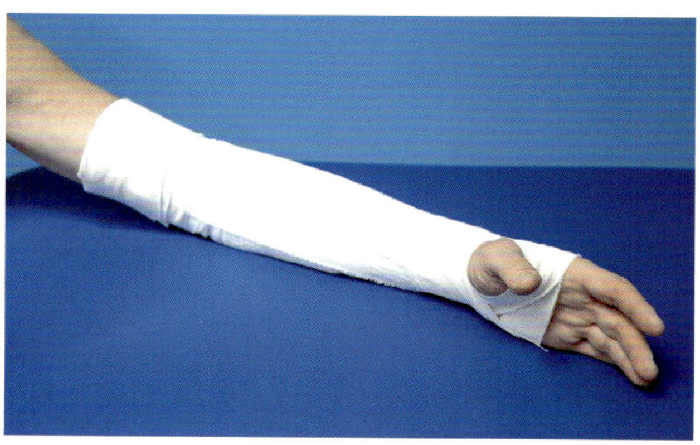
7

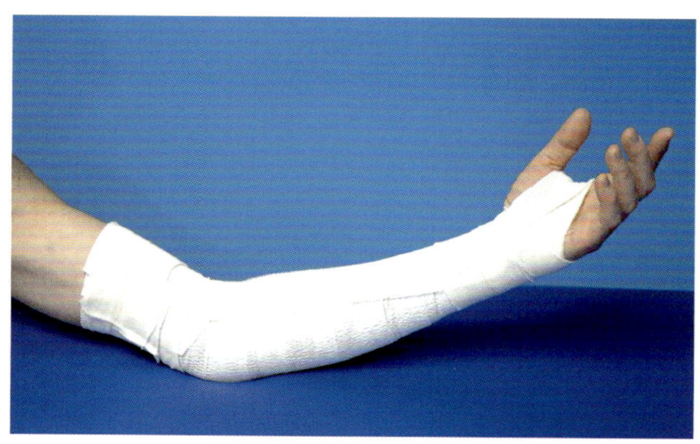
8

Stabilization, limitation of extension and supination

MATERIAL

✓ Elastic cohesive bandage
✓ Cotton fabric porous elastic adhesive bandage that can be stretched lengthwise, 5 or 7.5 cm in width

APPLICATION

1 Using the cohesive bandage, base bandaging is made in a distal-proximal direction, covering the forearm and the arm with spiral wrappings (see page 50).

2-3 The subject flexes the elbow 20-30 degrees. A reinforced elastic adhesive bandage is positioned so as to limit extension and cover the inner space of the elbow.

The reinforced bandage must be made by overlapping two strips of mono-extensible elastic adhesive bandage of the proper length.

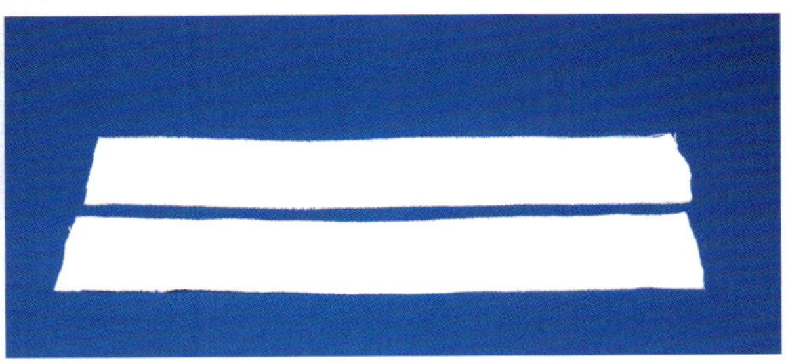

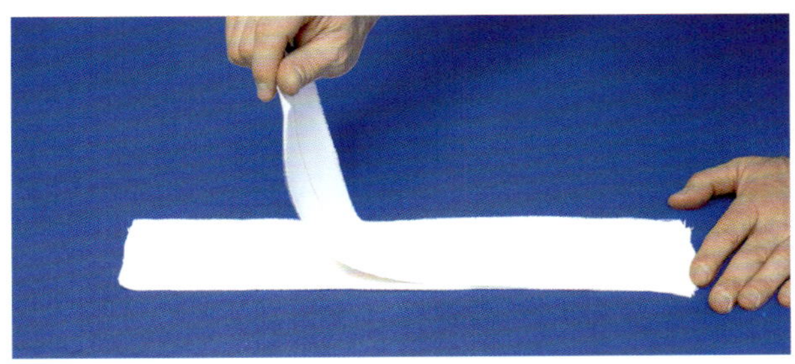

4 In order to limit the supination of the forearm and instead favor its pronation, a bandage is applied on the forearm beginning posteriorly on the distal third of the arm and directed toward the radial styloid.

5-6 The free extremity of the bandage is cut distally, dividing it into two equal strips that are wrapped around the thumb and affixed at the wrist.

7 The bandaging is set with two wraps of adhesive elastic bandage, one applied on the distal third of the arm and wrapping the axis of the humerus, and the other on the distal third of the forearm in order to stabilize the wrist.

8 Bandaging is complete.

INDICATIONS

✓ *Epicondylitis*

ELBOW JOINT

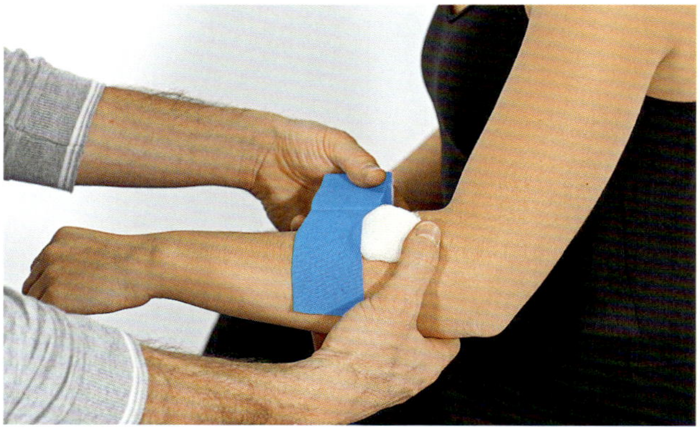

1

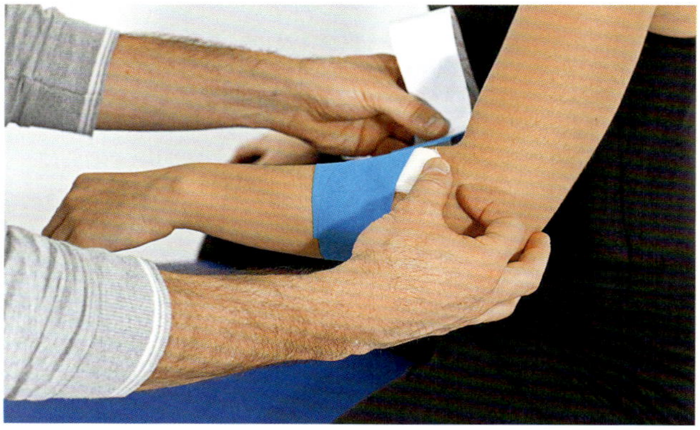

2

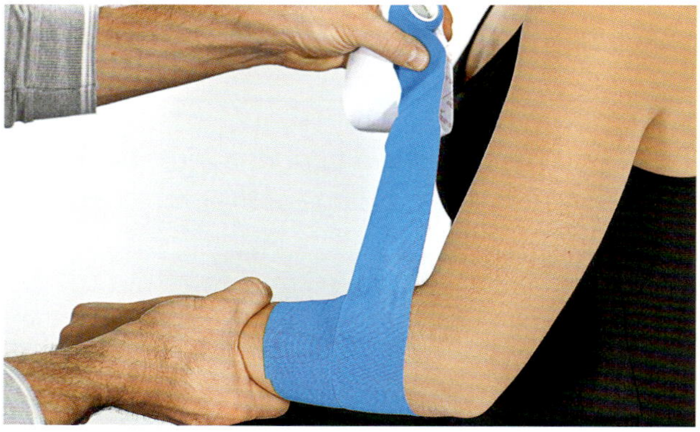

3

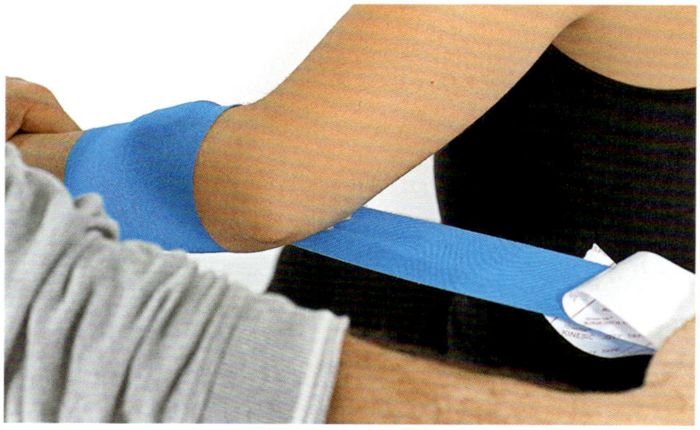

4

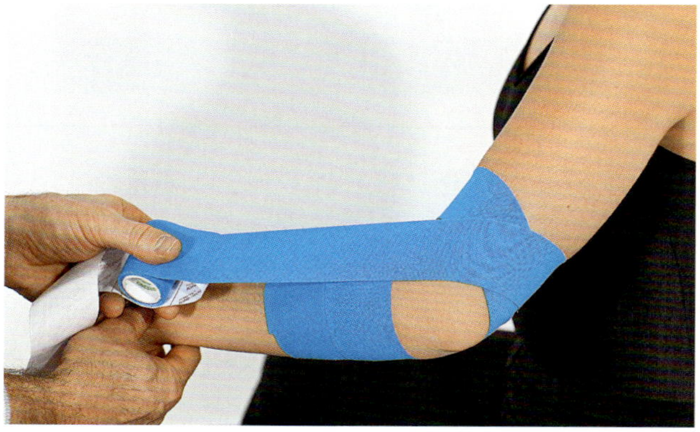

5

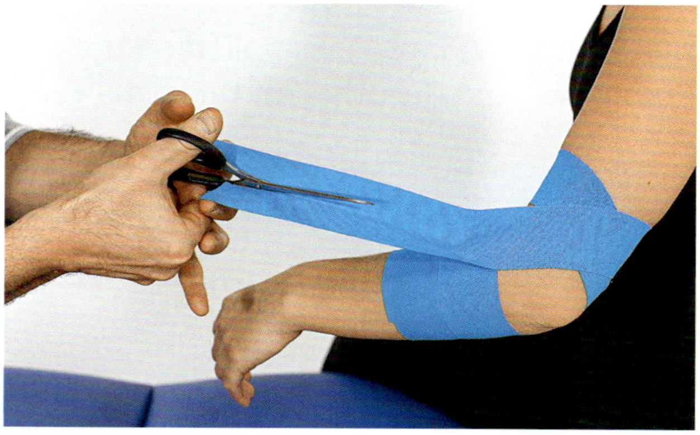

6

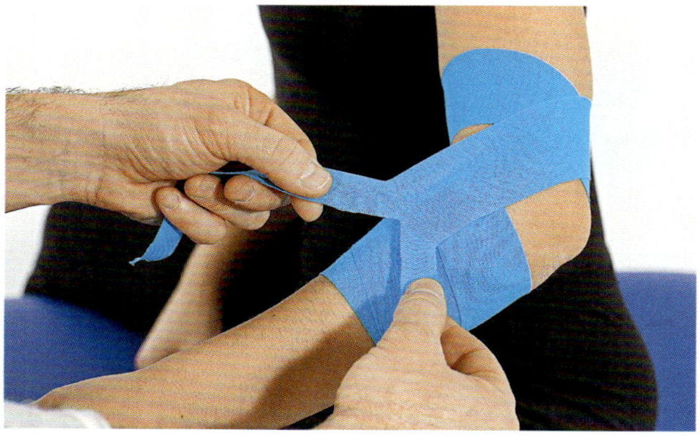

7

Muscular and tendinous unloading

MATERIAL

- ✓ Elastic adhesive tape, extensible lengthwise, 5 cm in width
- ✓ Foam rubber or pre-tape compress for creating a compressive pad
- ✓ 5 cm wide inelastic adhesive tape to affix bandaging

APPLICATION

1 The subject is in a seated position, with the limb to be treated in elbow flexion of 90 degrees and the forearm pronated; the elastic adhesive tape is applied to the medial third of the forearm beginning from the skin projection of the ulna. An oval-shaped compress is positioned on the belly of the supinator muscle.

2-3 The tape is applied with spiral wrappings in a distal-proximal direction in order to cover the pad and favor the pronation of the forearm, limiting its supination.

4 The tape, once reaching the proximal third of the forearm, is made to pass posteriorly above the elbow.

5 With a full wrap done at the distal third of the arm, the tape is put under tension and directed over the posterior surface of the forearm.

6-7 Beginning from its free end, the tape is longitudinally cut into two equal parts so as to obtain two pieces that may be used to affix the distal anchoring point.

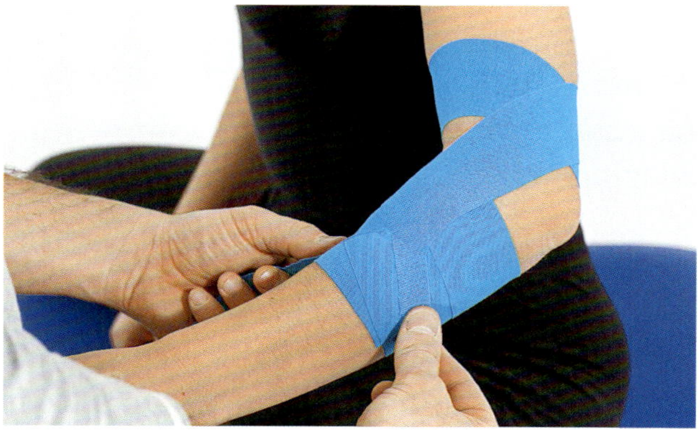
8

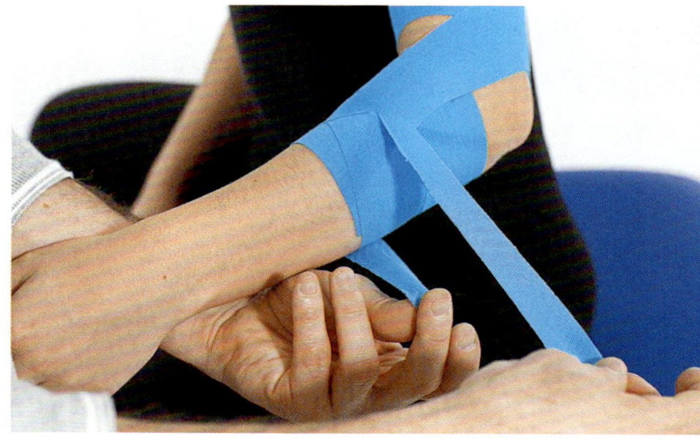
9

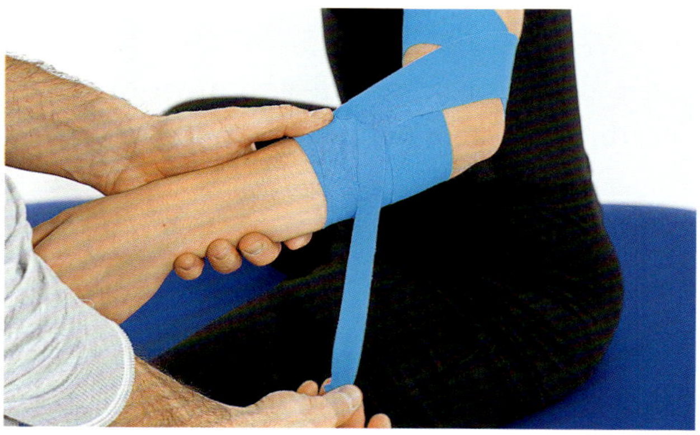
10

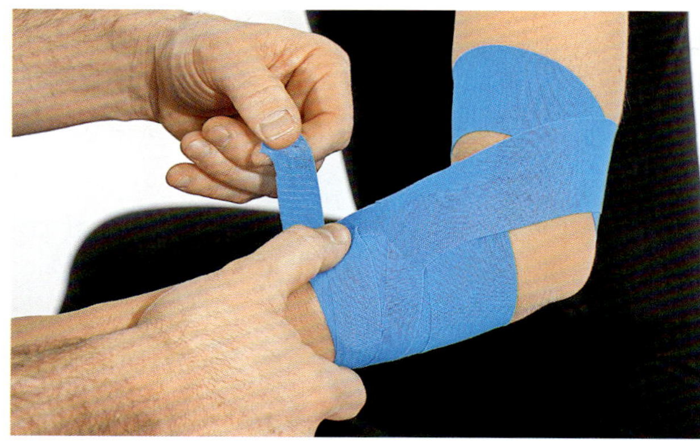
11

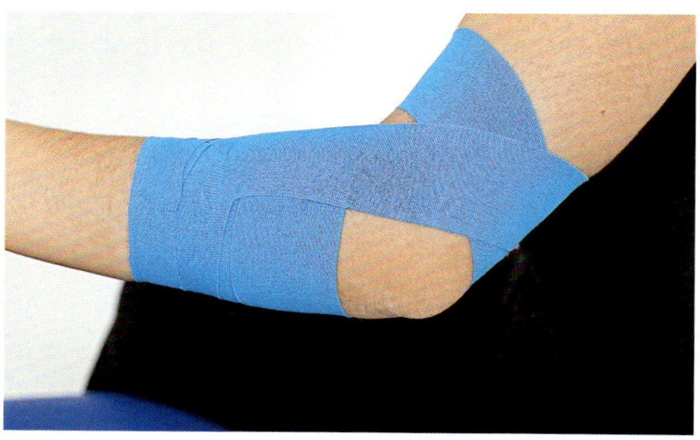
12

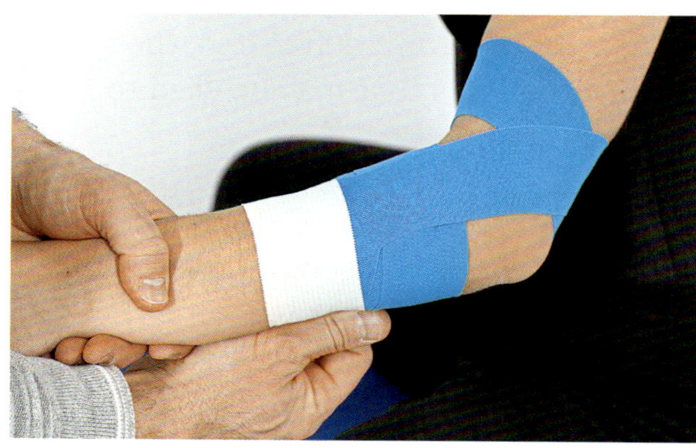
13

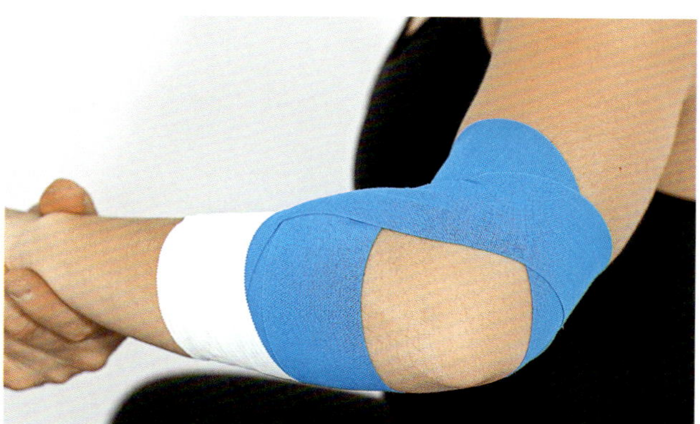
14

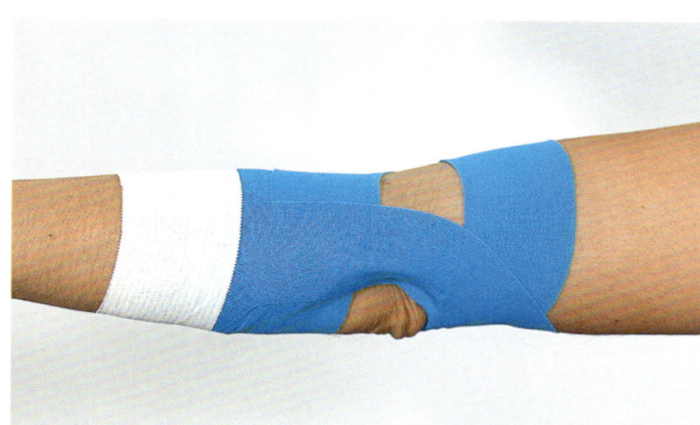
15

Muscular and tendinous unloading

8-9-10-11-12 The two pieces of elastic adhesive tape are affixed by adhering them around the forearm, first one and then the other.

13 The distal anchoring point is finished with the application of a strip of inelastic adhesive tape.

14-15 Bandaging is complete.

INDICATIONS

✓ *Epicondylar pain of myotendinous origin*

SUPINATOR MUSCLE

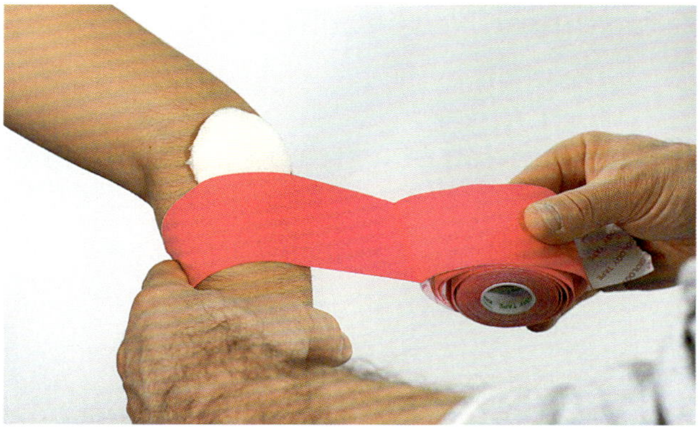
1

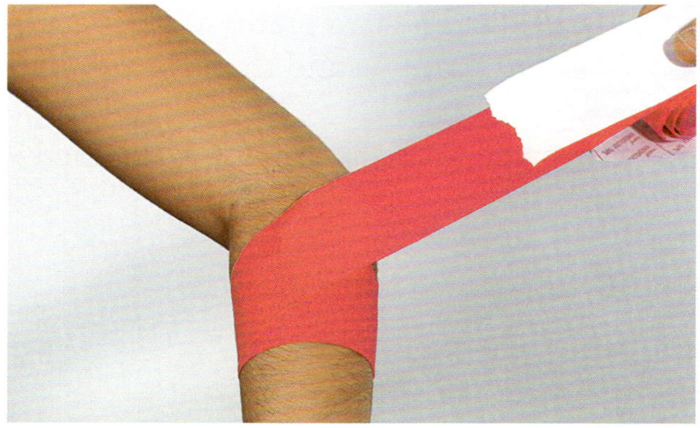
2

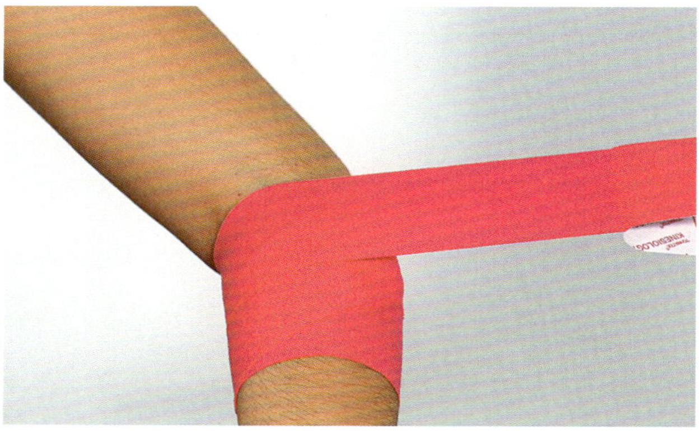
3

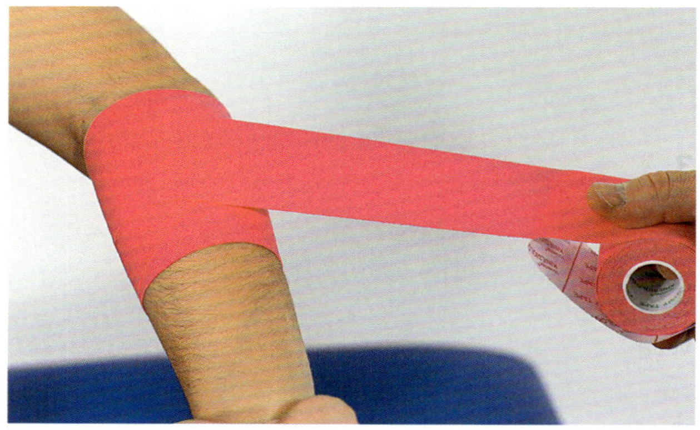
4

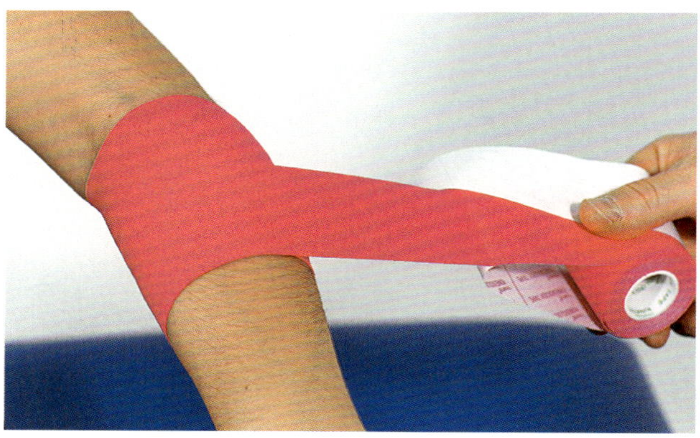
5

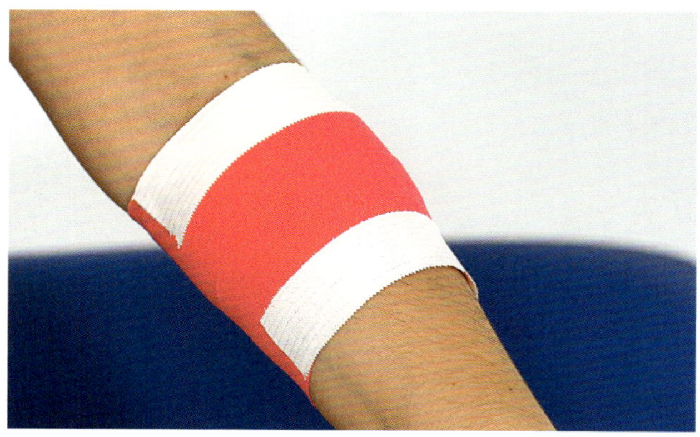
6

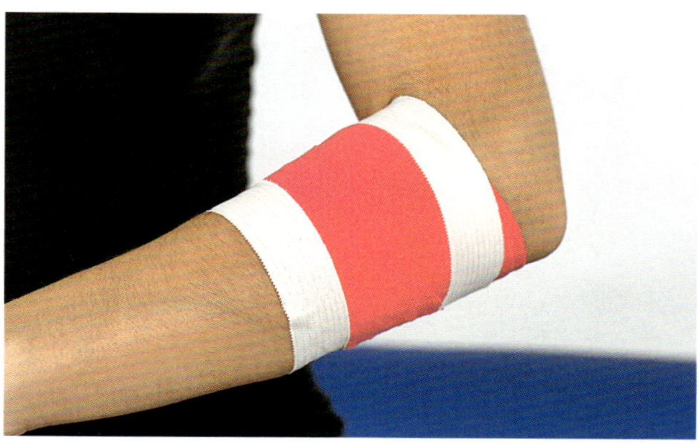
7

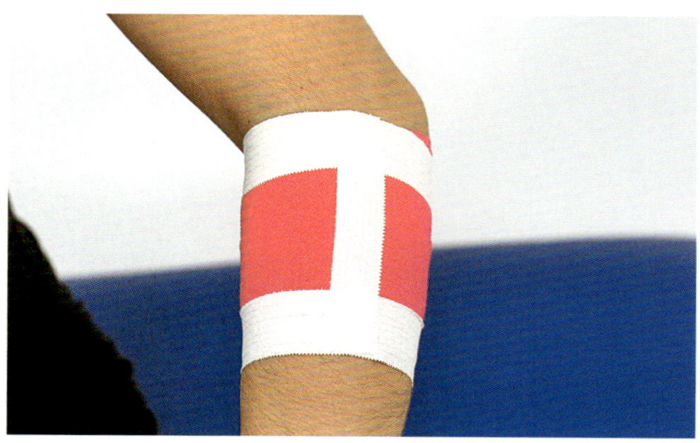
8

Muscular unloading

MATERIAL

- ✓ Elastic adhesive tape, extensible lengthwise, 5 cm in width
- ✓ Inelastic adhesive tape of various widths: 1 cm, 2.5 cm, 5 cm
- ✓ Foam rubber compress for creating a compressive pad

APPLICATION

1 The subject slightly flexes the upper limb at the elbow and positions the forearm in pronation. A foam rubber compress, shaped into an oval, is positioned on the belly of the supinator muscle. A wrap of elastic adhesive bandage is applied on the distal third of the compress.

2 Bring the bandage in a diagonal direction to reach the proximal third of the compress.

3 Next, a complete wrapping of the bandage is made to cover the proximal third of the compress.

4 The bandage descends again to the distal third of the compress, crossing the previous wrapping.

5 An additional wrapping of the bandage is applied around the distal third of the compress.

6-7 Two 2.5 cm wide strips of inelastic adhesive tape are applied in a semicircle in order to provide the proximal and distal anchoring points.

8 A third 2.5 cm wide strip of inelastic adhesive tape is placed over the compress from the distal anchoring point to the proximal one.

SUPINATOR MUSCLE

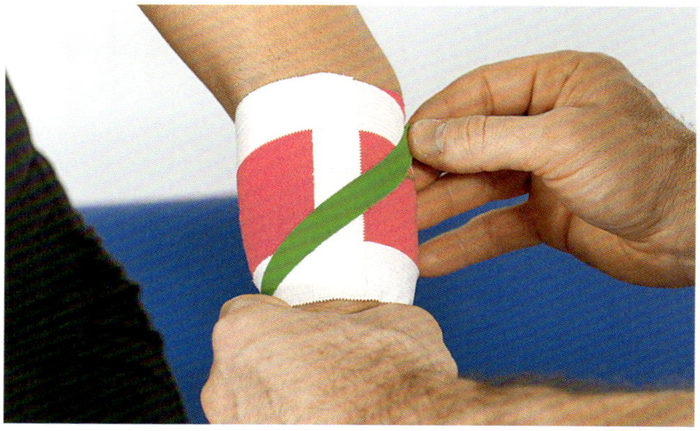
9

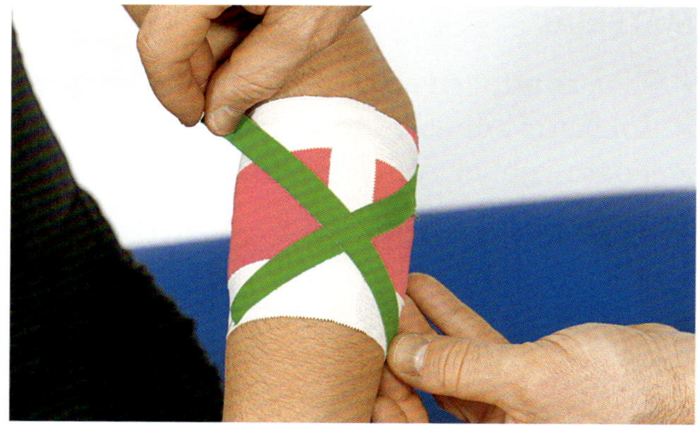
10

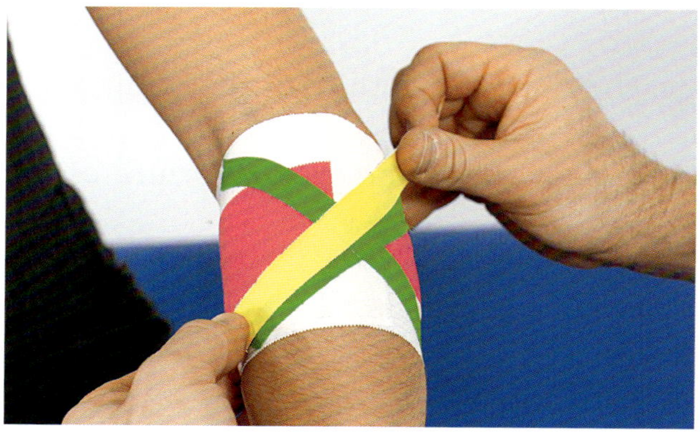
11

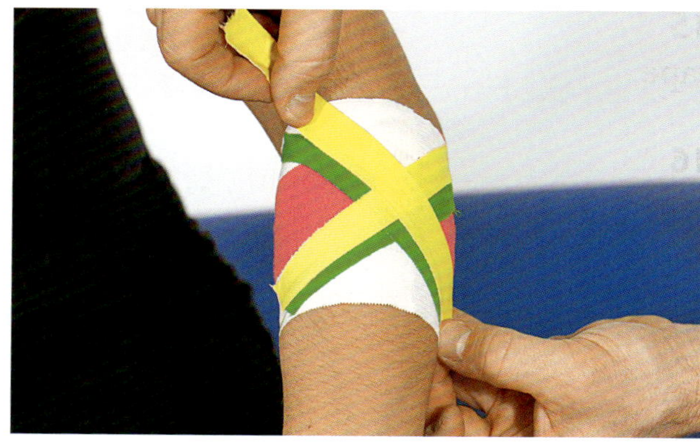
12

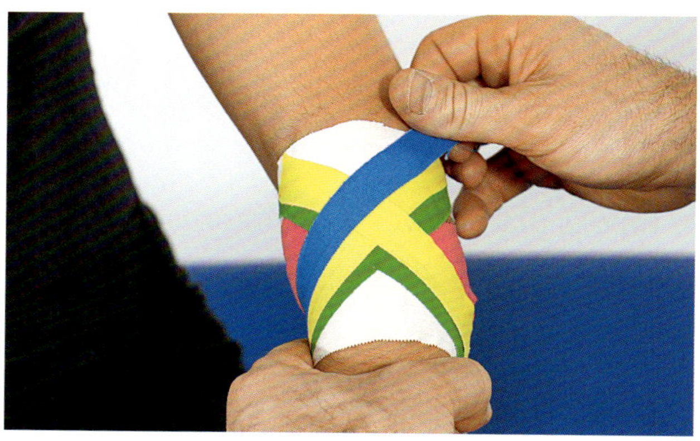
13

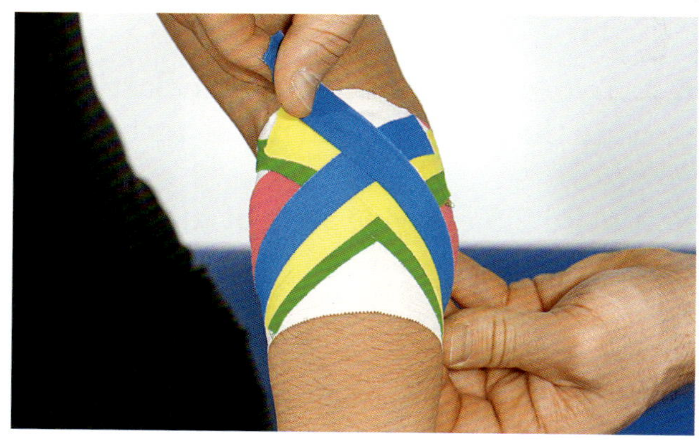
14

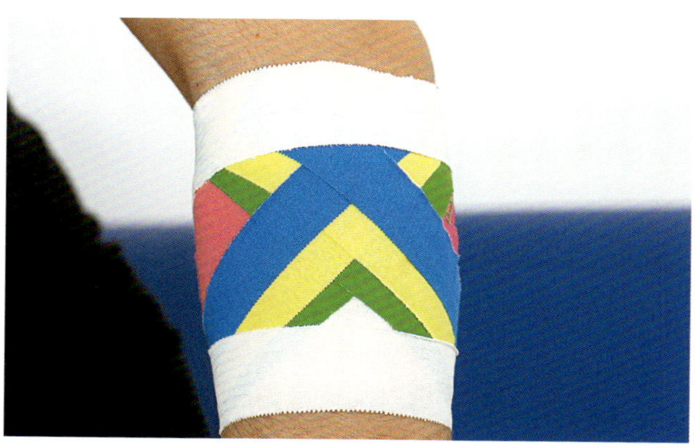
15

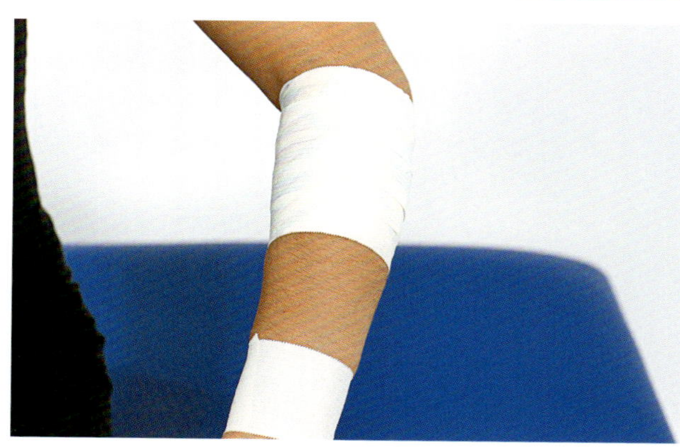
16

Muscular unloading

9-10 An X-shaped bandage is made with two 1 cm wide strips of inelastic adhesive tape, beginning from the distal anchoring point and reaching the proximal one. The tapes should cross one another at the distal end of the compress.

11-12 Bandaging then proceeds by applying another X-shaped formation on the central part of the compress.

13-14 Finally, a third X-shaped bandaging formation is made in the area of the proximal part of the compress.

15 The bandaging is affixed proximally and distally with the 2.5 cm wide inelastic adhesive tape.

16 To finish, the strips of inelastic adhesive tape are applied in a semicircle so as to cover all of the bandaging. The radioulnar joint is stabilized with a wrapping of 5 cm wide inelastic adhesive tape at the wrist.

INDICATIONS

✓ *Epicondylar pain of muscular origin*

RADIOCARPAL JOINT

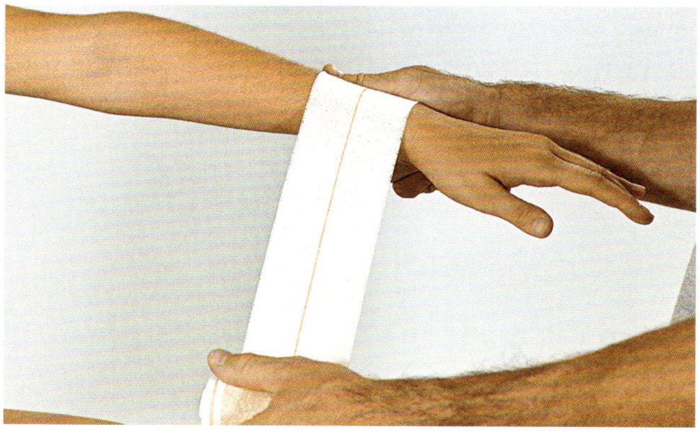

1

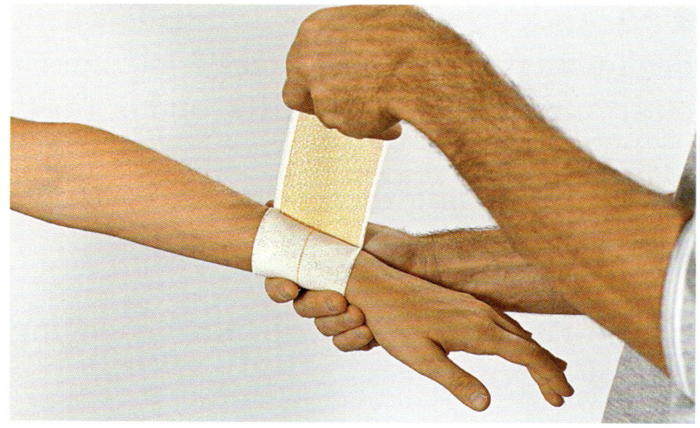

2

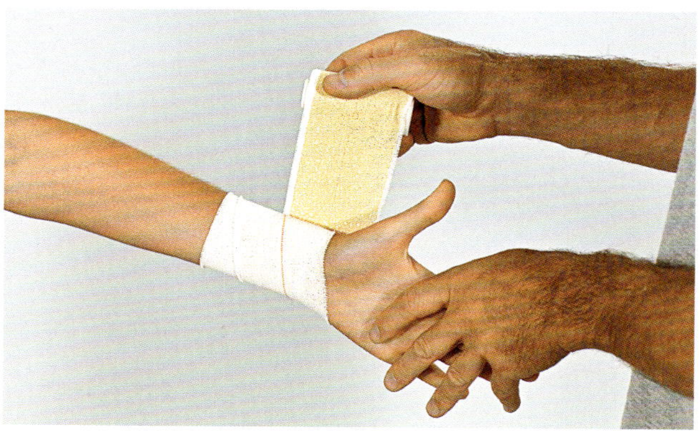

3

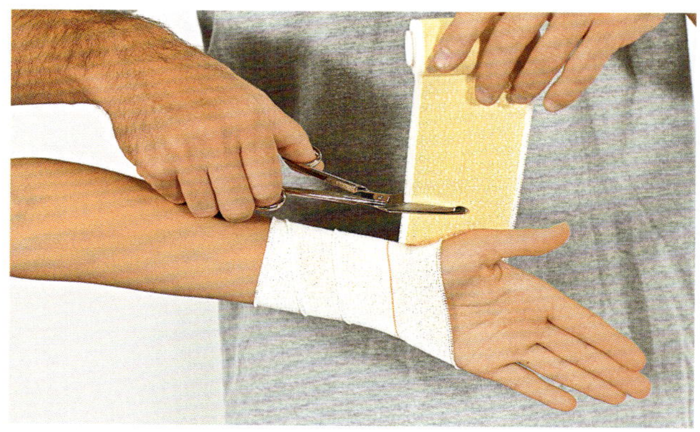

4

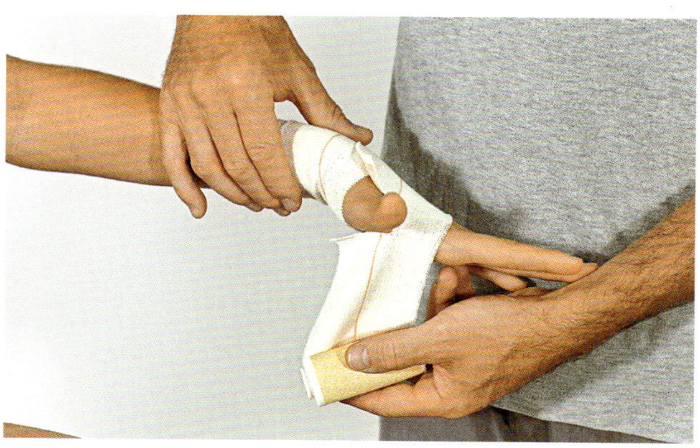

5

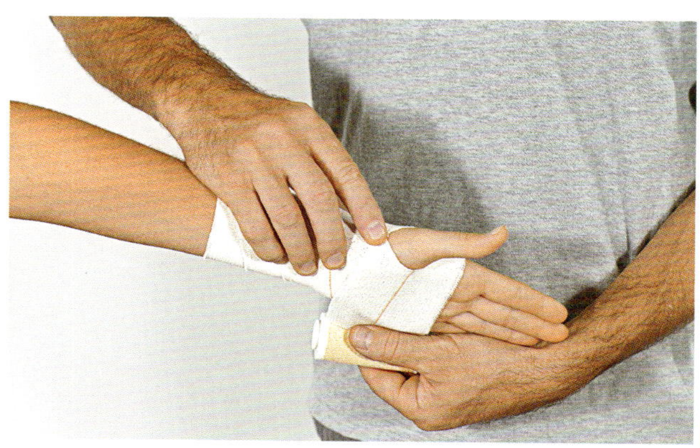

6

Base bandaging

MATERIAL

- ✓ Cotton fabric porous elastic adhesive bandage that can be stretched lengthwise, 7.5 cm in width
- ✓ Inelastic adhesive tape for preparing anchoring points

APPLICATION

1 To begin, a full wrap of bandage is applied, beginning over the dorsal projection of the distal third of the forearm in the ulnar-radial direction.

2-3 Bandaging proceeds with two spiral wrappings around the forearm, moving in a proximal-distal direction and with about 50% overlap over the previous bandage.

4 At the dorsal part of the metacarpophalangeal joint of the thumb, make a 3-4 cm long transverse cut of the bandage.

5-6 The two pieces of bandage are adhered so as to wrap the base of the thumb.

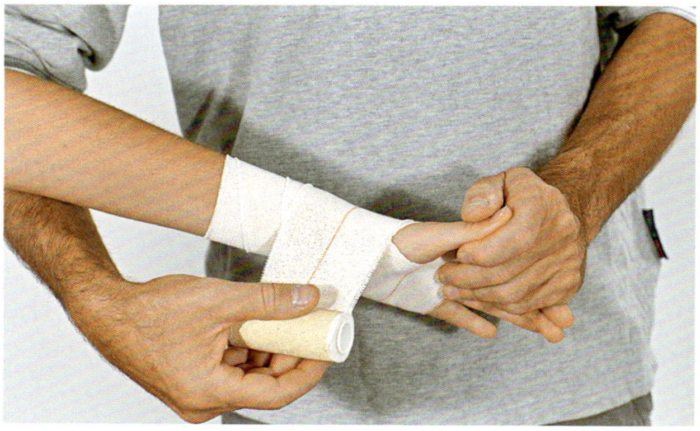

7

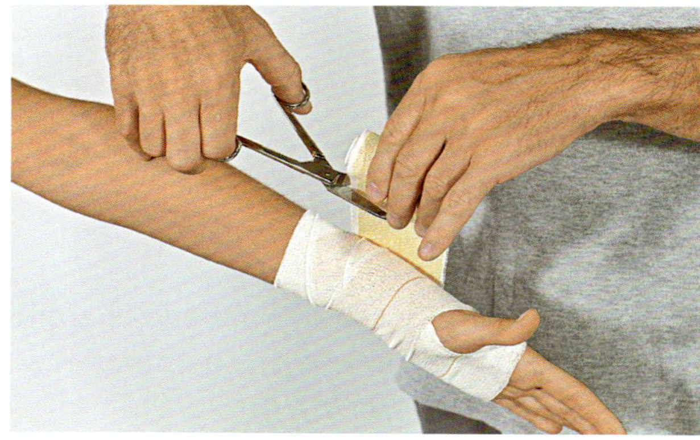

8

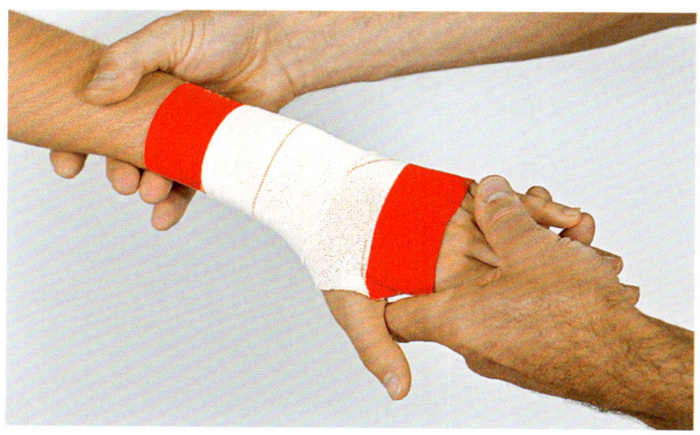

9

Base bandaging

7-8 At this point, a spiral wrapping is done around the forearm, moving in the distal-proximal direction.

9 The bandaging is concluded with the application of the proximal and distal anchoring points made with inelastic adhesive tape.

INDICATIONS

✓ *Sprain trauma*
✓ *Effects of fracture*
✓ *Joint support*

RADIOCARPAL JOINT

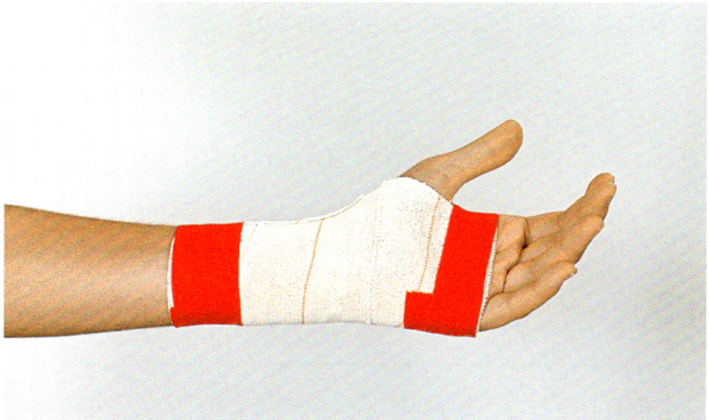

1

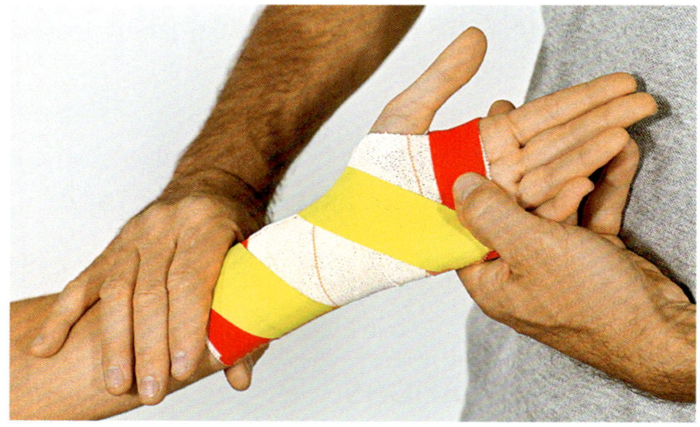

2

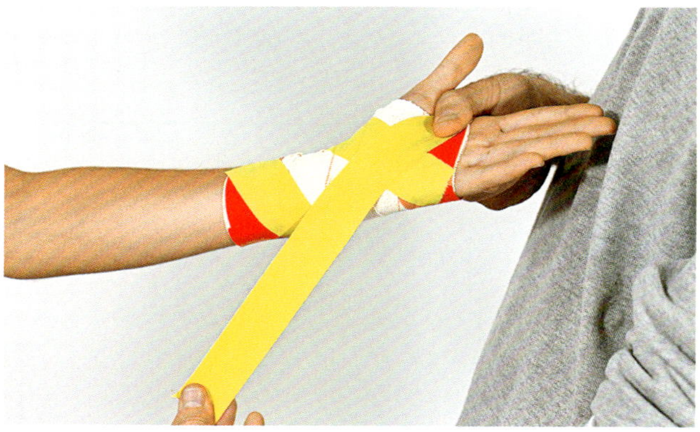

3

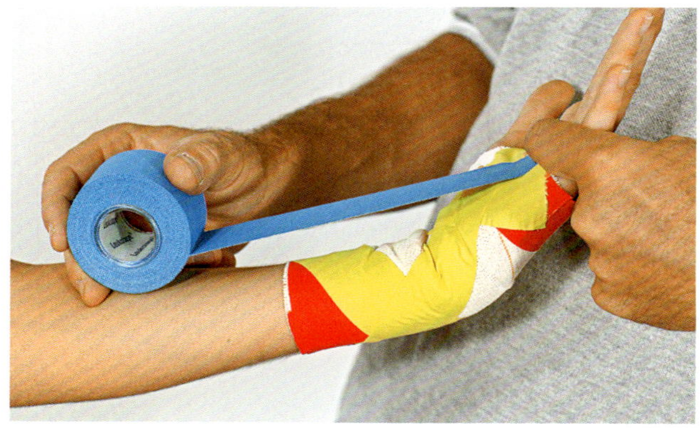

4

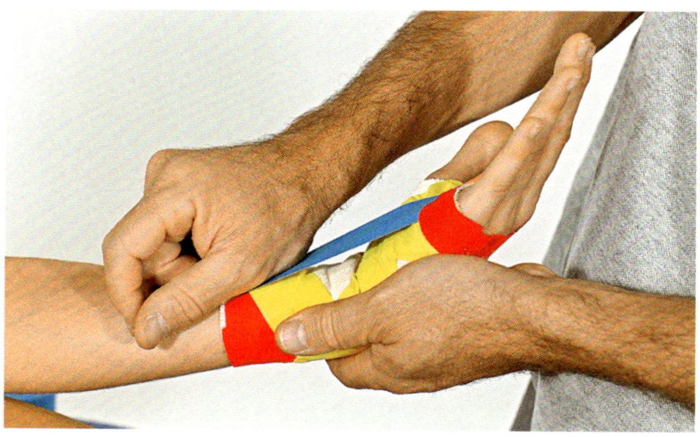

5

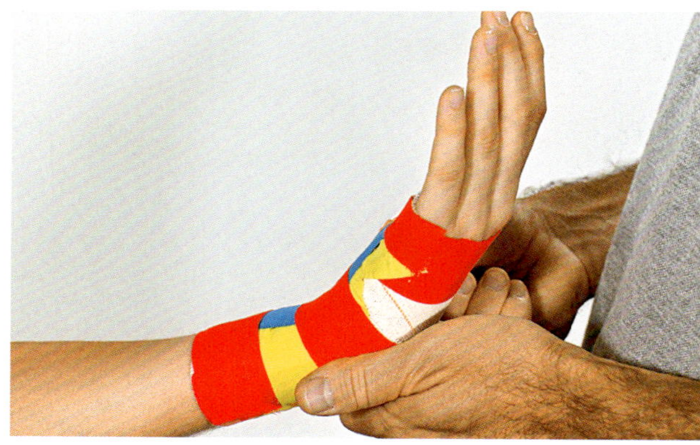

6

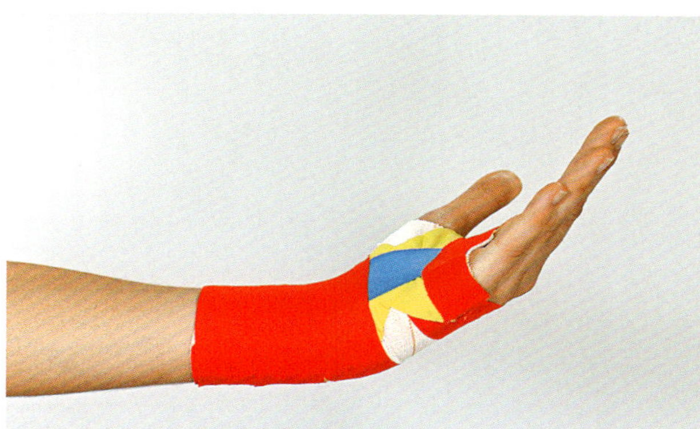

7

Limitation of extension on base bandaging

MATERIAL

✓ Inelastic adhesive tape, 2 to 5 cm in width
✓ 7.5 cm wide cotton fabric porous elastic adhesive bandage for base bandaging

APPLICATION

1 This type of bandaging is done over base bandaging of the radiocarpal joint (see pages 64-67), completed by the distal and proximal anchoring points.

2 To begin, a strip of inelastic adhesive tape is applied, beginning from the distal anchoring point at the fifth metacarpal bone and then directed toward the skin projection of the radial styloid process. Here, the bandage makes a spiral wrap around the forearm and is adhered to the palmar side of the proximal anchoring point.

3 A second strip of inelastic adhesive tape is applied, beginning from the distal anchoring point, this time at the second metacarpal bone, and is then directed toward the skin projection of the ulnar styloid process. The tape, after wrapping around the forearm, is affixed on the palmar side of the proximal anchoring point.

4 A strip of inelastic adhesive tape is now applied to the distal anchoring point at the skin projections of the third and fourth metacarpal bones and is directed longitudinally to the axis of the forearm toward the proximal anchoring point.

5 After this strip is affixed with a wrap of tape on the distal anchoring point, the wrist is placed in palmar flexion.

6 After having affixed the strip to the proximal anchoring point as well, a piece of tape is applied at the radioulnar and radiocarpal joints for stabilization.

7 The bandaging finishes with the application of other strips of inelastic adhesive tape, perpendicular to the longitudinal axis of the forearm.

INDICATIONS

✓ *Pain during dorsal extension of the hand*
✓ *Effects of surgery*
✓ *Sprain trauma*
✓ *Effects of fracture*
✓ *Capsuloligamentous instability*

RADIOCARPAL JOINT

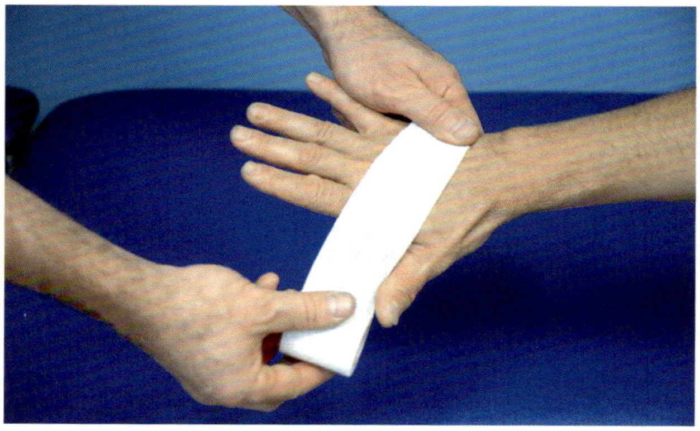
1

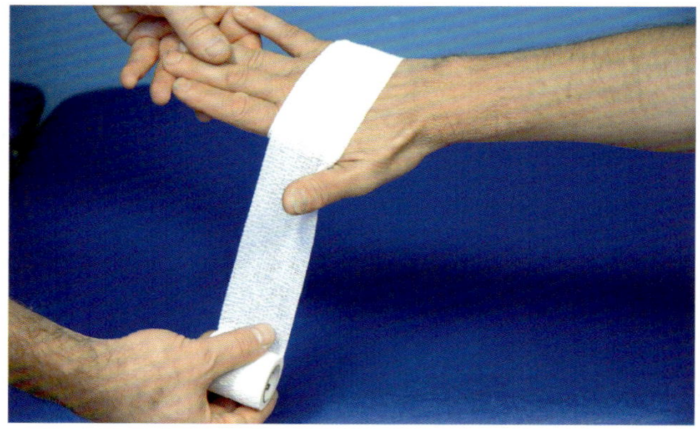
2

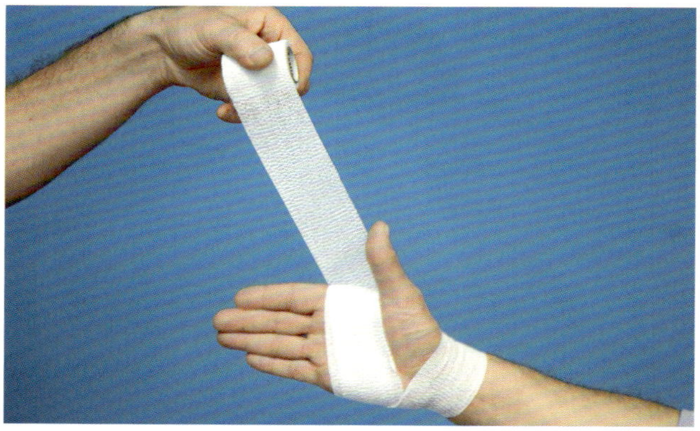
3

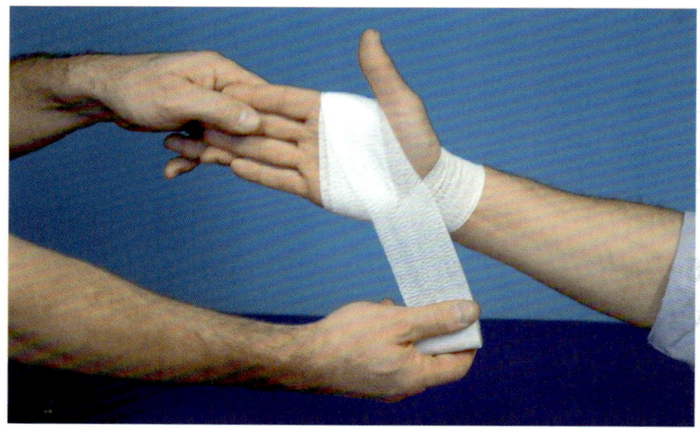
4

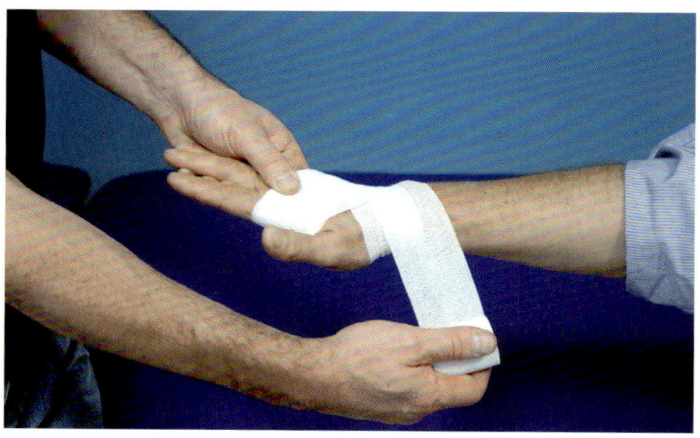
5

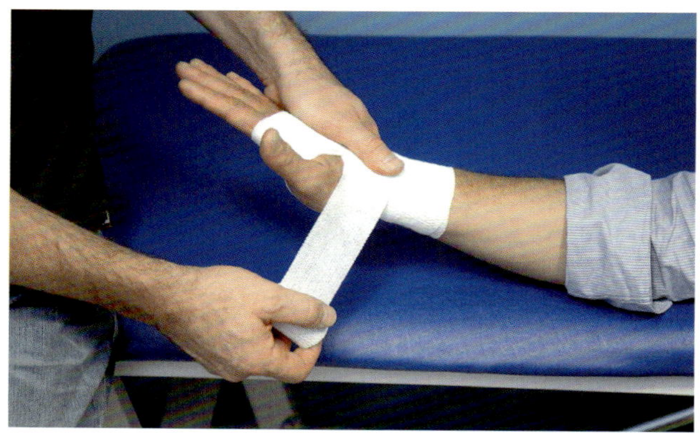
6

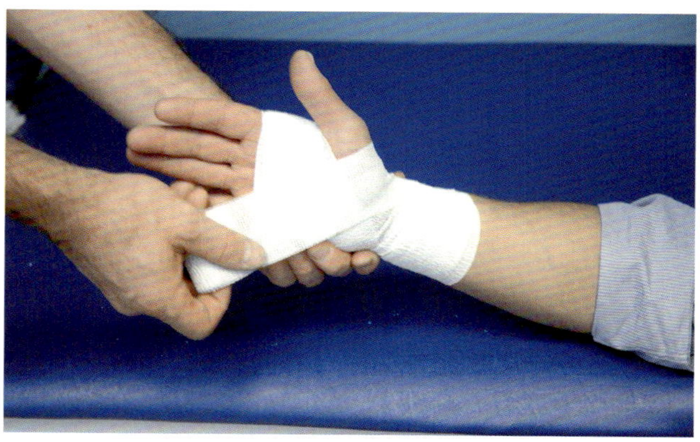
7

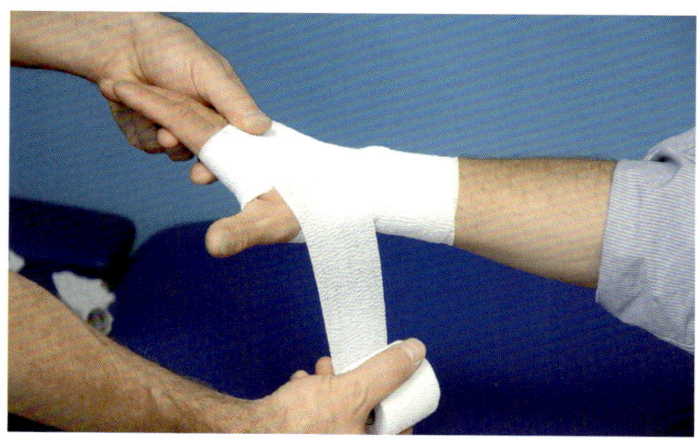
8

Support and limitation of extension

MATERIAL

✓ 2.5 or 5 cm wide elastic cohesive bandage
✓ Inelastic cohesive tape, 2 cm in width

APPLICATION

1-2 Base bandaging is done with the cohesive bandage, covering the entire hand and wrist. To begin, a complete wrap of the bandage is done around the hand.

3 Bandaging proceeds, wrapping the wrist.

4 The bandage is passed between the thumb and index finger, and then obliquely over the palm of the hand.

5 The distal third of the forearm is covered with several spiral wrappings of the bandage.

6-7-8 Bandaging proceeds, covering the empty spaces and reinforcing joint support at the wrist with several strips of bandage.

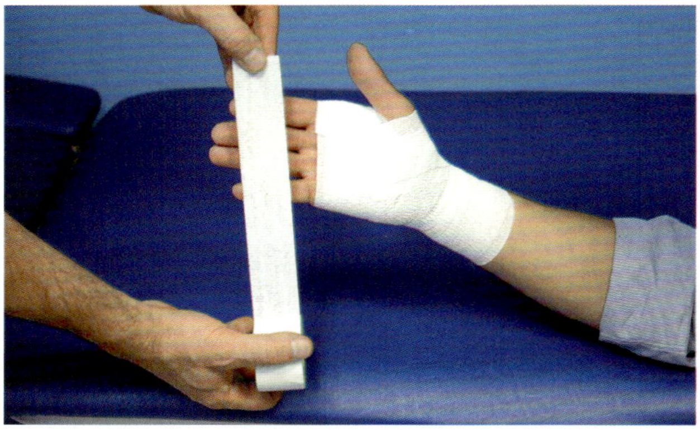
9

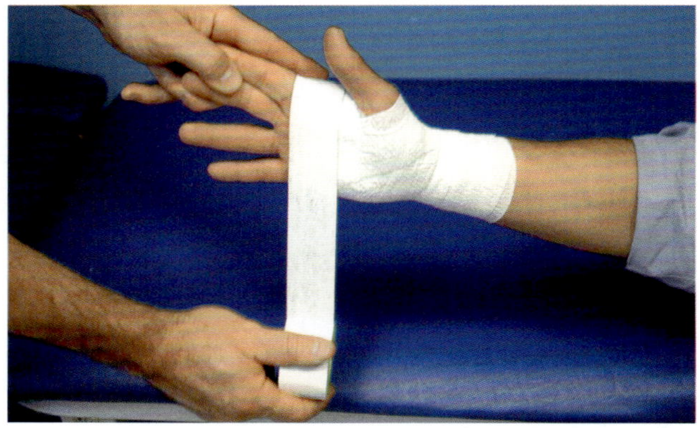
10

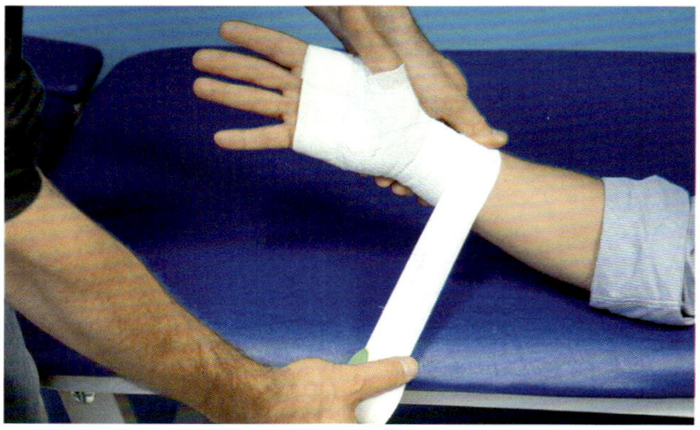
11

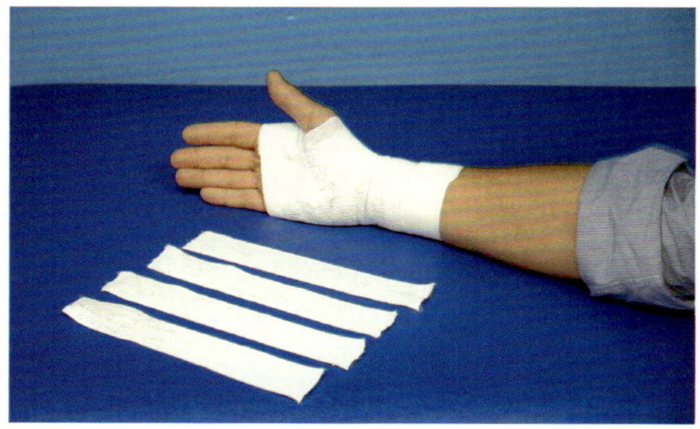
12

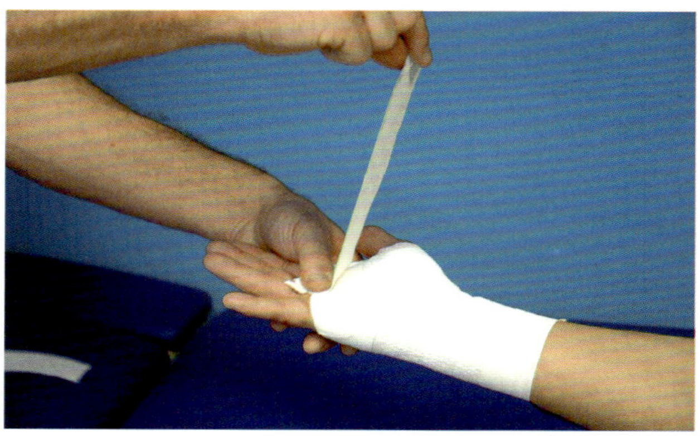
13

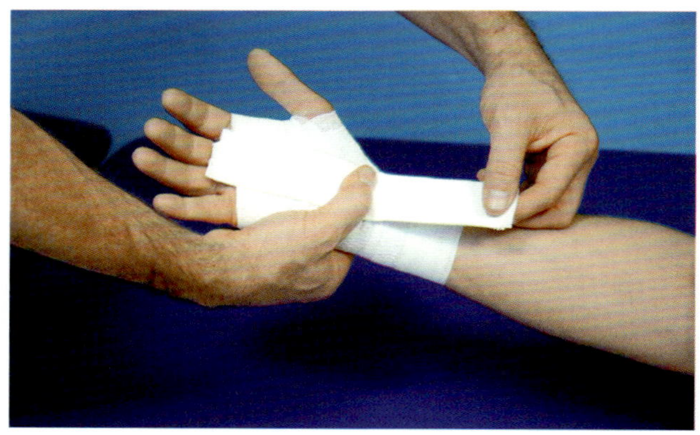
14

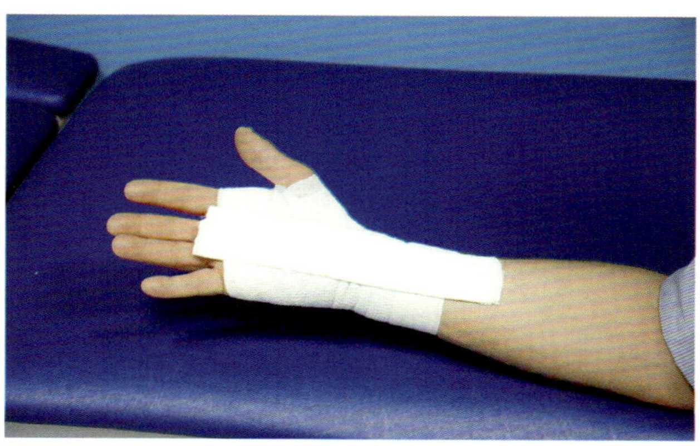
15

Support and limitation of extension

9-10 Distal anchoring points are prepared with a full wrap of inelastic bandage around the hand.

11 A proximal anchoring point is prepared with a full wrap of inelastic bandage around the forearm.

12 Four reinforced fasteners are prepared by applying two strips of inelastic bandage, one on top of the other.

13 The first fastener is applied, starting from the distal anchoring point in the region between the third and fourth finger.

14-15 Keeping the wrist in slight palmar flexion (10 degrees), the fastener is adhered over the base bandaging and then affixed to the proximal anchoring point as well.

RADIOCARPAL JOINT

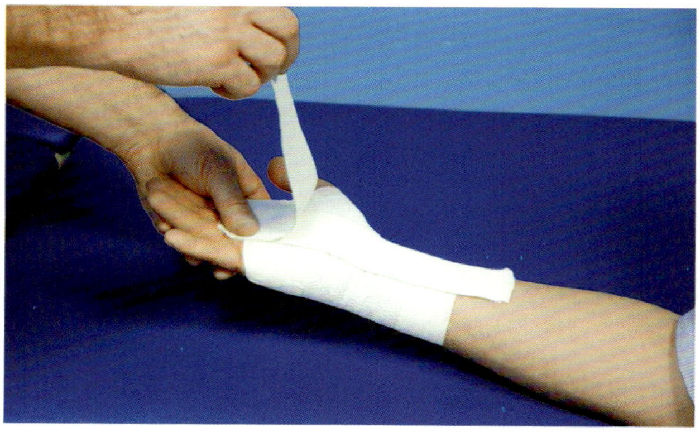
16

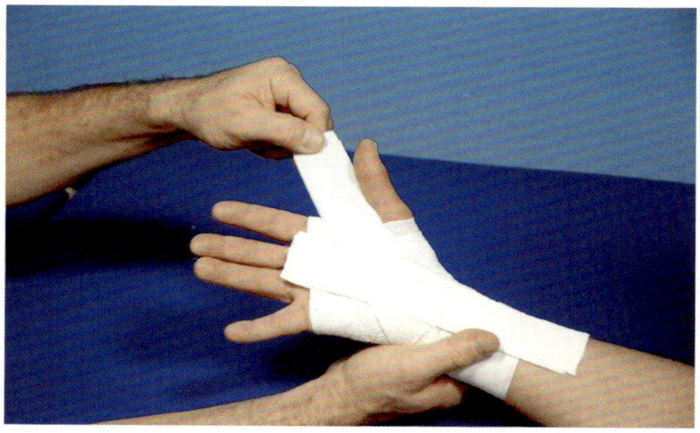
17

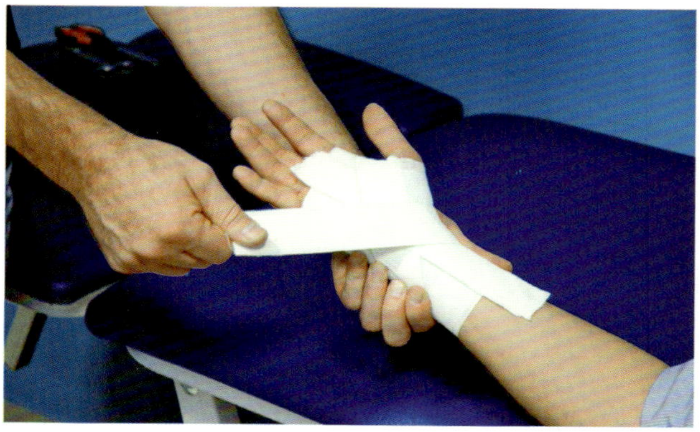
18

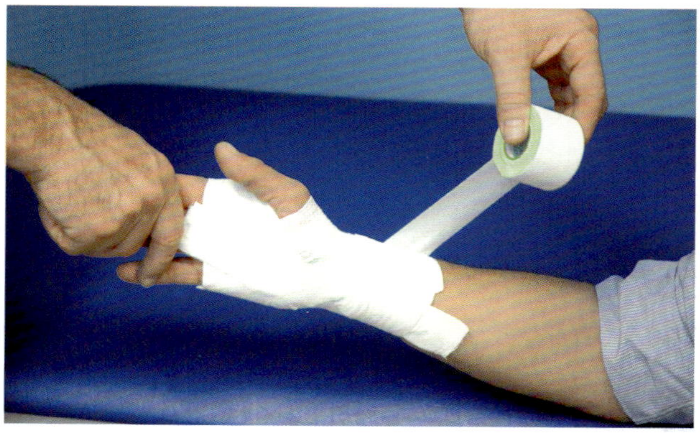
19

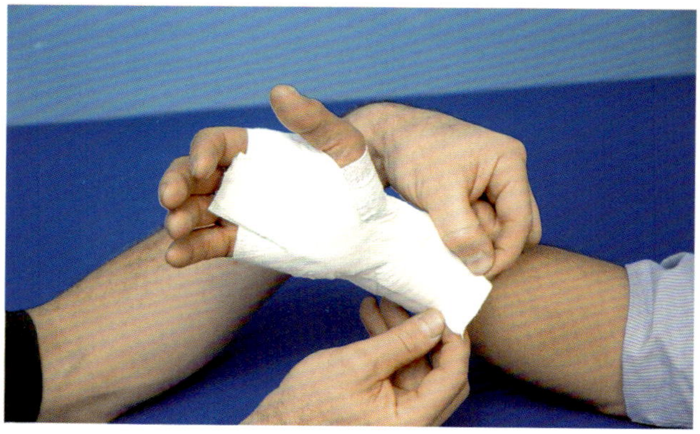
20

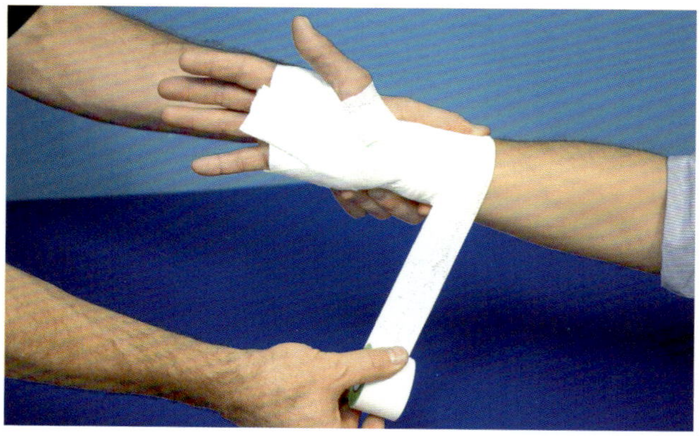
21

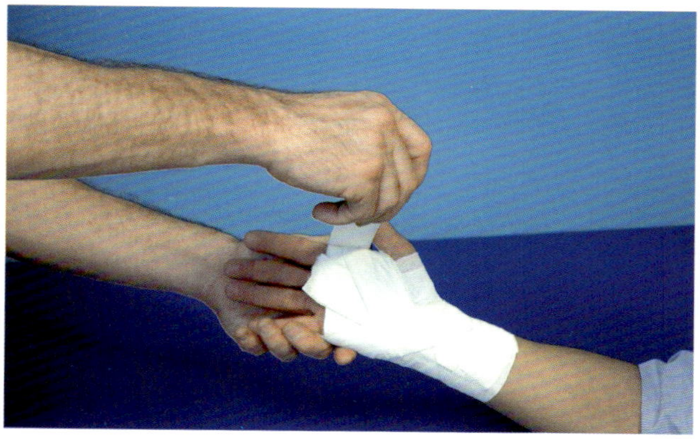
22

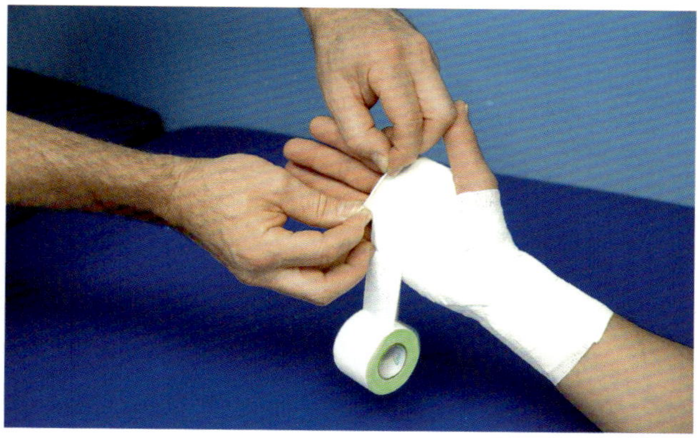
23

Support and limitation of extension

16 The bandage is reinforced by positioning the second fastener exactly over the first.

17 The third fastener is applied, starting from the proximal anchoring point on the projection of the ulnar styloid and proceeding to the distal anchoring point close to the second finger.

18 The fourth fastener is applied, starting from the proximal anchoring point on the projection of the radial styloid and proceeding to the distal anchoring point close to the fifth finger.

19 The fasteners are held in place with a wrap of bandage that covers the proximal anchoring point, but leaves the edges of the first two fasteners free.

20-21 The free edges of the first two fasteners are folded over themselves and held in place with another wrap of the bandage.

22 The distal anchoring point must also be covered with a wrap of bandage; the edges of the first two fasteners must remain free.

23 The free edges of the first two fasteners are folded over themselves.

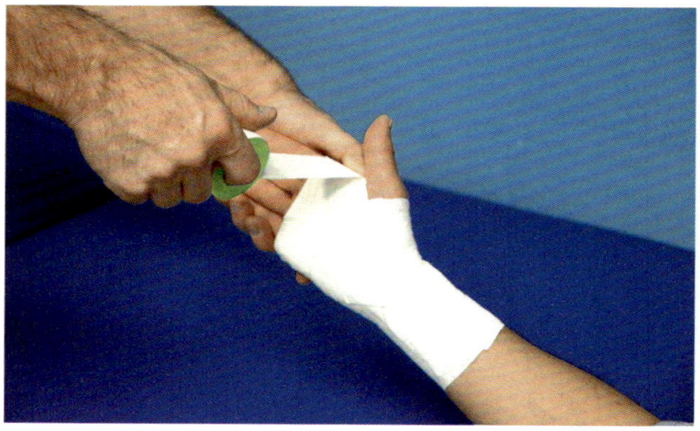

24

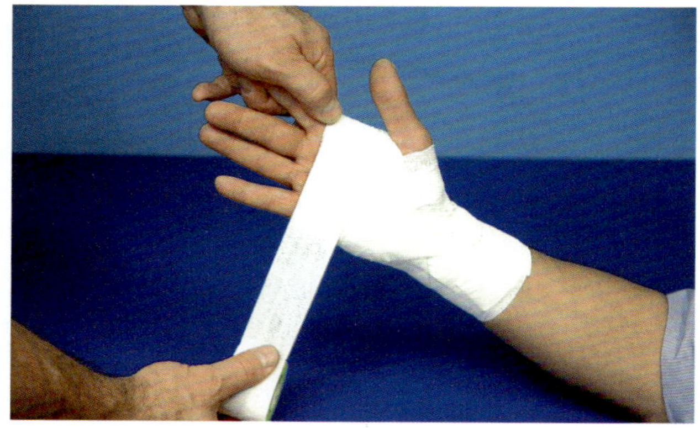

25

Support and limitation of extension

24-25 The bandaging is finished with another wrap of the bandage.

It is possible to reinforce the bandaging with additional applications of inelastic bandage in an X-shape or figure eight, in order to support the joints of the wrist.

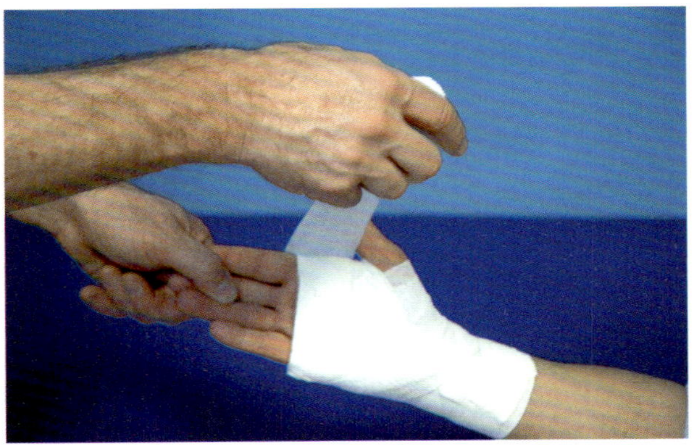

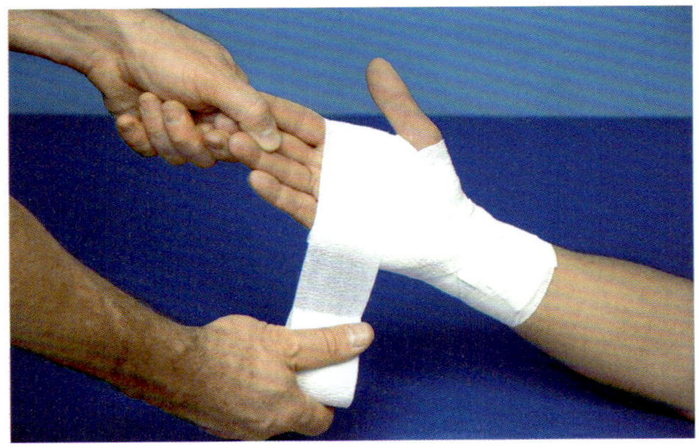

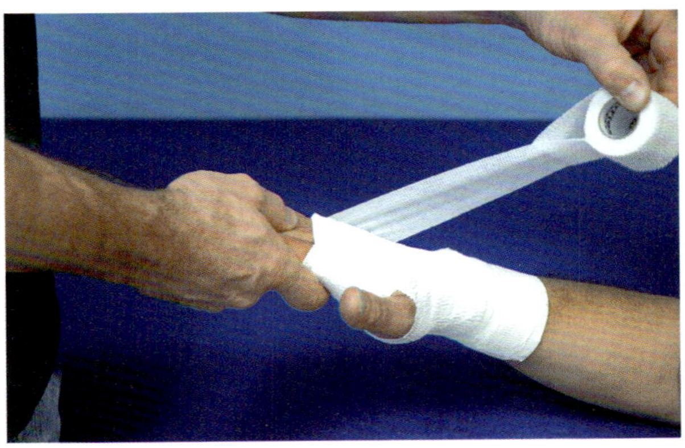

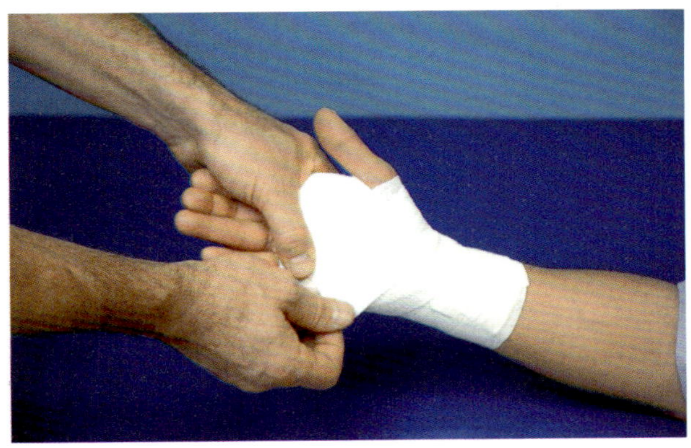

INDICATIONS

- ✓ *Posttraumatic conditions*
- ✓ *Preventative sports treatment*

RADIOCARPAL JOINT

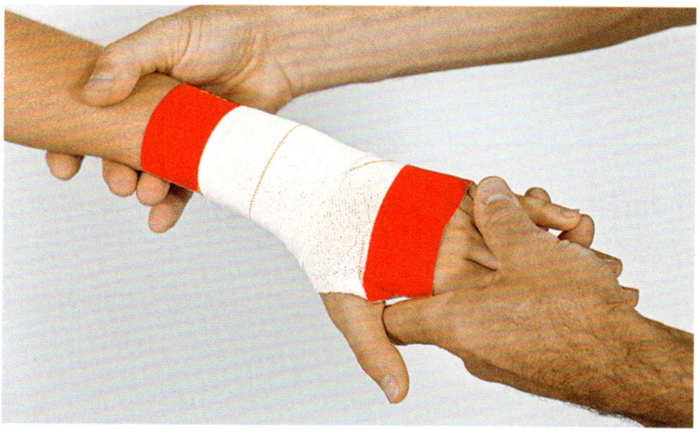
1

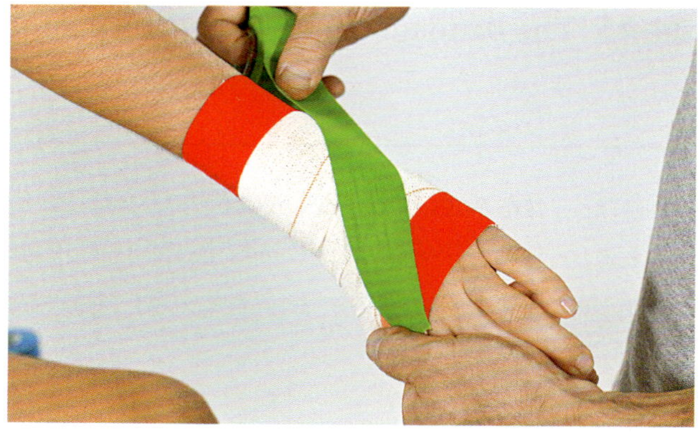
2

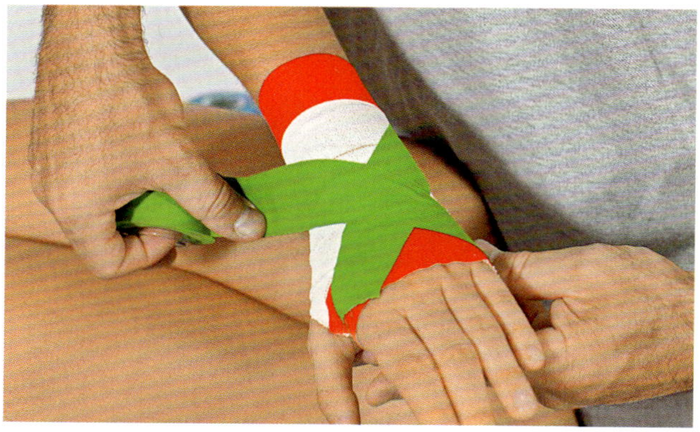
3

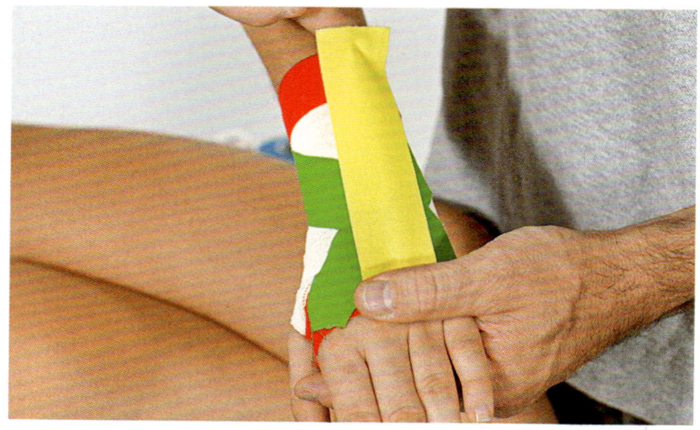
4

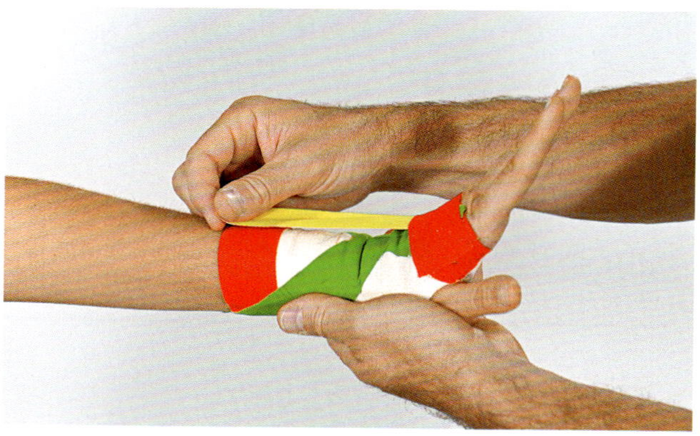
5

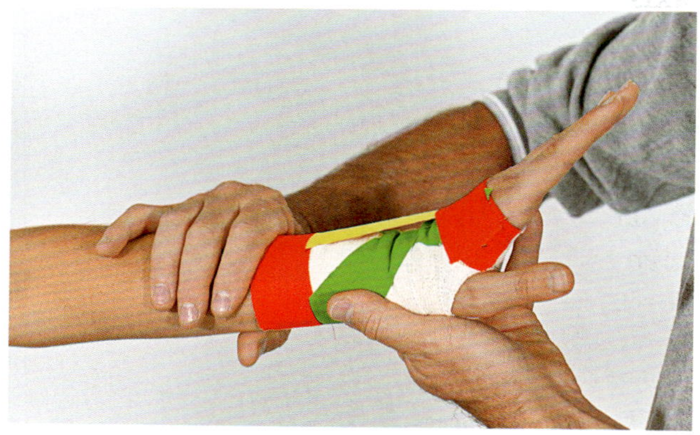
6

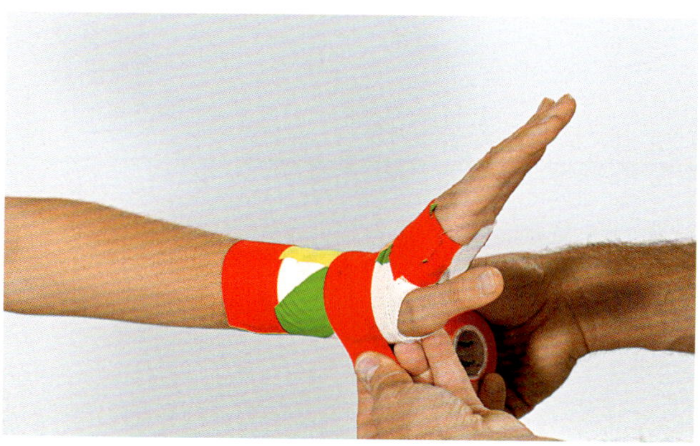
7

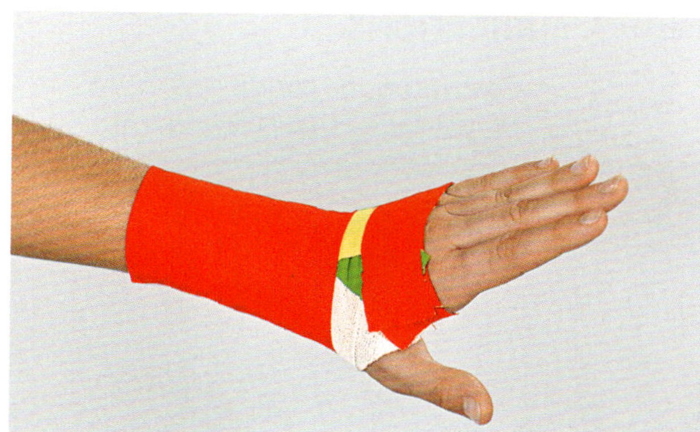
8

Limitation of flexion on base bandaging

MATERIAL

- ✓ Inelastic adhesive tape, 2 to 5 cm in width
- ✓ 7.5 cm wide cotton fabric porous elastic adhesive bandage for base bandaging

APPLICATION

1 This type of bandaging is done over base bandaging of the radiocarpal joint (see pages 64-67), completed by the distal and proximal anchoring points.

2 A strip of inelastic adhesive tape is applied, beginning from the distal anchoring point at the second metacarpal bone and directed toward the skin projection of the ulnar styloid process.

3 A second strip of inelastic adhesive tape is applied, beginning from the distal anchoring point at the fifth metacarpal bone and directed toward the skin projection of the radial styloid process. The two pieces of tape must adhere well to the palmar side of the proximal anchoring point.

4 A third strip of inelastic adhesive tape is applied to the distal anchoring point at the skin projections of the third and fourth metacarpal bones and is longitudinally directed to the axis of the forearm, toward the proximal anchoring point.

5 After this strip is affixed with a wrap of inelastic adhesive tape on the distal anchoring point, the wrist is placed in dorsal extension.

6 The strip is affixed to the proximal anchoring point with another wrap of inelastic adhesive tape.

7 Next, tape is applied at the radioulnar and radiocarpal joints for stabilization.

8 The bandaging finishes with the application of other strips of inelastic adhesive tape perpendicular to the longitudinal axis of the forearm.

INDICATIONS

- ✓ *Sprain trauma*
- ✓ *Effects of fracture*
- ✓ *Effects of surgery*
- ✓ *Pain during palmar flexion of the hand*
- ✓ *Capsuloligamentous instability*

RADIOCARPAL JOINT

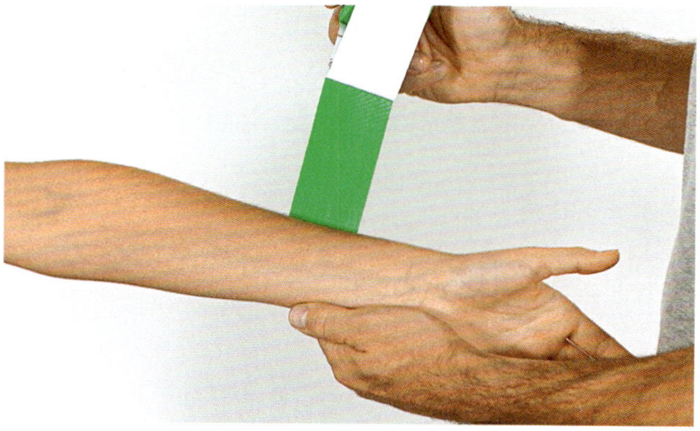

1

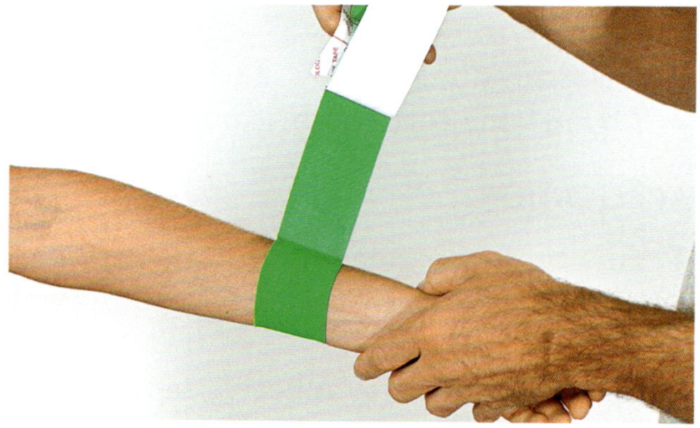

2

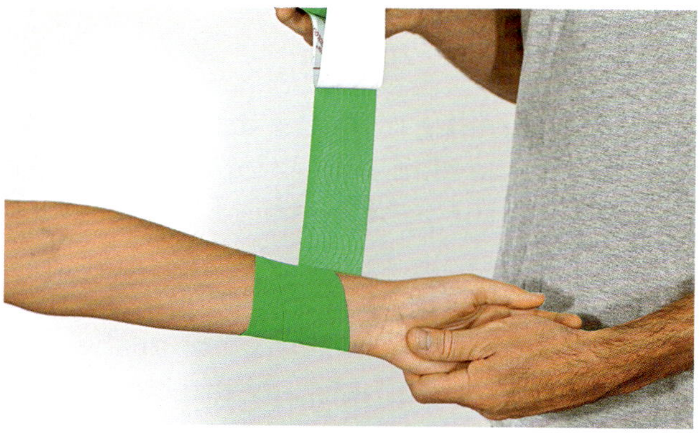

3

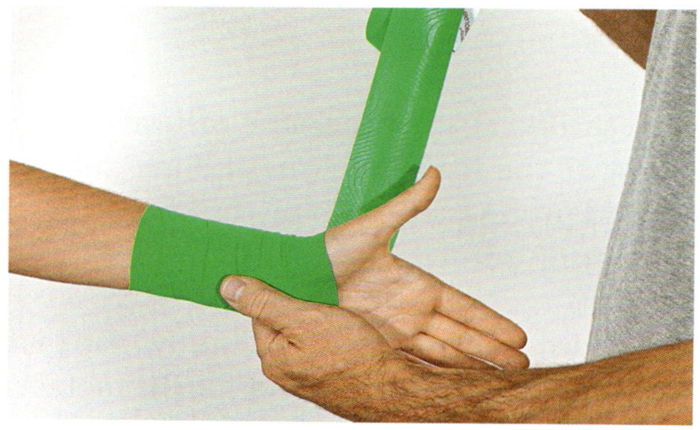

4

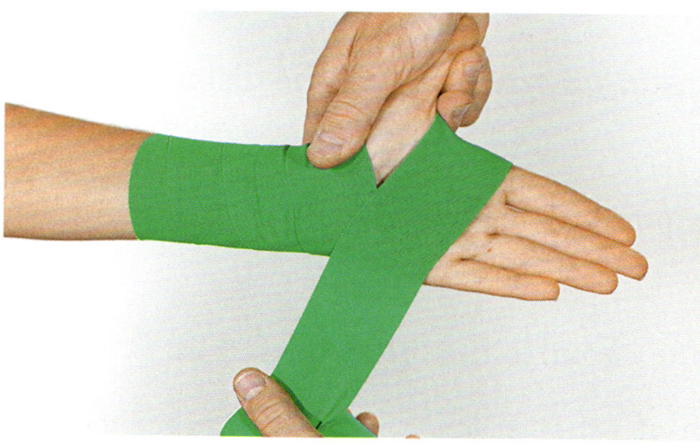

5

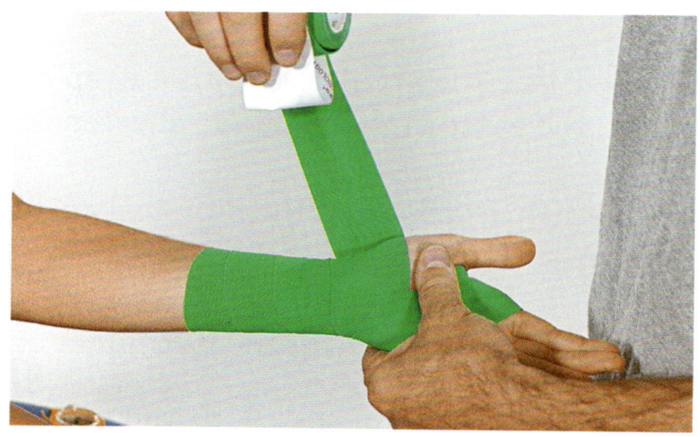

6

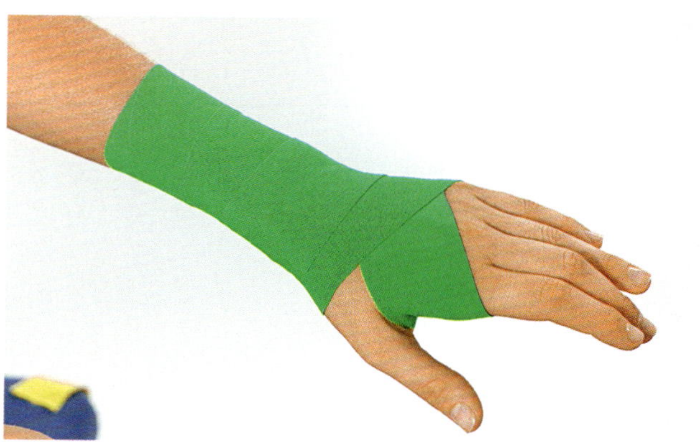

7

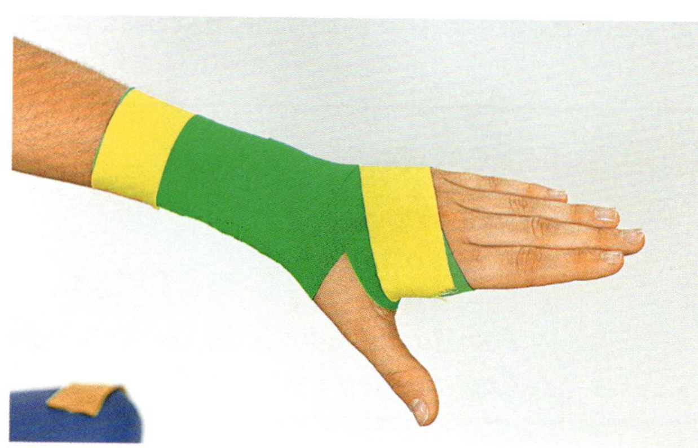

8

Limitation of flexion on tape base bandaging

MATERIAL

- ✓ Elastic adhesive tape, extensible lengthwise, 5 cm in width
- ✓ 5 cm wide inelastic adhesive tape to affix bandaging

APPLICATION

1 The elastic adhesive tape is applied on the dorsal side of the middle third of the forearm such that it may be unrolled in an ulnar-radial direction.

2 To begin, a complete wrap of the tape is made.

3-4 The forearm is wrapped in a spiral, moving in the proximal-distal direction and with an overlap of about 50%.

5 The hand is also wrapped, at the metacarpals, with the tape passing first over the dorsum of the hand and then over the palm, leaving the thumb free.

6 The tape passes again over the dorsum of the hand and reaches the radial styloid process.

7 Several spiral wraps are done in the distal-proximal direction, until reaching the middle third of the forearm where the bandaging began.

8 Next, the proximal and distal anchoring points are prepared using inelastic adhesive tape.

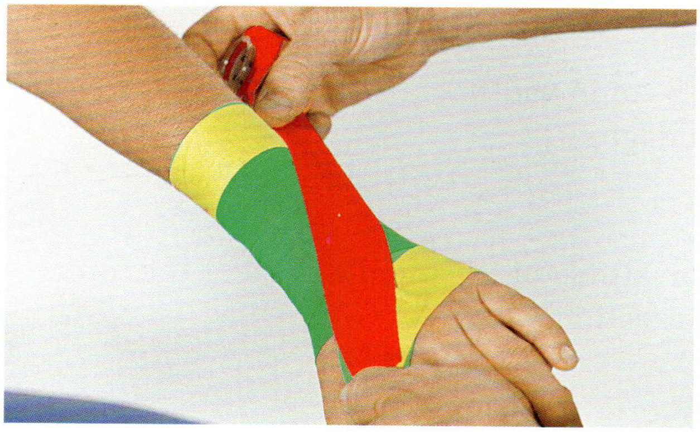
9

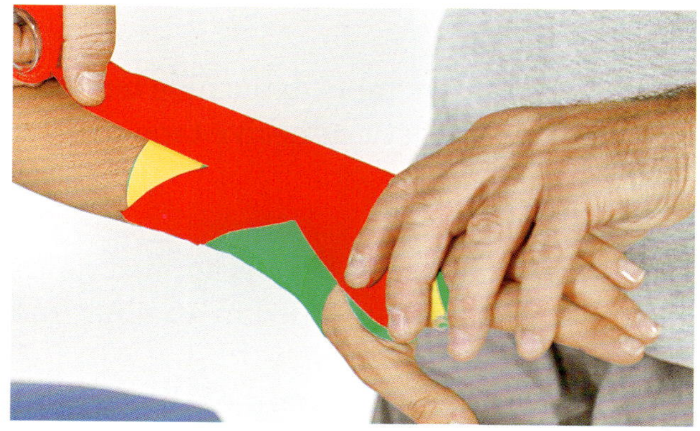
10

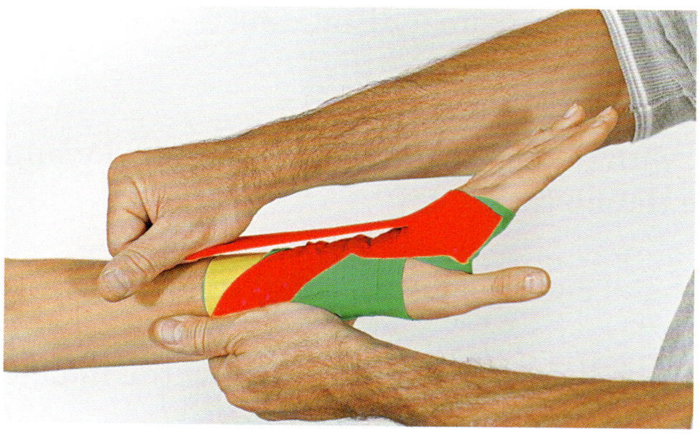
11

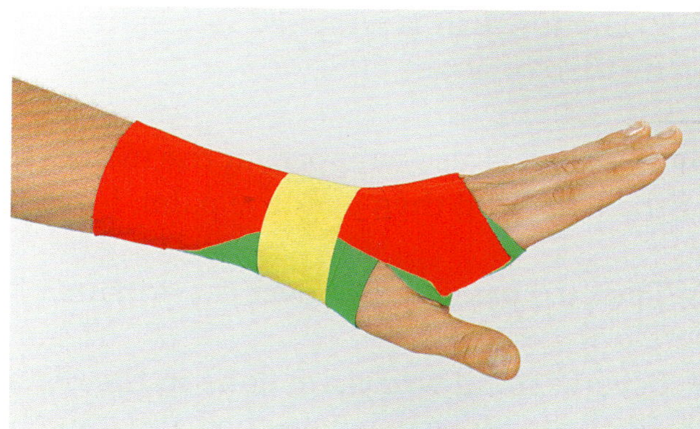
12

Limitation of flexion on tape base bandaging

9-10-11 The bandaging is reinforced with the application of three pieces of tape. The first starts from the distal anchoring point at the second metacarpal bone, and then is brought obliquely over the skin projection of the ulnar styloid process. The second piece of tape begins from the distal anchoring point at the fifth metacarpal bone, and is brought obliquely over the skin projection of the radial styloid process. The third piece of tape begins from the central part of the distal anchoring point and, following the longitudinal axis of the forearm, is pulled in the distal-proximal direction. All three pieces of tape are affixed over the proximal anchoring point with a strip of elastic adhesive tape applied in a semicircle.

12 Bandaging concludes with the application of a strip of inelastic adhesive material that wraps and stabilizes the distal radioulnar, radiocarpal, and midcarpal joints.

INDICATIONS

✓ *Sprain trauma*
✓ *Effects of fracture*
✓ *Effects of surgery*
✓ *Pain during palmar flexion of the hand*
✓ *Capsuloligamentous instability*

RADIOCARPAL JOINT

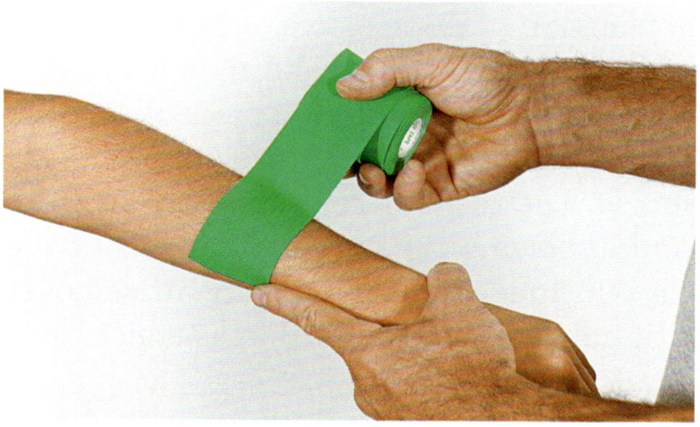
1

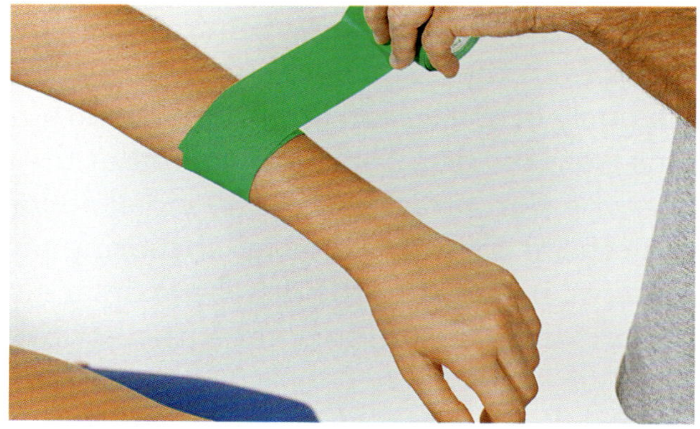
2

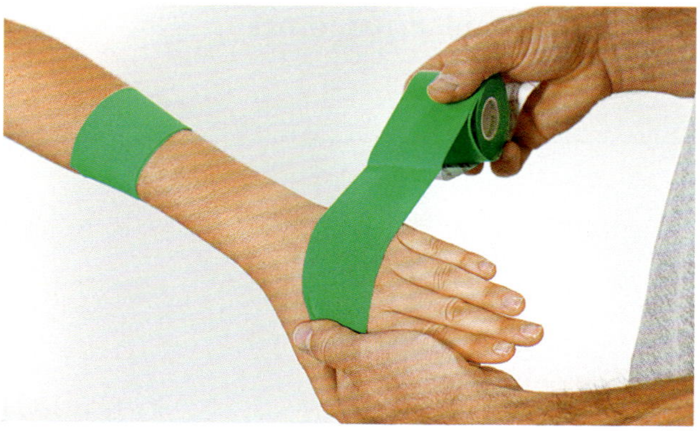
3

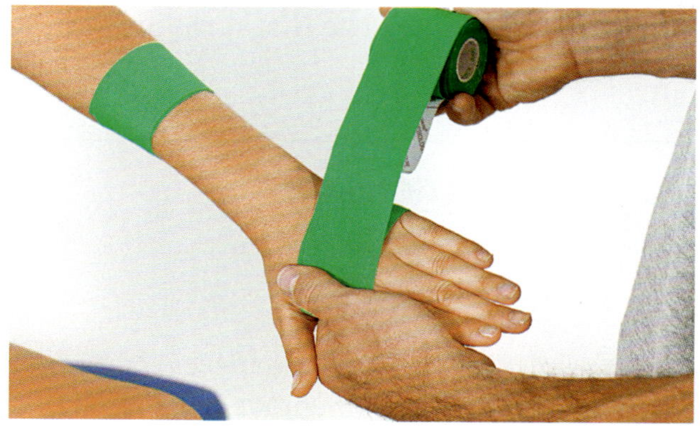
4

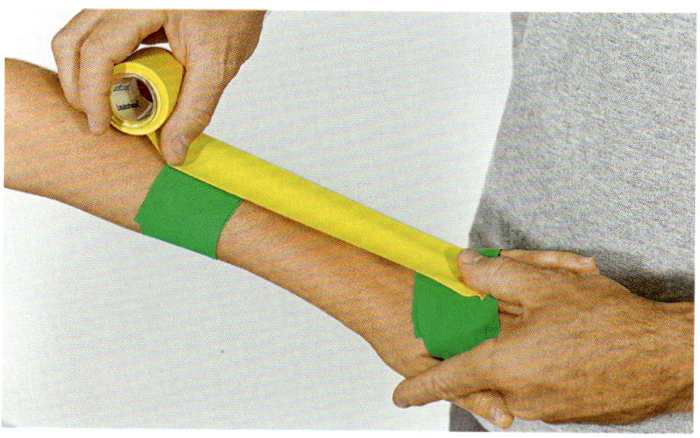
5

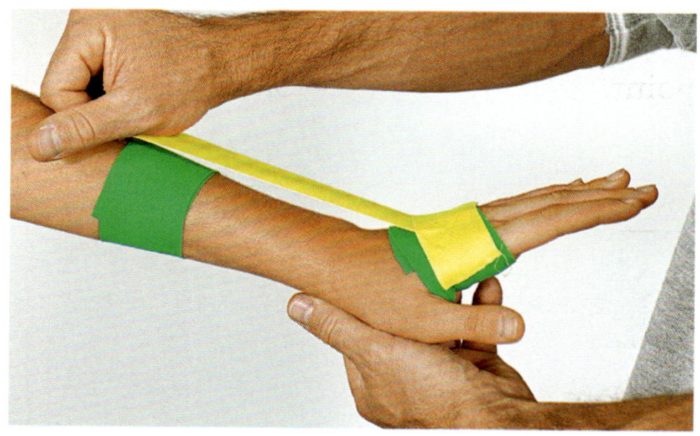
6

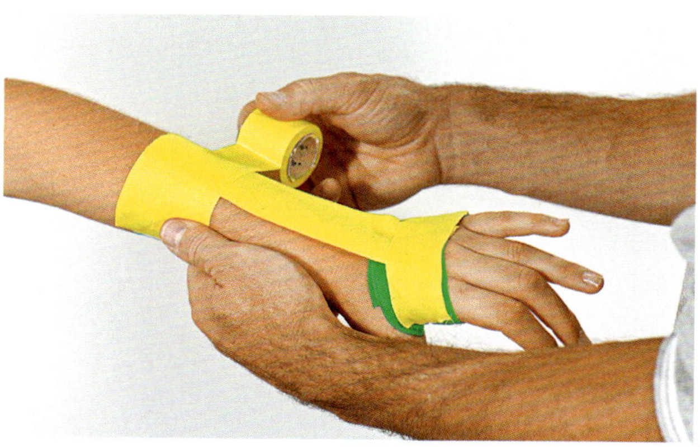
7

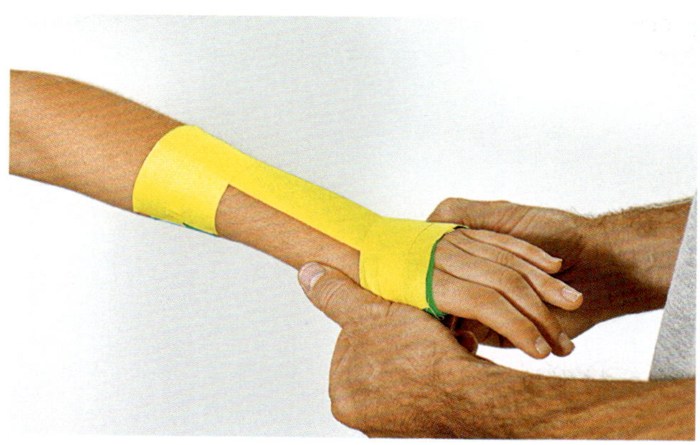
8

Limitation of flexion

MATERIAL

✓ Inelastic adhesive tape, 2.5-5 cm in width
✓ Elastic adhesive tape, extensible lengthwise, 5 or 7.5 cm in width, to prepare anchoring points

APPLICATION

1-2 To begin, the proximal anchoring point is prepared on the middle third of the forearm using a complete wrap of elastic adhesive tape.

3-4 The distal anchoring point is created with a wrap of elastic adhesive tape at the metacarpal area.

5 A piece of inelastic adhesive tape is applied to the distal anchoring point.

6 After affixing the tape to the distal anchoring point, the hand is pulled into light dorsal flexion.

7 The tape is also affixed to the proximal anchoring point with two strips applied in a semicircle.

8 Another strip of tape is applied at the metacarpal region to reinforce the distal anchoring point.

An alternative method of creating the anchoring points uses a cotton fabric porous elastic adhesive bandage, extensible lengthwise.
In order to ensure greater flexibility of the wrist, instead of the inelastic adhesive tape, a strip of 5 cm wide adhesive tape may be used, put under traction.
For better holding and greater efficacy, it is possible to cover and finish the bandaging with an elastic cohesive bandage.

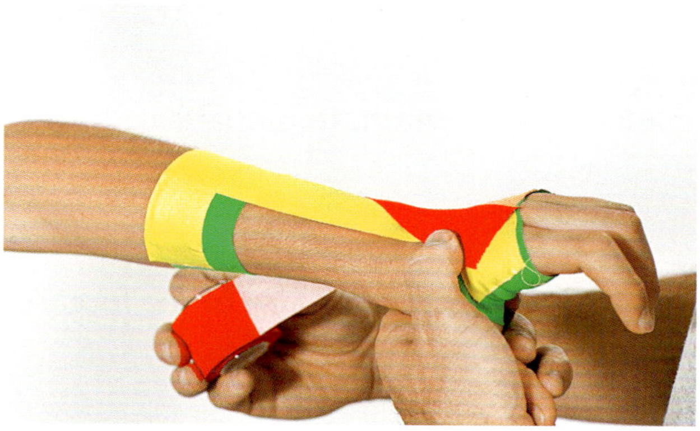
9

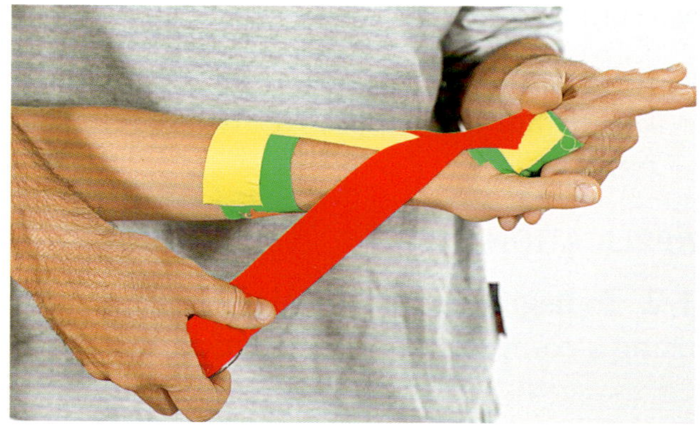
10

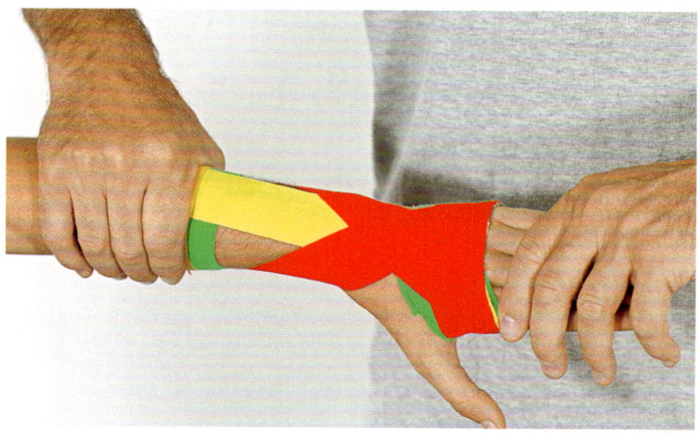
11

Limitation of flexion

9-10 The bandaging is reinforced with the application of two more pieces of tape; the first starts from the distal anchoring point at the skin projection of the second metacarpal bone and reaches, keeping an oblique trajectory, the skin projection of the radial styloid process; the second piece of tape starts from the distal anchoring point at the projection of the fifth metacarpal bone and reaches, keeping an oblique trajectory, the skin projection of the ulnar styloid process. Both pieces of tape end on the palmar side of the proximal anchoring point.

11 Bandaging is complete.

INDICATIONS

- ✓ *Sprain trauma*
- ✓ *Effects of fracture*
- ✓ *Effects of surgery*
- ✓ *Pain during palmar flexion of the hand*
- ✓ *Capsuloligamentous instability*

METACARPOPHALANGEAL JOINTS

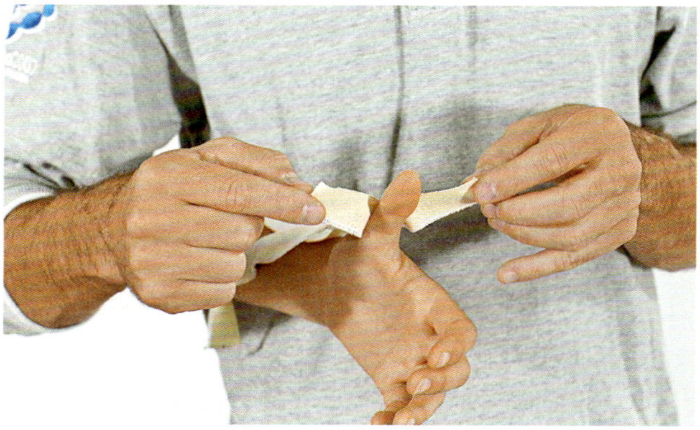

1

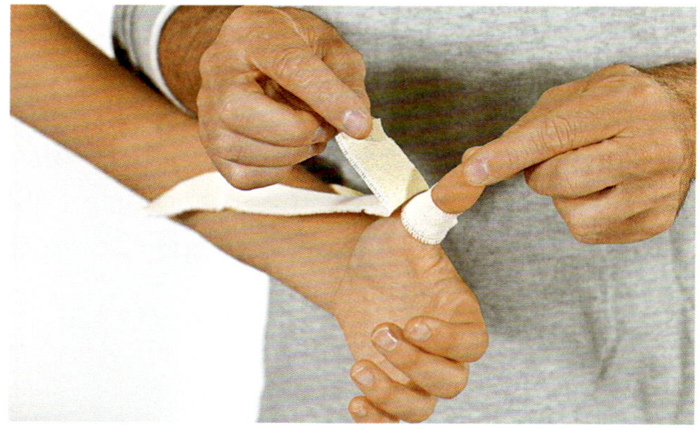

2

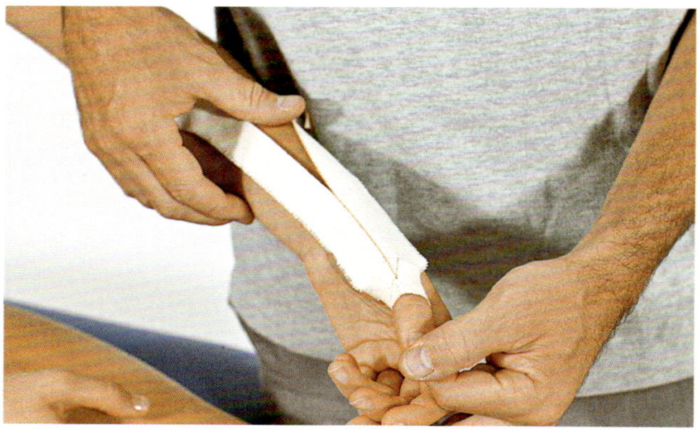

3

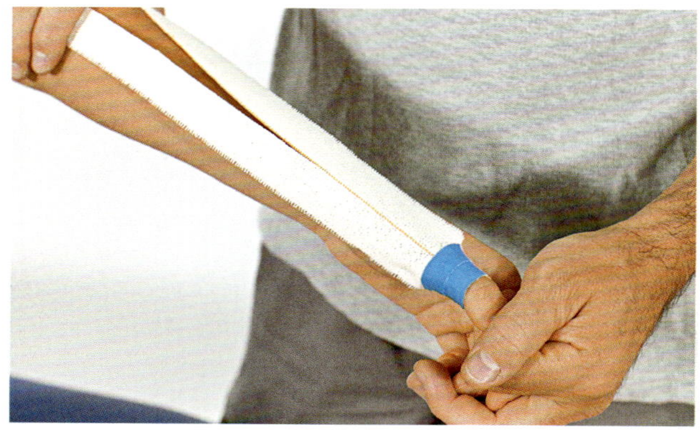

4

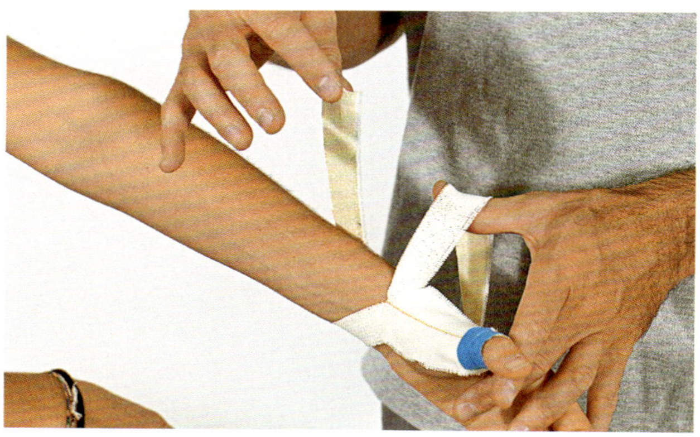

5

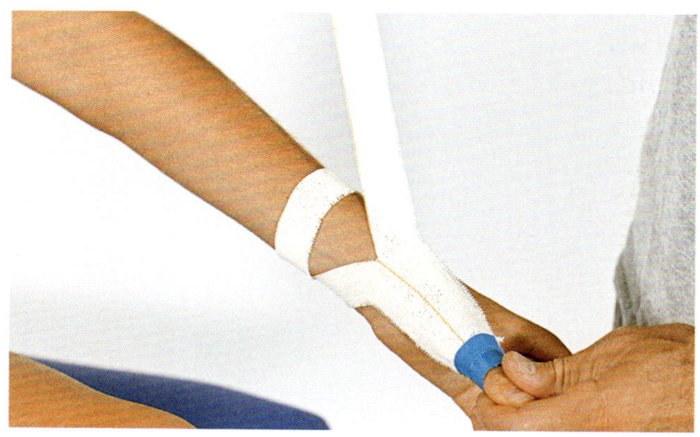

6

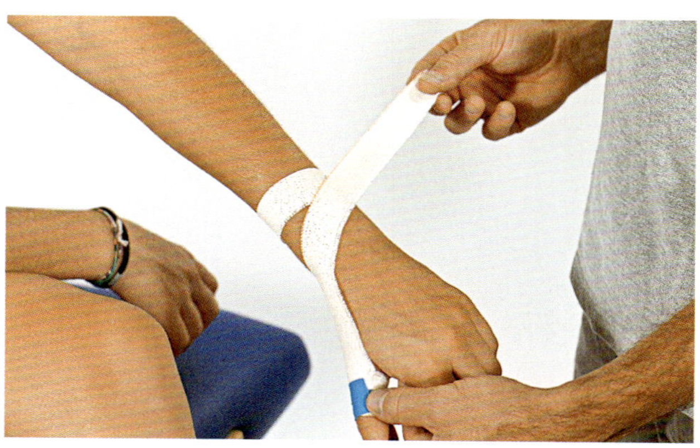

7

Unloading and protection of the thumb

MATERIAL

- ✓ Cotton fabric porous elastic adhesive bandage that can be stretched lengthwise, 5 cm in width
- ✓ Inelastic adhesive tape, 2 cm in width

APPLICATION

1-2-3 A strip of elastic adhesive bandage is cut longitudinally from both ends, leaving an uncut part of the bandage in the center of about 7-8 cm in length. The two pieces of one of the ends are applied in order to wrap the phalanx of the first finger above the metacarpo-phalangeal joint.

4 The distal anchoring point is reinforced with a strip of inelastic adhesive bandage.

5-6-7 The proximal parts of the bandage are pulled in the distal-proximal direction and then applied in order to wrap the distal third of the forearm.

The base bandage can be reinforced by applying one or more pieces of 2 cm wide inelastic adhesive tape in order to wrap the base of the first finger: the pieces of tape must follow the path of the base bandaging.
A wrapping of 5 cm wide inelastic adhesive tape may also be applied so as to wrap the radioulnar joint and the carpal joints.

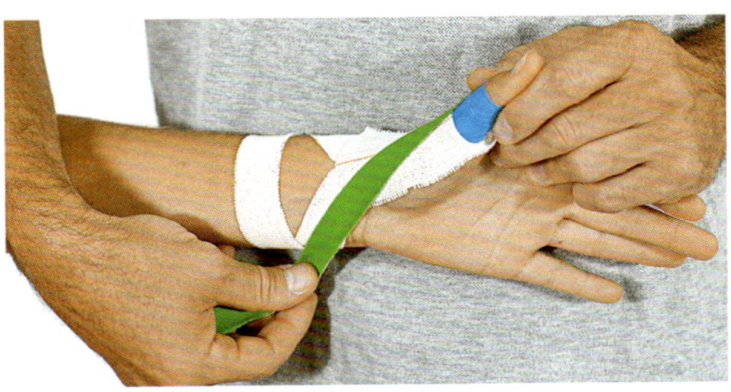

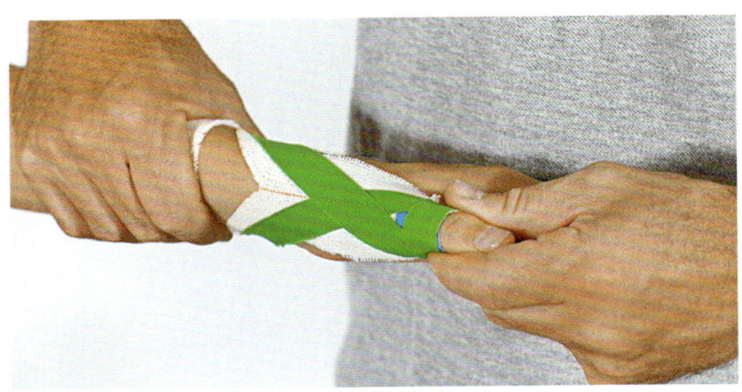

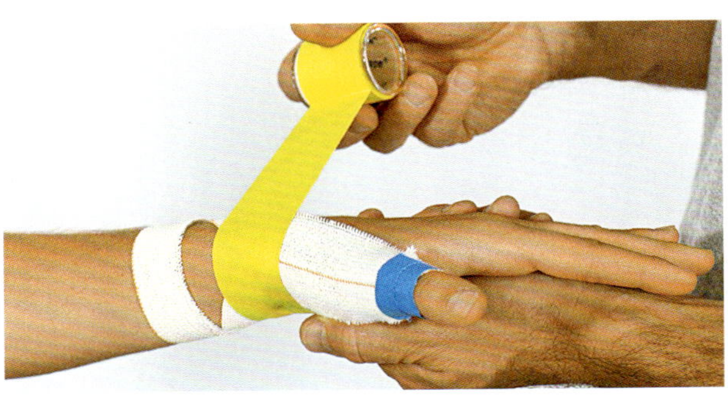

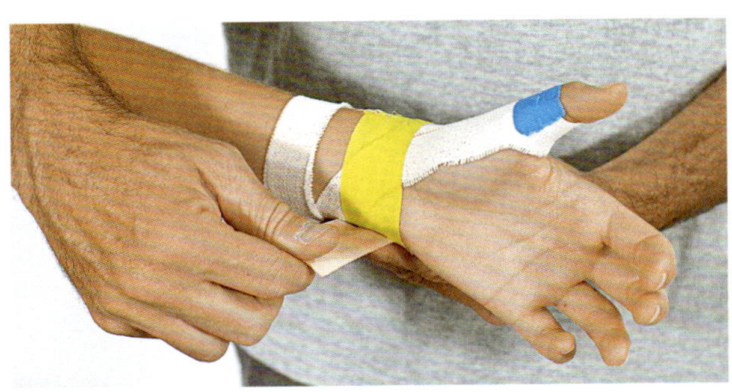

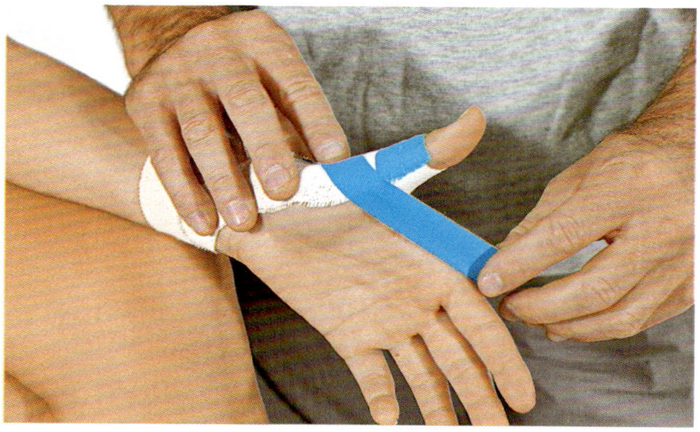
8

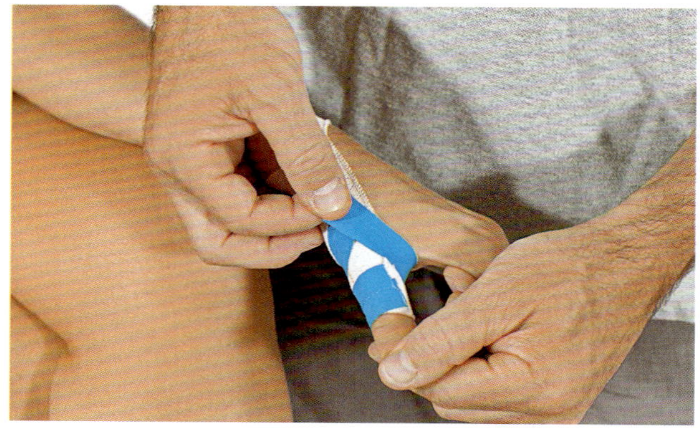
9

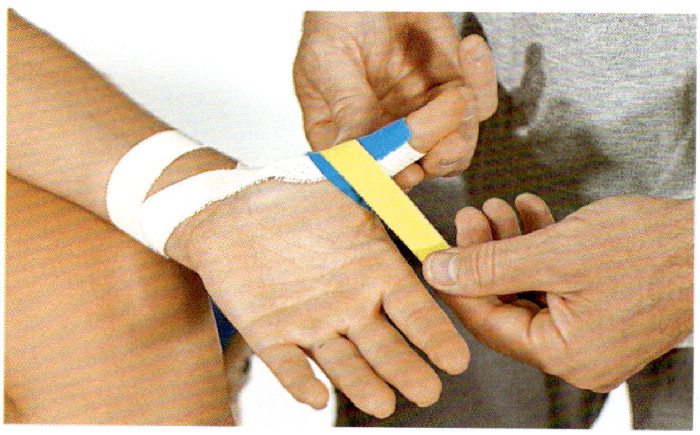
10

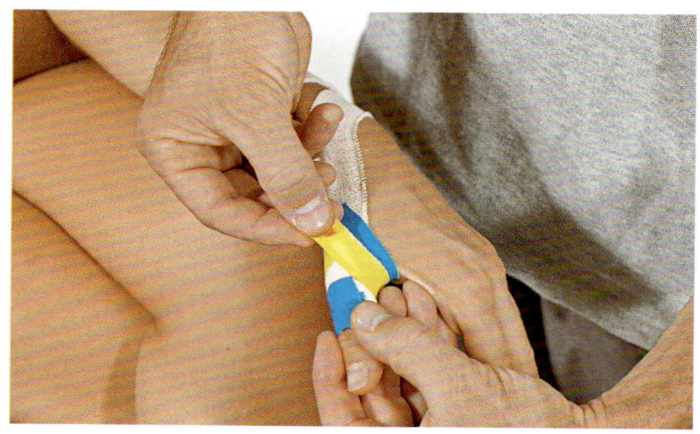
11

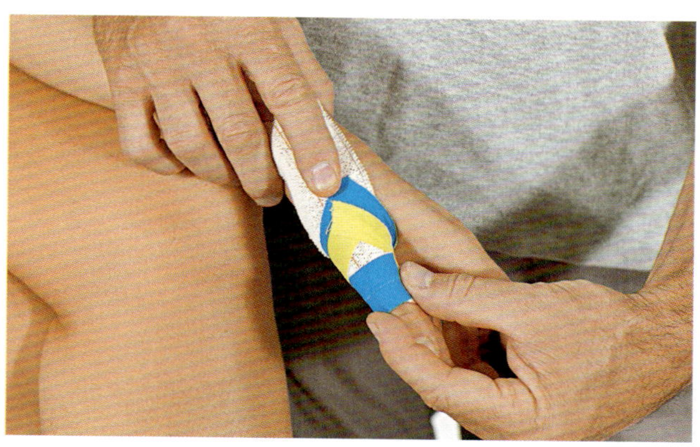
12

Unloading and protection of the thumb

8-9-10-11 It is possible to reinforce the support of the joint with the application of several strips of 2 cm wide inelastic adhesive tape to wrap the base of the first finger. The strips must overlap by 50%.

12 Bandaging is complete.

INDICATIONS

✓ *Traumatic sprain injuries*
✓ *Inflammation*

METACARPOPHALANGEAL JOINTS

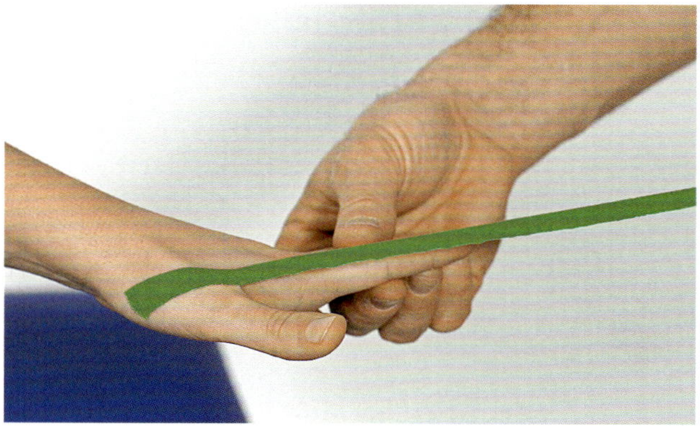

1

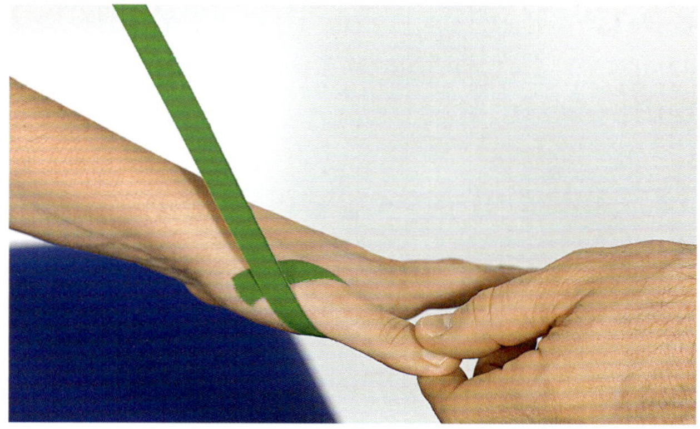

2

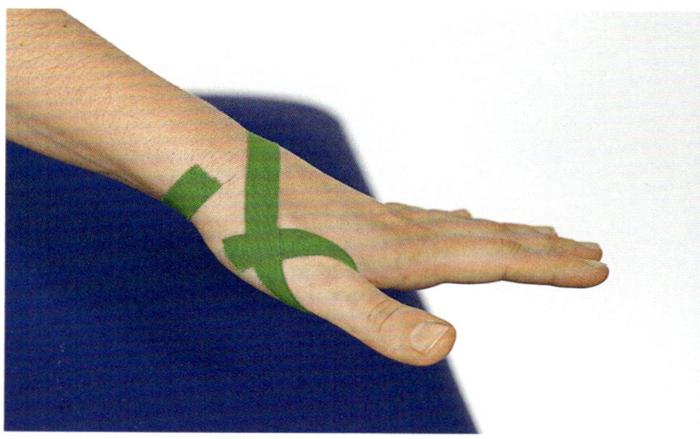

3

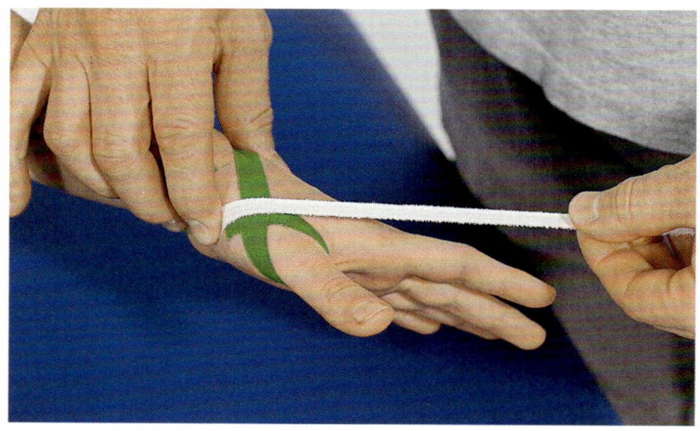

4

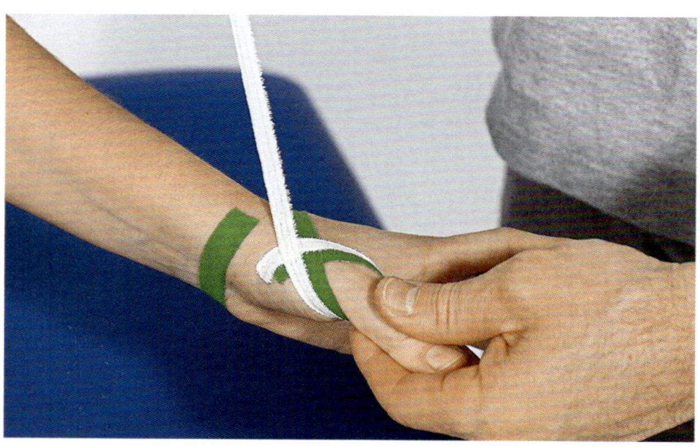

5

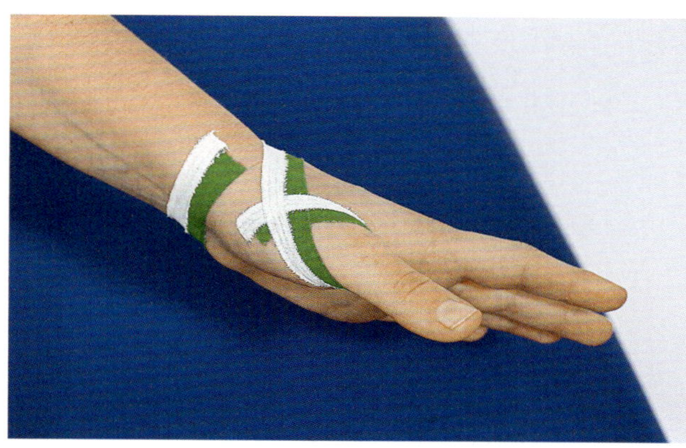

6

Stabilization of the thumb

MATERIAL

✓ Inelastic adhesive tape, 1 cm in width
✓ 2.5 cm wide inelastic adhesive tape to affix bandaging

APPLICATION

1 A strip of 1 cm wide inelastic adhesive tape is applied along the dorsal projection of the first metacarpal bone.

2 The tape is directed between the thumb and index finger, wrapped around the metacarpophalangeal joint of the thumb, and brought to cross dorsally.

3 The tape passes over the ulnar styloid process and ends at the projection of the radial styloid process.

4 A second inelastic adhesive strip is applied in the distal-proximal direction, covering 50% of the previous tape.

5-6 Again, the tape passes between the thumb and index finger, wraps around the metacarpophalangeal joint of the thumb, crosses dorsally, then passes over the ulnar styloid process and ends at the projection of the radial styloid process.

METACARPOPHALANGEAL JOINTS

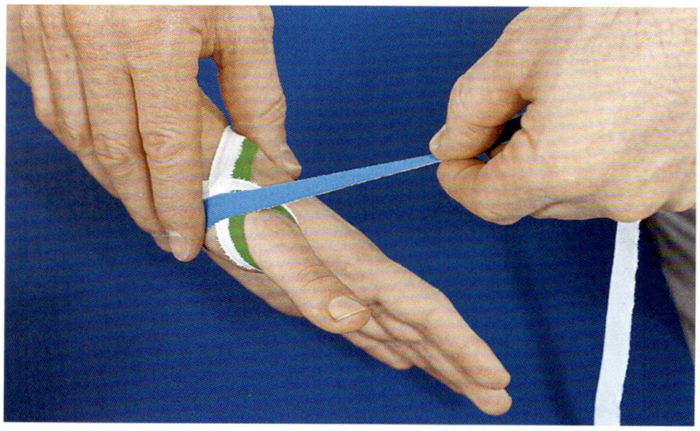

7

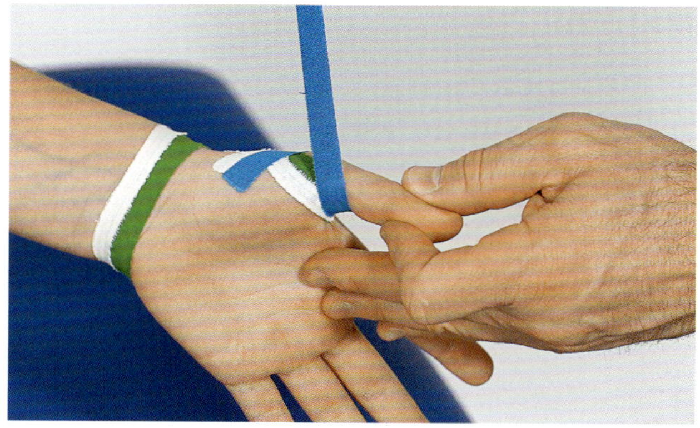

8

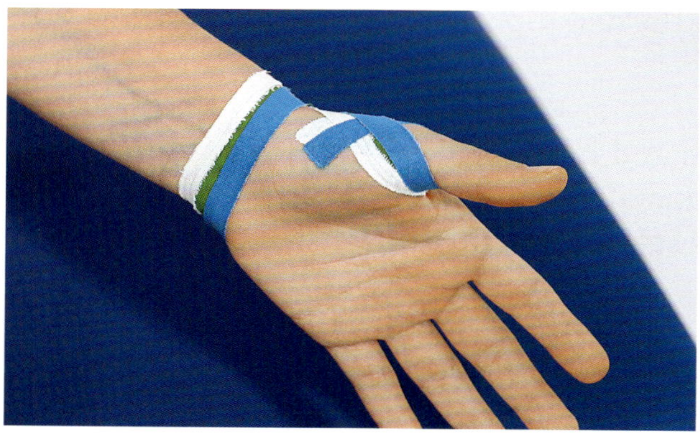

9

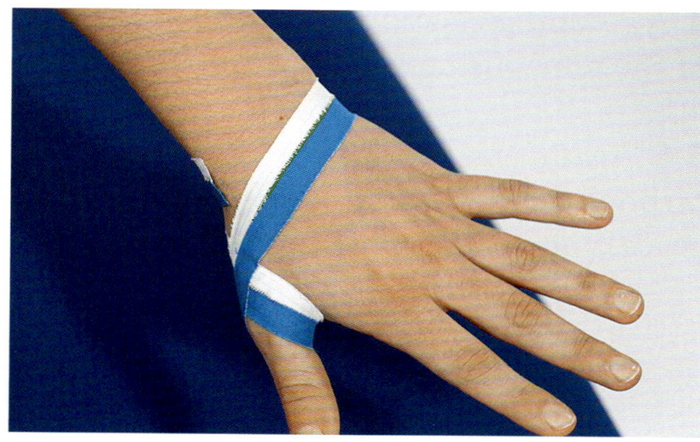

10

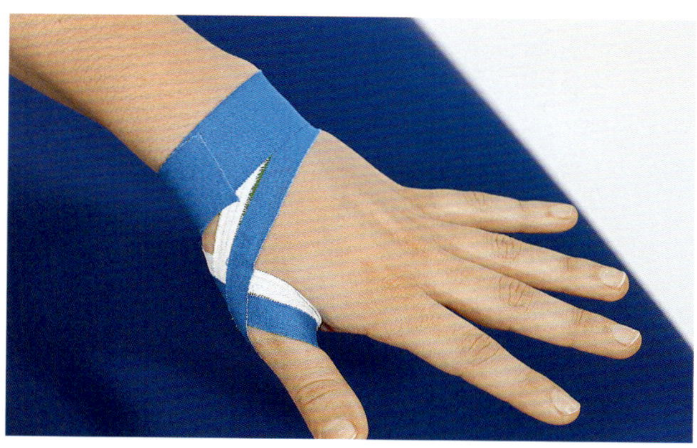

11

Stabilization of the thumb

7-8-9-10 Moving in the proximal-distal direction, it goes on to cover the remaining uncovered portion of the first tape. A third inelastic adhesive strip is applied, and the paths of the previous pieces of tape are repeated with it.

11 The bandaging is affixed at the wrist with a wrapping of 2.5 cm wide inelastic adhesive bandage.

INDICATIONS

✓ *Sprain trauma*
✓ *Preventative sports treatment*

METACARPOPHALANGEAL JOINTS

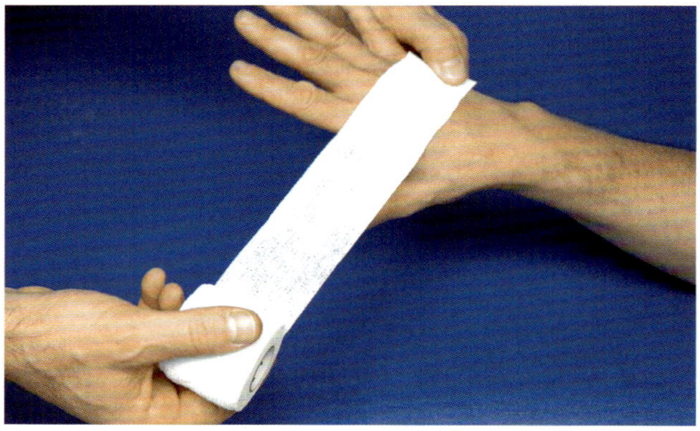
1

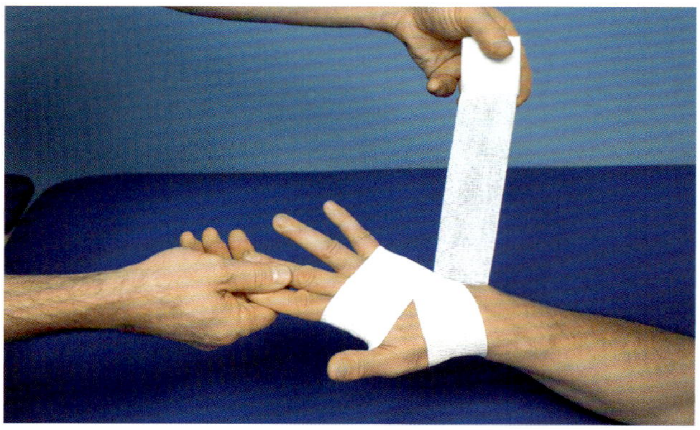
2

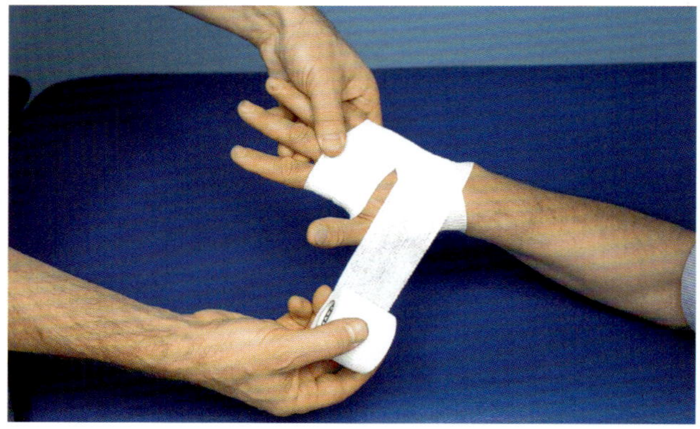
3

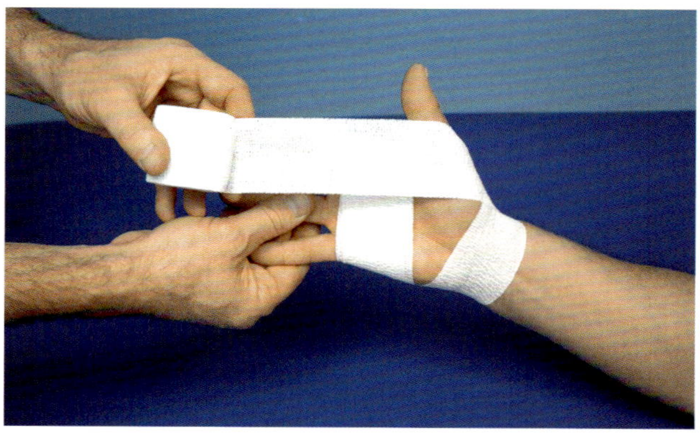
4

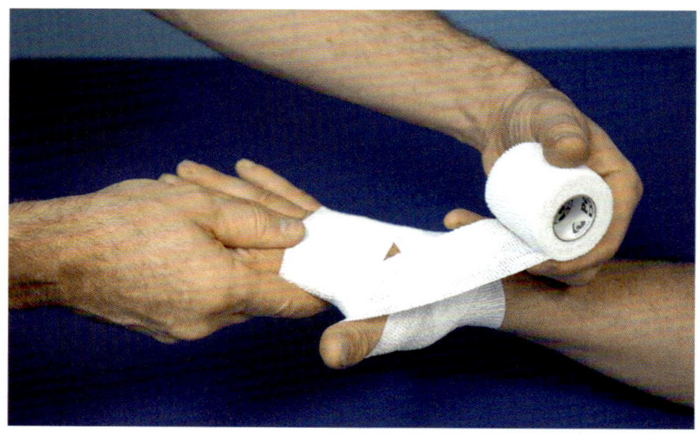
5

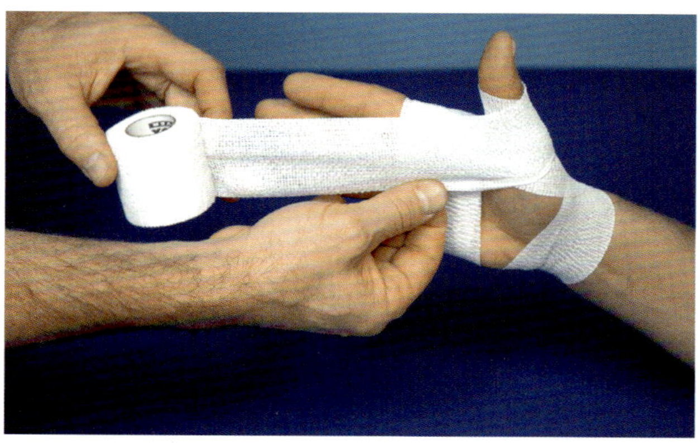
6

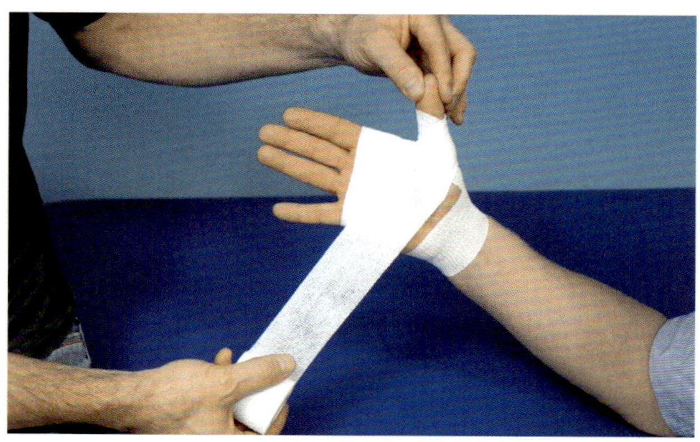
7

Limitation and stabilization of abduction and extension of the thumb

MATERIAL

✓ 2.5 or 5 cm wide elastic cohesive bandage
✓ Inelastic cohesive tape, 2 cm in width

APPLICATION

1 Bandaging proceeds by preparing, before all else, the base bandaging. A wrap of cohesive bandage is made to cover the dorsal and palmar regions of the hand.

2-3 The bandage covers the metacarpophalangeal joint of the first finger and then wraps the carpometacarpal and radioulnar joints.

4-5 The bandage then wraps the metacarpophalangeal joint and the phalanx of the thumb.

6 A full wrap of the bandage is made around the phalanx of the first finger.

7 The bandage is directed over the palm of the hand.

METACARPOPHALANGEAL JOINTS

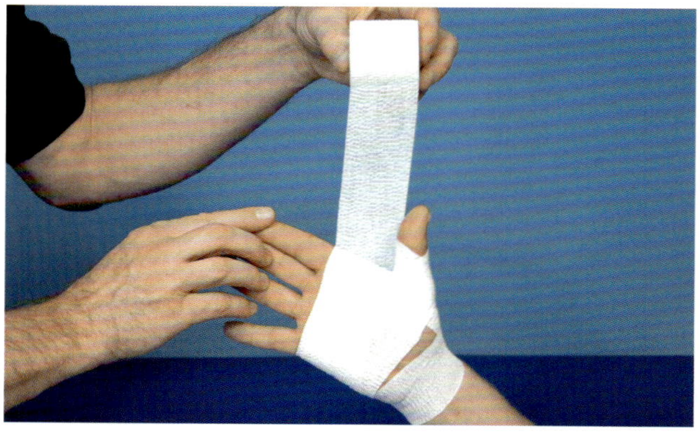

8

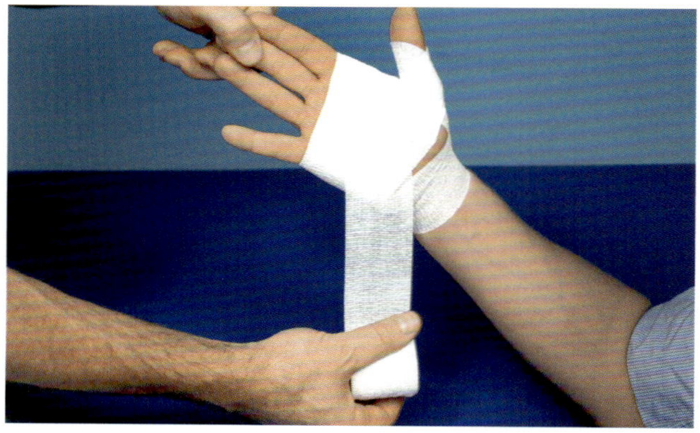

9

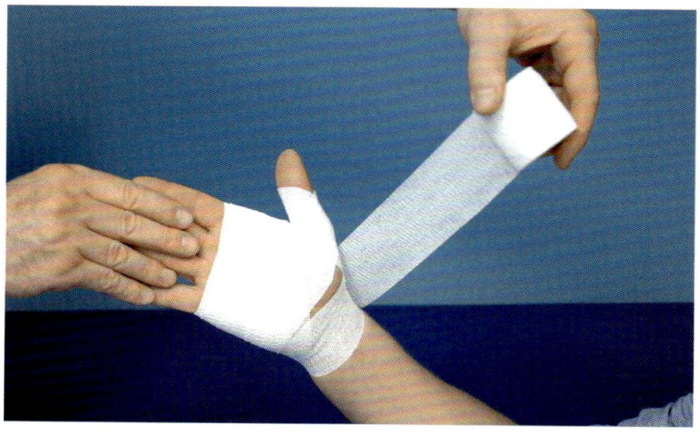

10

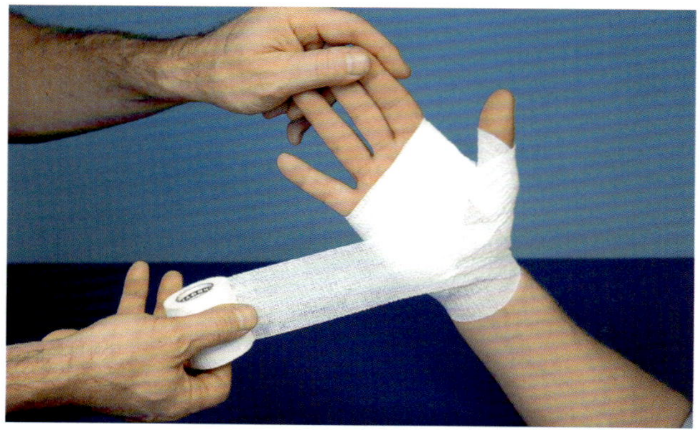

11

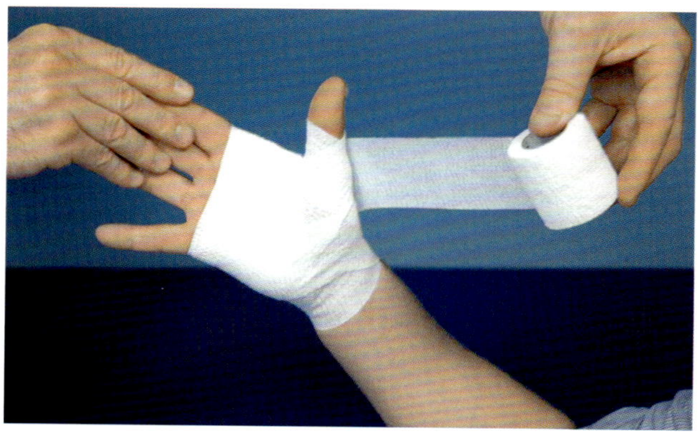

12

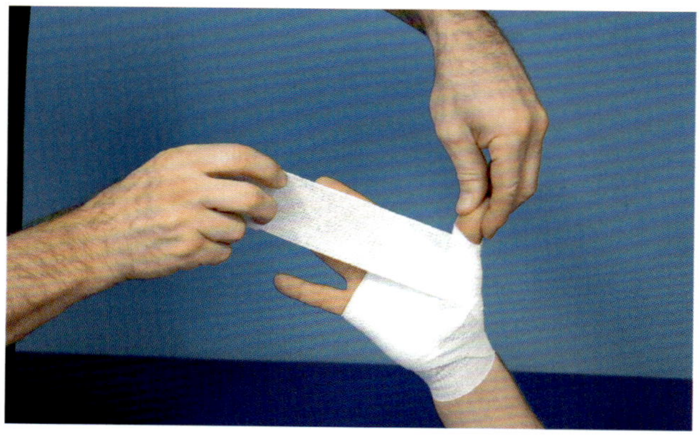

13

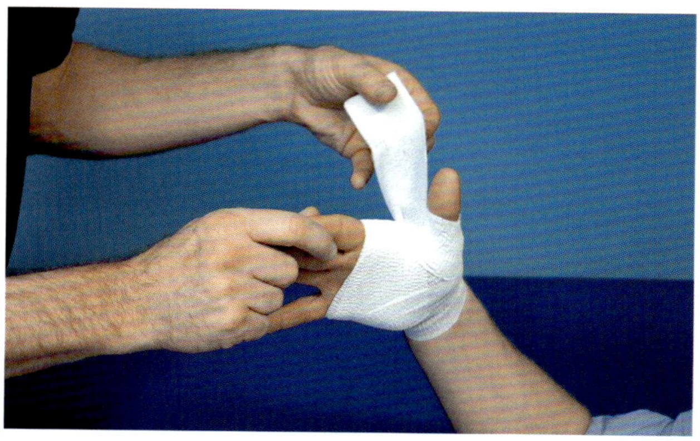

14

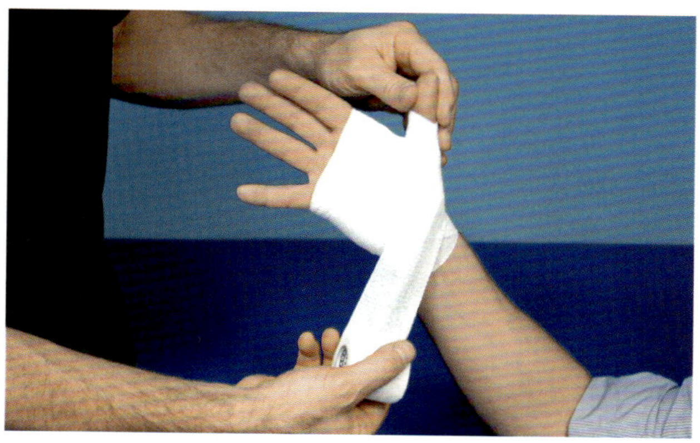

15

Limitation and stabilization of abduction and extension of the thumb

8-9-10-11-12-13-14-15 Bandaging proceeds, covering and carefully stabilizing all of the spaces left on the hand and the wrist.

METACARPOPHALANGEAL JOINTS

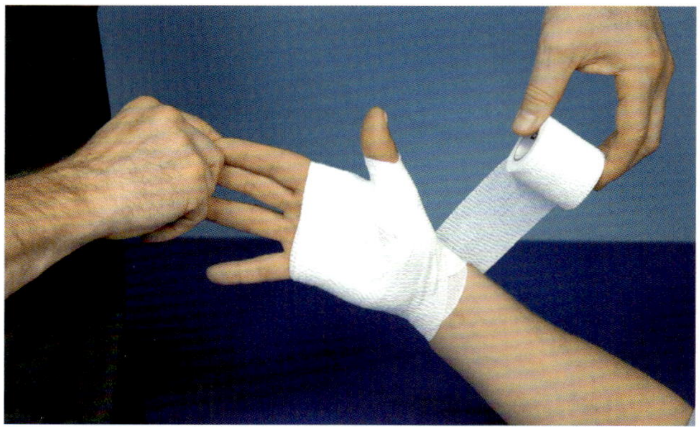
16

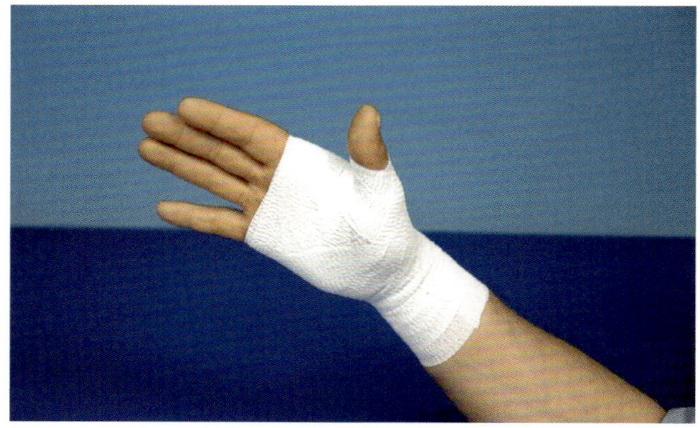
17

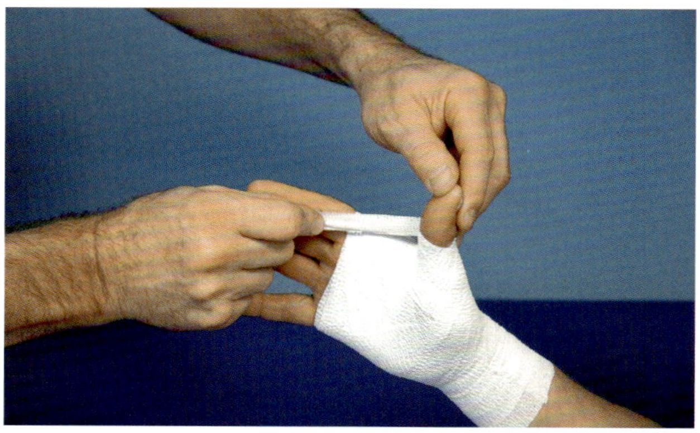
18

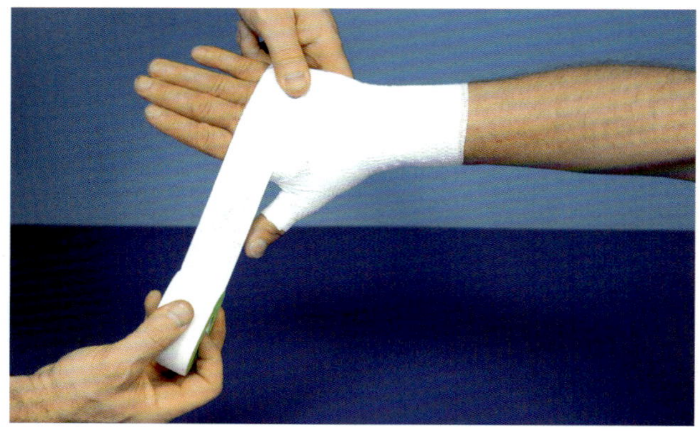
19

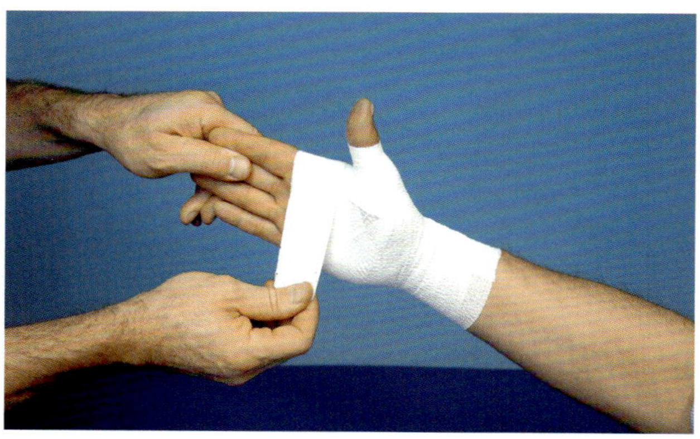
20

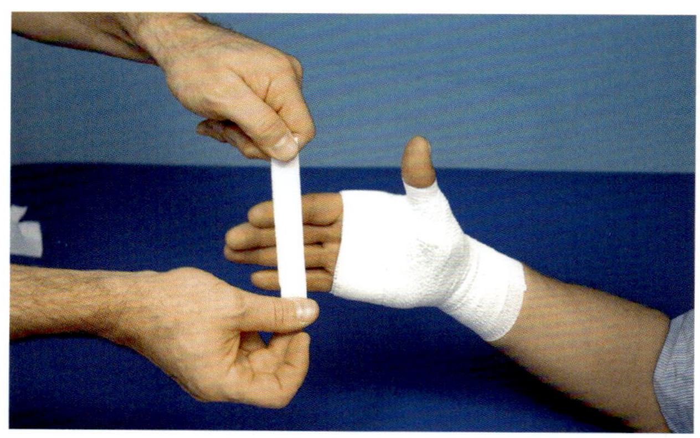
21

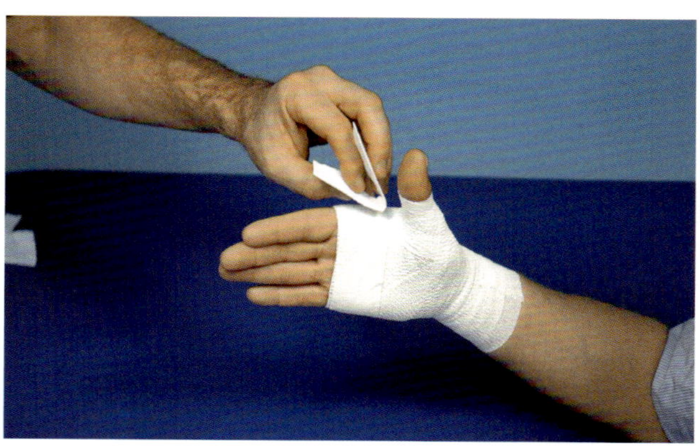
22

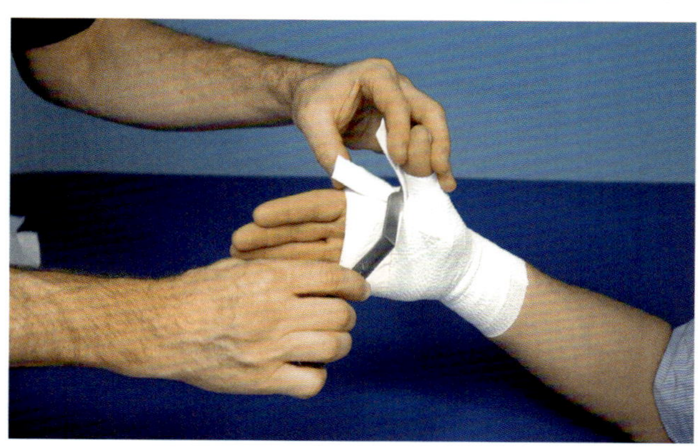
23

Limitation and stabilization of abduction and extension of the thumb

16-17 The base bandaging is finished with several wrappings around the wrist at the radioulnar joint.

18 Using a strip of inelastic bandage, an anchoring point is positioned on the first finger.

19-20 Always using inelastic bandages, an anchoring point is also made on the hand.

21 A fastener of inelastic material is cut to 1 cm in width.

22-23 The fastener is positioned between the thumb and the index finger.

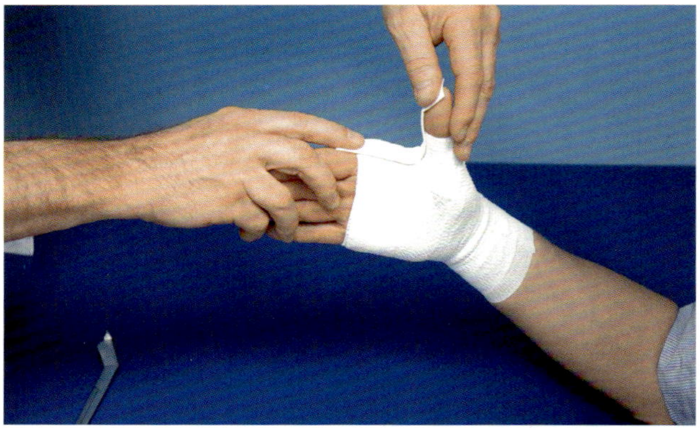

24

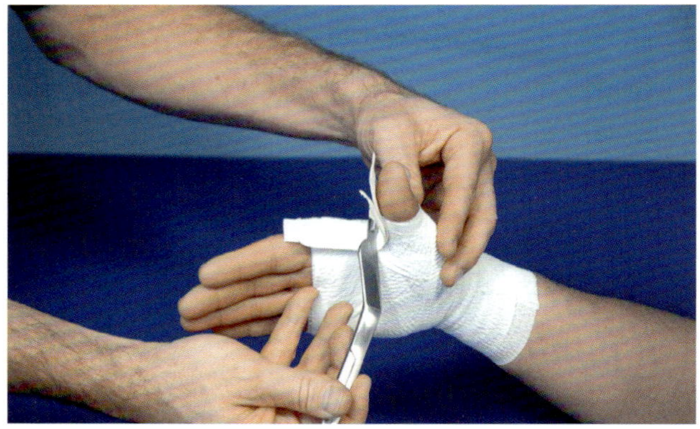

25

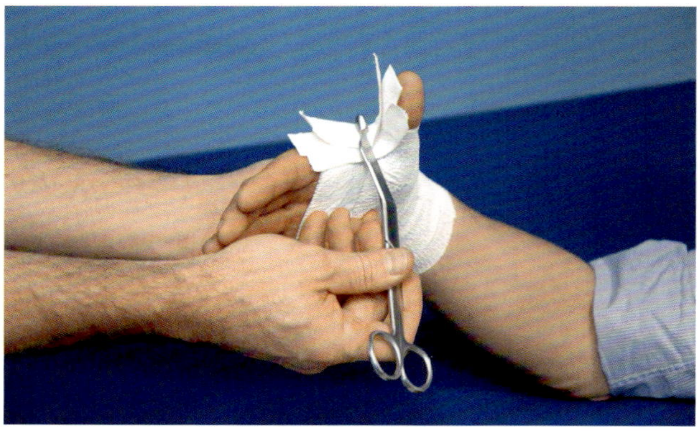

26

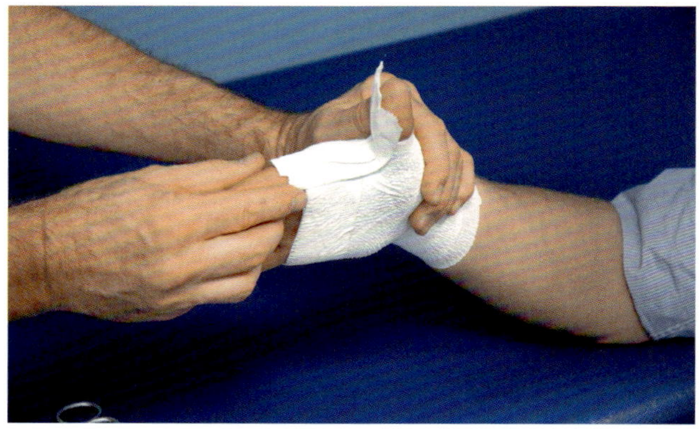

27

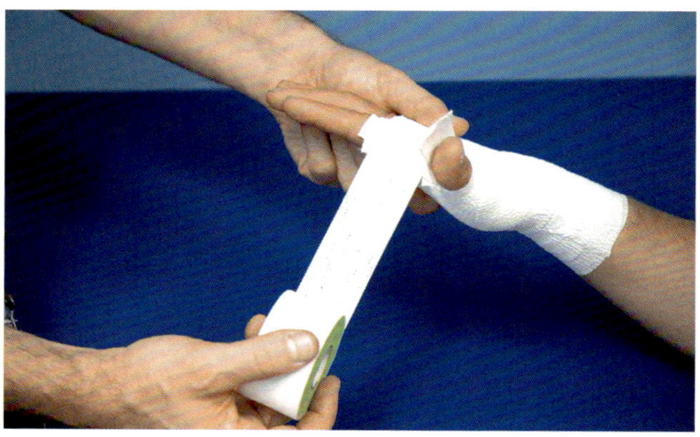

28

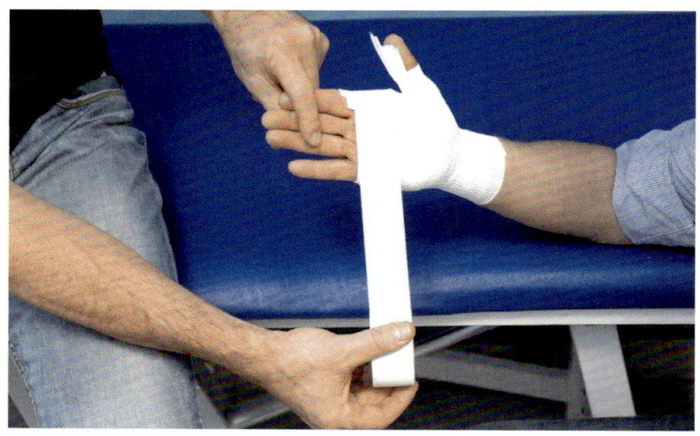

29

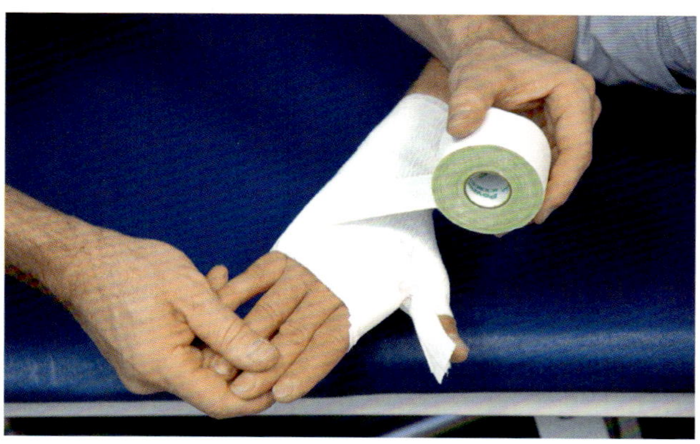

30

Limitation and stabilization of abduction and extension of the thumb

24-25-26 Bandaging proceeds, reinforced with the application of two more fasteners made of inelastic bandage positioned parallel to the first.

27 The thumb is positioned in slight flexion and opposition.

28-29-30 The ends of the fasteners that end on the index finger are held in place with a wrap of inelastic bandage around the hand.

METACARPOPHALANGEAL JOINTS

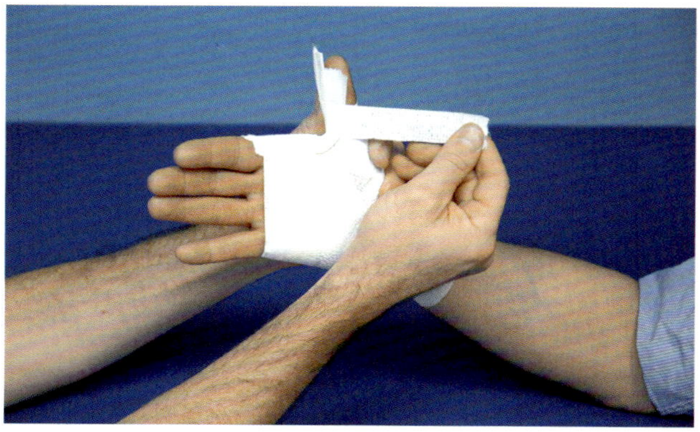
31

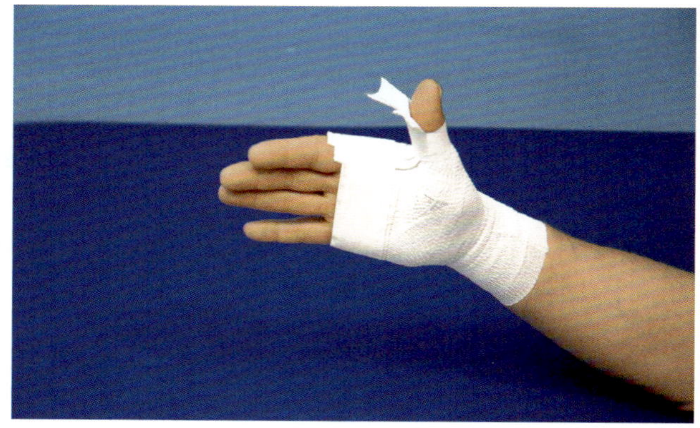
32

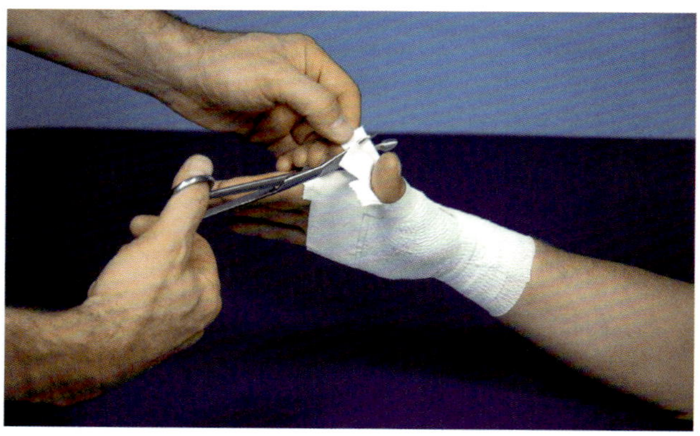
33

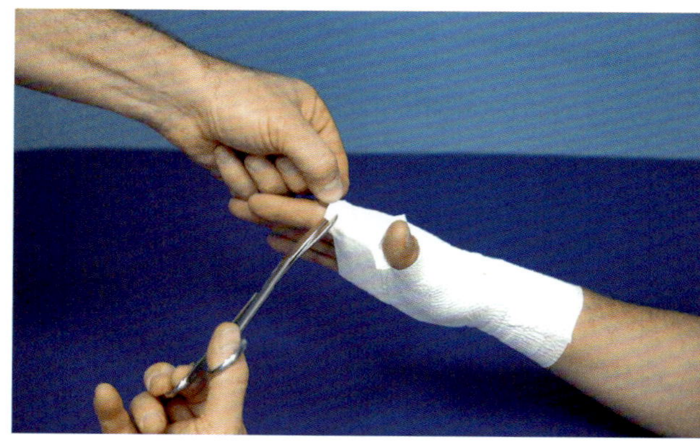
34

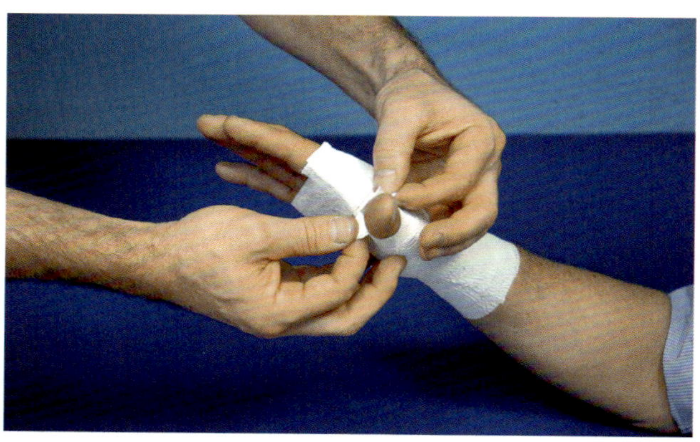
35

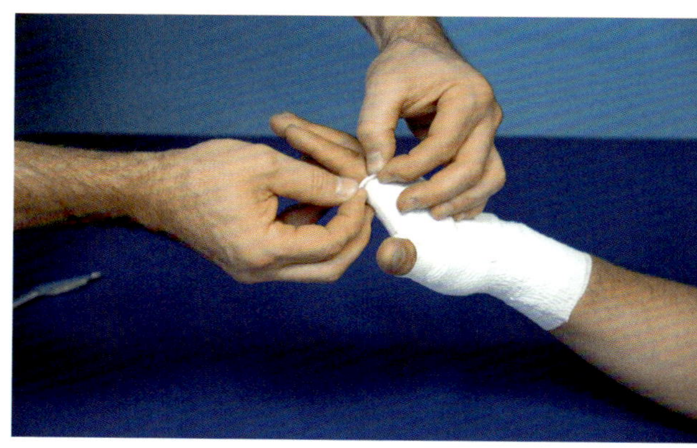
36

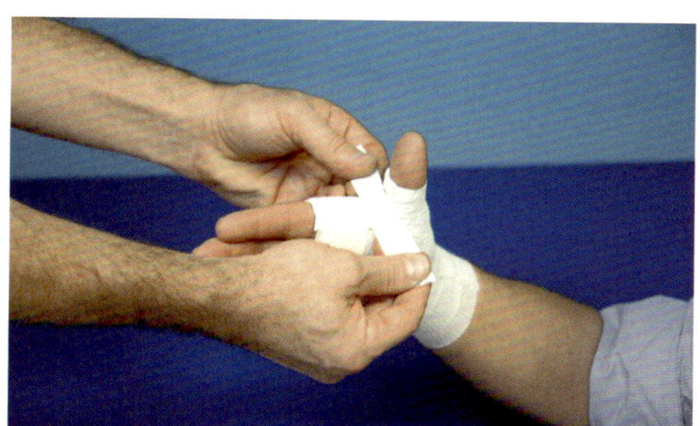
37

Limitation and stabilization of abduction and extension of the thumb

31-32 The ends of the fasteners that end on the thumb are held in place with a wrap of inelastic bandage around the phalanx of the first finger.

33-34 The excess pieces of bandage are shortened without getting rid of them completely.

35-36 The remaining excess pieces of bandage are folded over themselves.

37 The bandaging must be reinforced with a fastener positioned in the cavity between the thumb and index finger.

METACARPOPHALANGEAL JOINTS

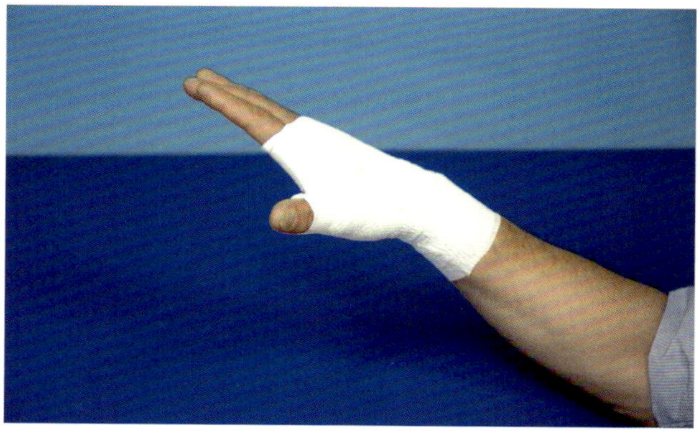

38

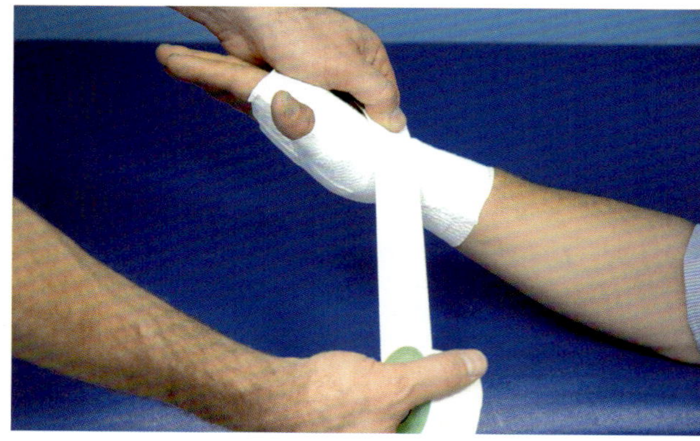

39

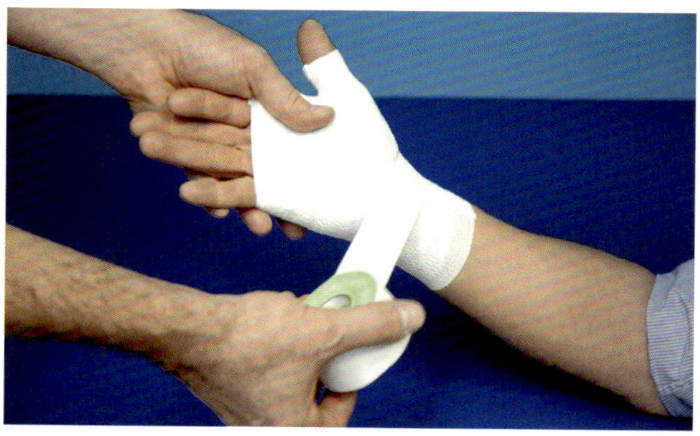

40

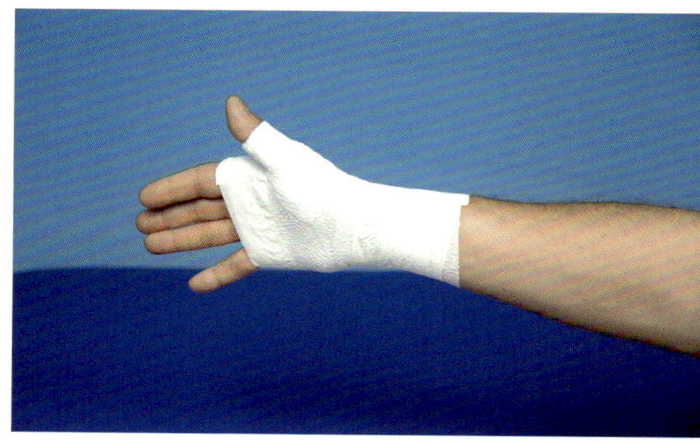

41

Limitation and stabilization of abduction and extension of the thumb

38-39-40 Bandaging is concluded with the application of a series of strips of inelastic bandage that hold in place and reinforce the bandaging.

41 Bandaging is complete.

INDICATIONS

✓ *Posttraumatic conditions*
✓ *Preventative sports treatment*

METACARPOPHALANGEAL JOINTS

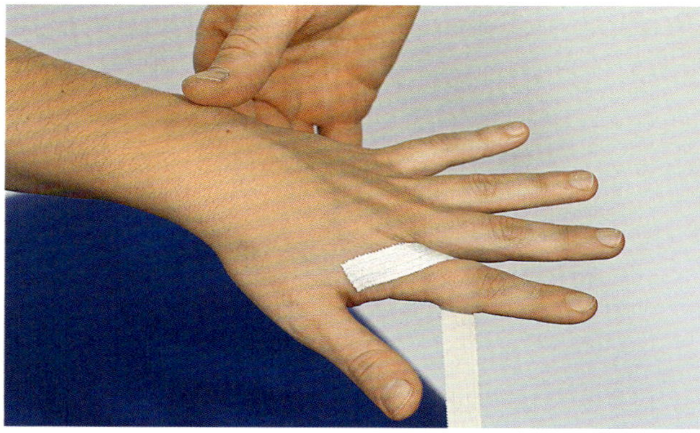
1

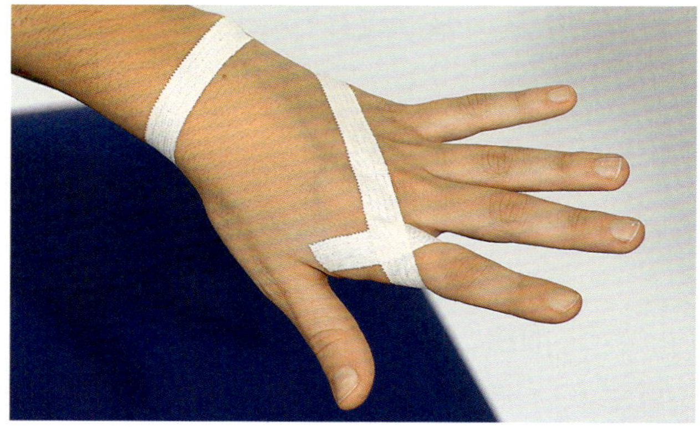
2

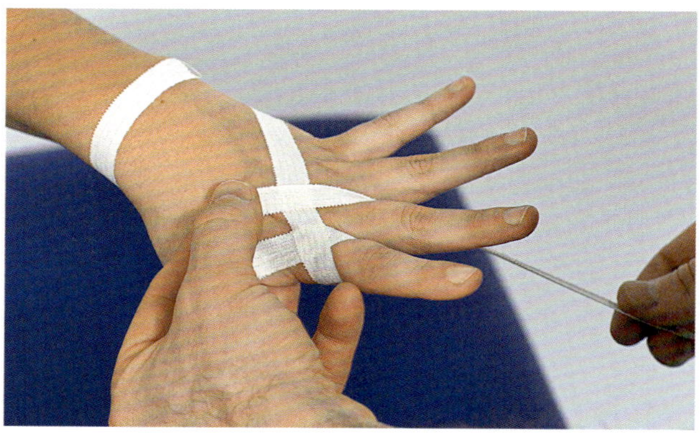
3

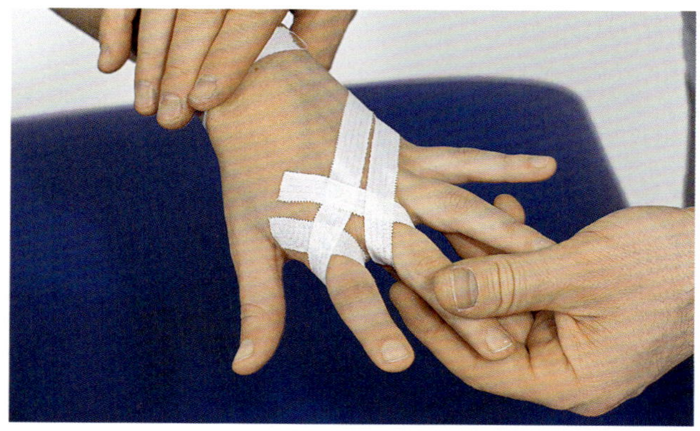
4

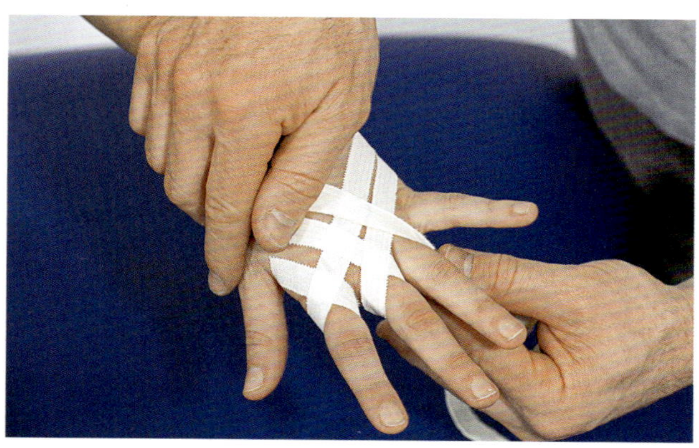
5

Stabilization of the fingers

MATERIAL

✓ Inelastic adhesive tape, 1 cm in width

APPLICATION

1 The end of a strip of inelastic adhesive tape is affixed to the dorsal surface of the hand in the region between the first and second metacarpal bones.

2 The tape wraps around the metacarpophalangeal joint of the index finger, crosses the dorsum of the hand, then fully wraps around the wrist, passing first over the palmar side and then over the dorsal side.

3-4-5 The same paths are repeated for the middle and ring fingers.

INDICATIONS

✓ *Sprain trauma*

METACARPOPHALANGEAL JOINTS

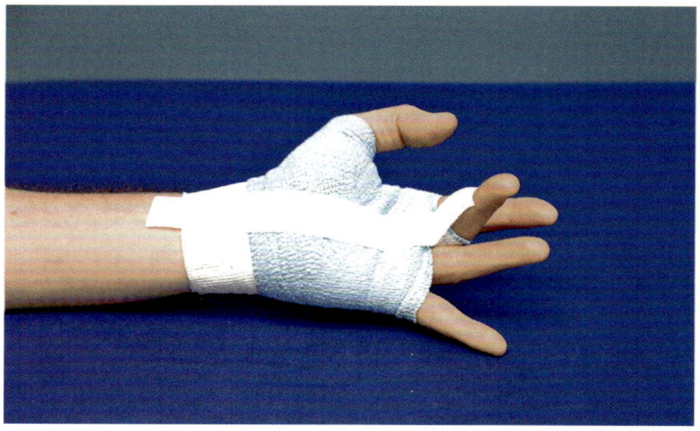

1

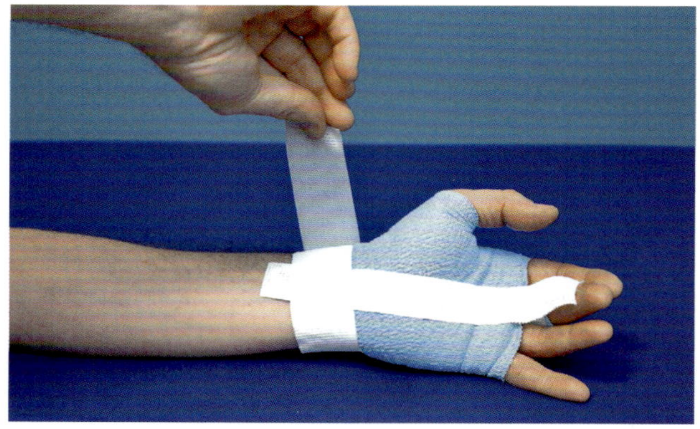

2

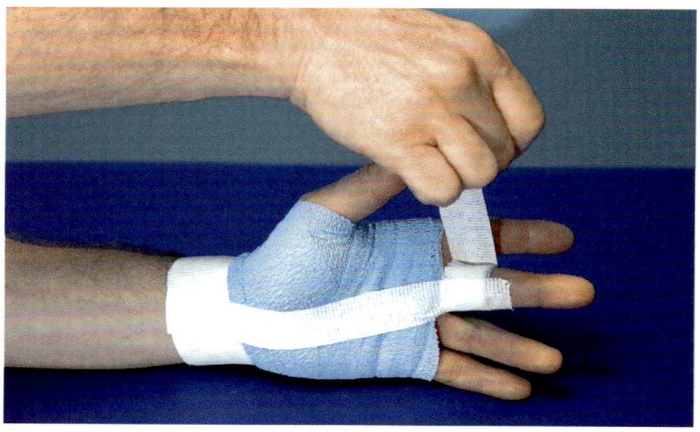

3

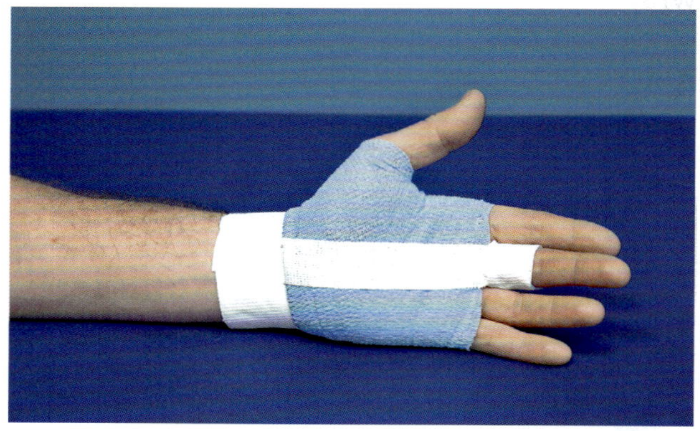

4

Limitation of the extension and flexion of the fingers

MATERIAL

✓ 2.5 cm wide elastic cohesive bandage for base bandaging
✓ Inelastic cohesive bandage, 1 cm in width

APPLICATION

1 To limit extension, bandaging is first done by wrapping the hand and the proximal phalanx of the finger to be stabilized with a cohesive elastic bandage. Next, the proximal anchoring points are made at the wrist, and the distal ones around the first phalanx of the finger. Along the finger, positioned in slight palmar flexion, and its projection on the palm, apply a fastener of inelastic cohesive bandage.

2-3 The fastener is affixed to the proximal and distal anchoring points with a complete wrap of inelastic cohesive bandage.

4 Bandaging is complete.

In order to limit flexion once the base bandaging with two anchoring points is made, a fastener of inelastic cohesive bandage is applied along the dorsum of the finger and is brought over the dorsum of the hand, beginning from the proximal anchoring point on the wrist and directed over the phalanx of the finger to be stabilized. The fastener is affixed with a complete wrap of inelastic cohesive bandage.

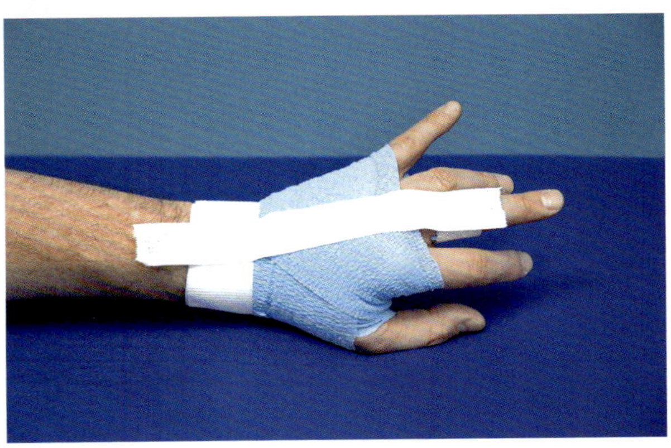

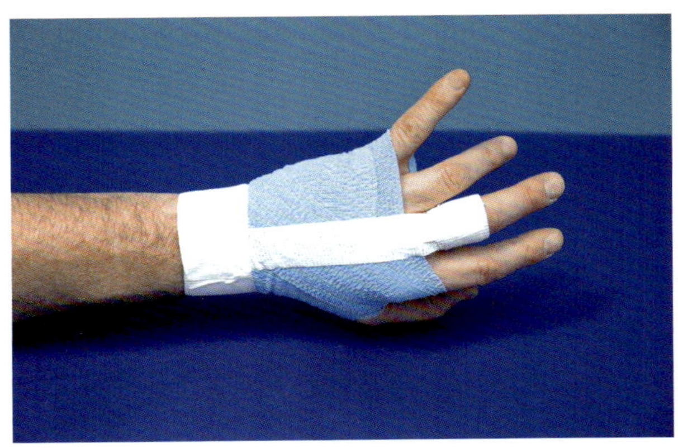

INDICATIONS

✓ *Sprain trauma*
✓ *Preventative sports treatment*

PROXIMAL INTERPHALANGEAL JOINTS

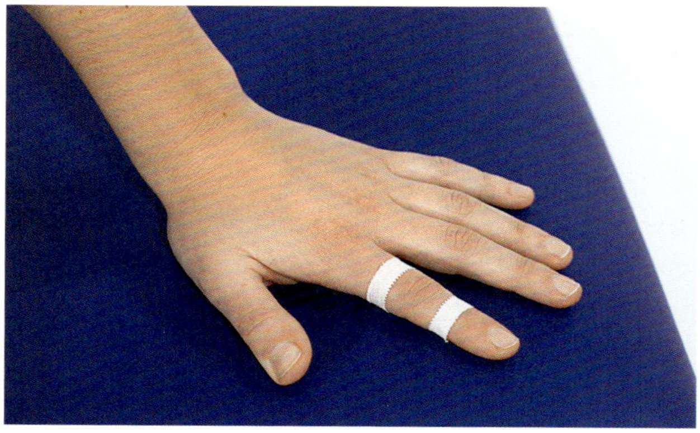

1

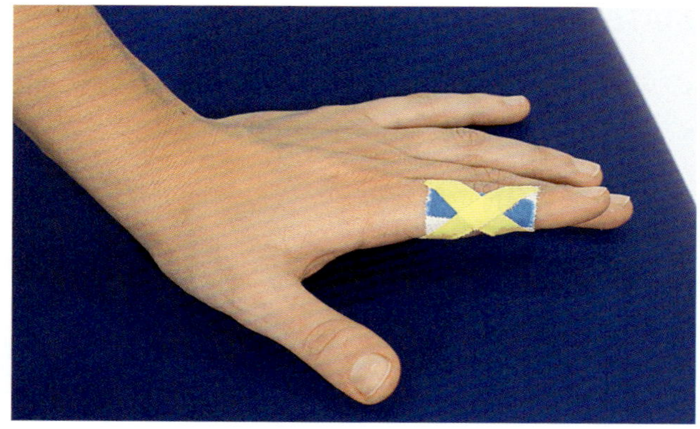

2

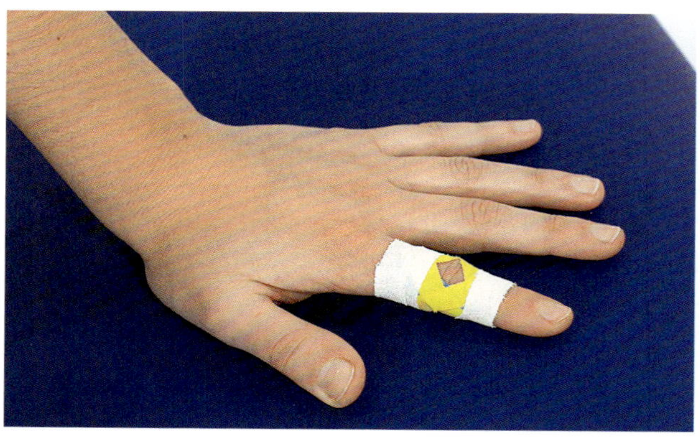

3

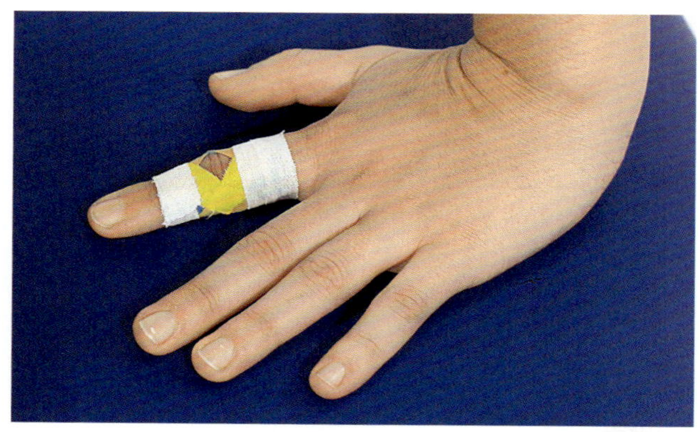

4

Lateral stabilization

MATERIAL

✓ Inelastic adhesive tape, 1 cm in width

APPLICATION

1 To begin, anchoring points are prepared by applying two wrappings of inelastic adhesive tape, one proximally and the other distally in regard to the joint.

2 Two strips of inelastic adhesive tape are applied along the longitudinal axis of the finger in its lateral and medial regions, beginning from the distal anchoring point and arriving at the proximal one. With four other strips of inelastic adhesive tape, two X-shaped bandages are made and passed over the center of the proximal interphalangeal joint, one on the medial surface of the finger and the other on the lateral one.

3-4 The bandaging is completed with the application of several wrappings of inelastic adhesive tape over the proximal and distal anchoring points.

Please note that the bandaging does not impede the flexion of the interphalangeal joint, but simply limits lateral excursion.

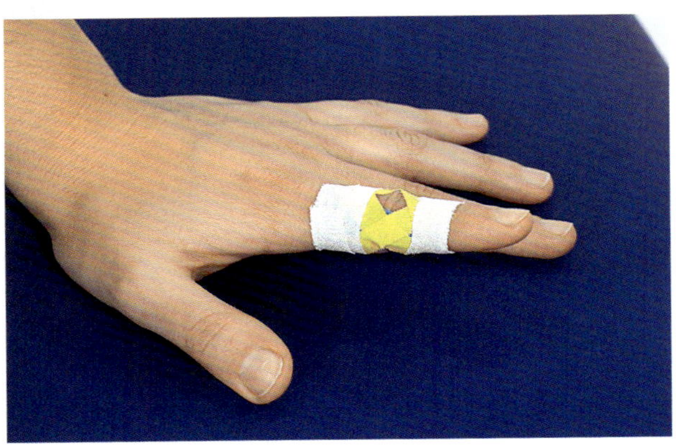

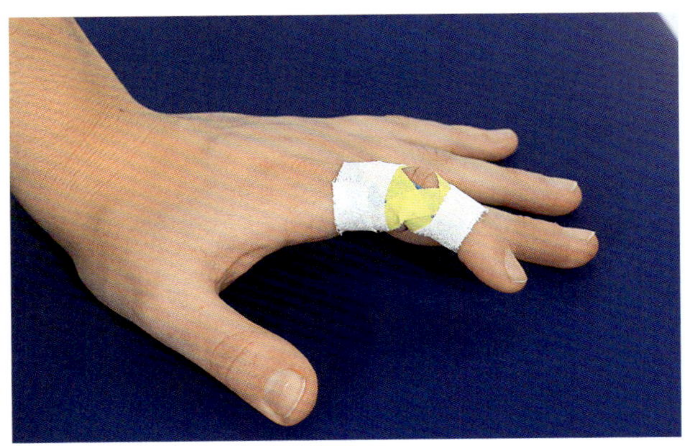

INDICATIONS

✓ *Sprain trauma*

PROXIMAL INTERPHALANGEAL JOINTS

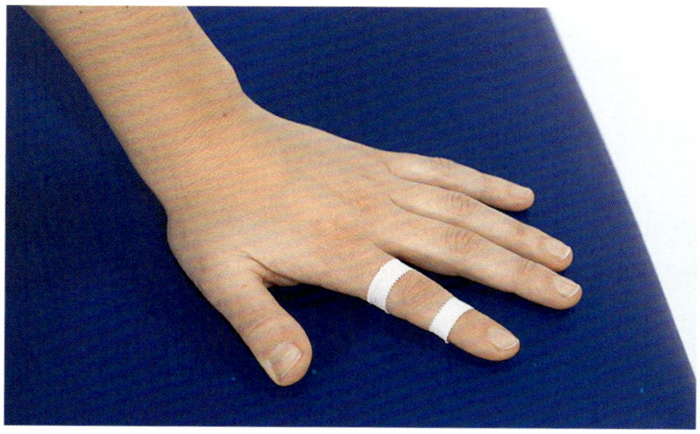

1

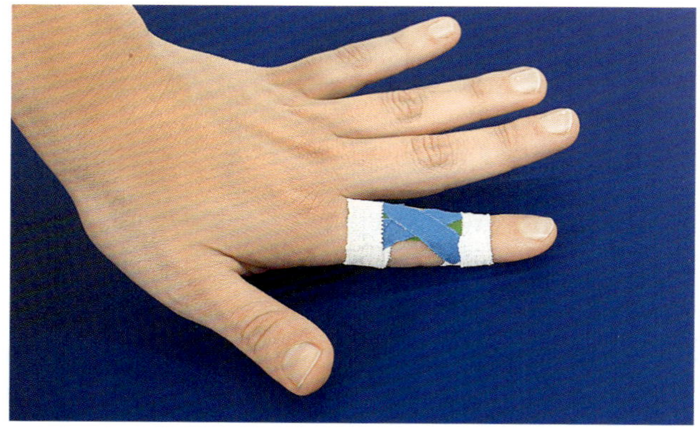

2

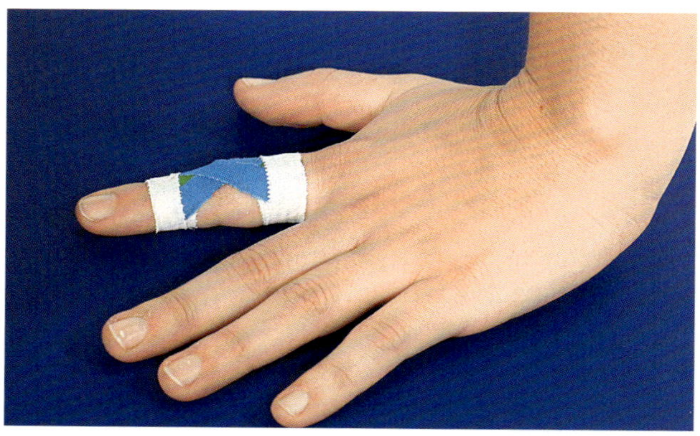

3

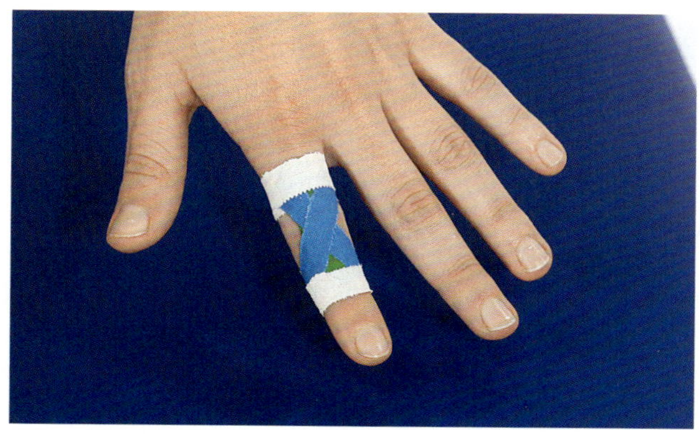

4

Stabilization and limitation of flexion

MATERIAL

✓ Inelastic adhesive tape, 1 cm in width

APPLICATION

1 To begin, anchoring points are prepared by applying two wrappings of inelastic adhesive tape, one proximally and the other distally in regard to the joint.

2 With two strips of inelastic adhesive tape, an X-shaped bandage is made and passed over the center of the joint at its dorsal skin projection. The bandaging is affixed with two wrappings of tape over the proximal and distal anchoring points.

3-4 Bandaging is complete.

INDICATIONS

✓ *Sprain trauma*

Lower limb

- **Medial muscles of the thigh**
- **Quadriceps femoris**
- **Rectus femoris**
- **Posterior muscles of the thigh**
- **Posterior muscles and joint of the knee**
- **Knee joint**
- **Posterior muscles of the lower leg**
- **Tibiotarsal joint**
- **Achilles tendon**
- **Plantar aponeurosis**
- **Metatarsophalangeal joints**

MEDIAL MUSCLES OF THE THIGH

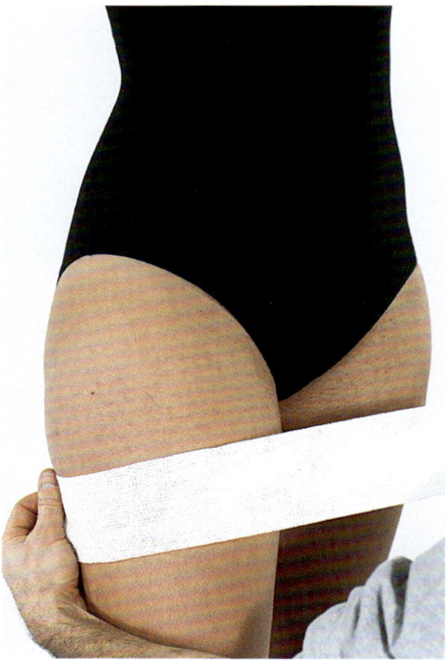

1

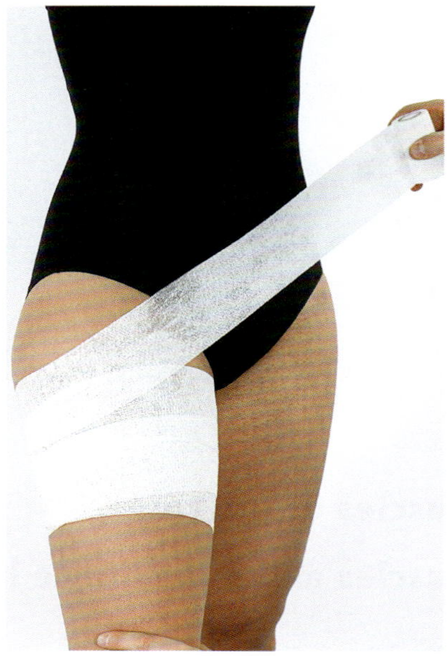

2

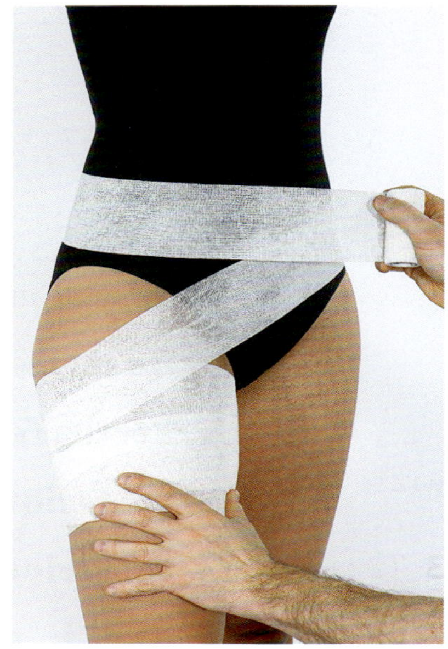

3

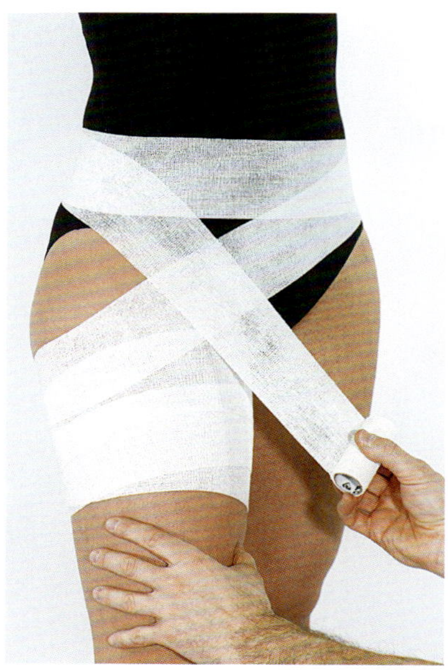

4

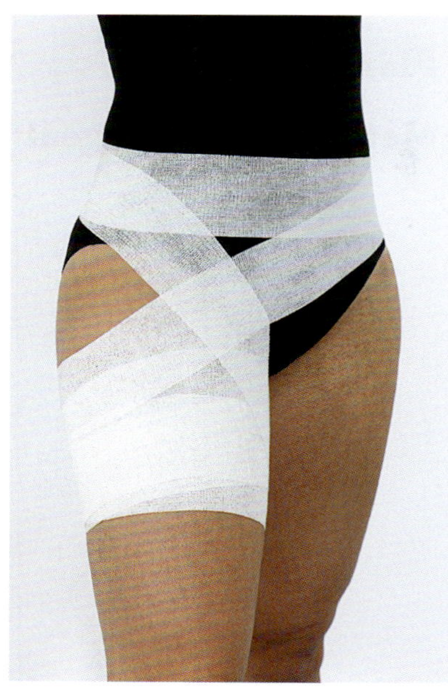

5

Unloading and limitation of abduction, extension, and outward rotation

MATERIAL

✓ 7.5 or 10 cm wide elastic cohesive bandage

APPLICATION

1 With the elastic bandage positioned at the lateral surface of the middle third of the thigh, make a complete bandage wrap, passing anteriorly over the thigh, in a lateral to medial direction.

2 Bandaging proceeds with several spiral wraps, moving in the distal-proximal direction toward the anterior superior iliac spine of the contralateral half of the pelvis; the bandage wraps should overlap by 25-50%.

3 The iliac crests and the anterior superior iliac spines are covered with a complete bandage wrap around the pelvis.

4 The bandage is directed diagonally in a proximal to distal direction until it covers the inguinal area.

5 Bandaging concludes with several spiral wrappings around the superior and medial thirds of the thigh.

INDICATIONS

✓ *Adductor muscle injuries*
✓ *Inguinal insertion pain*
✓ *Rectus adductor syndrome*

QUADRICEPS FEMORIS

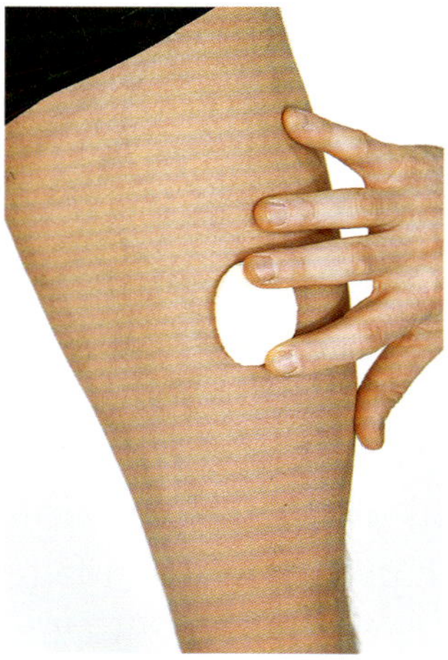

1

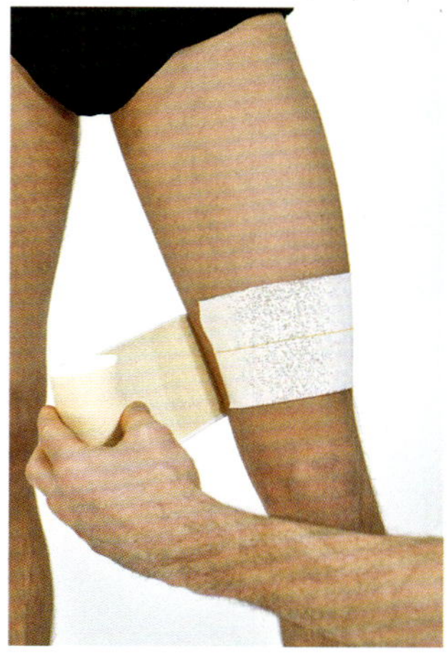

2

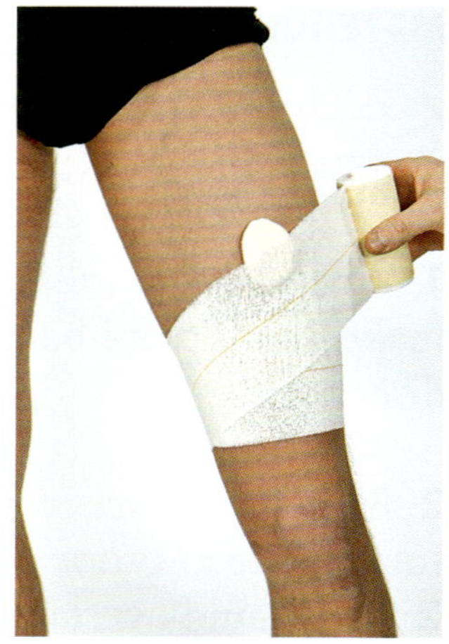

3

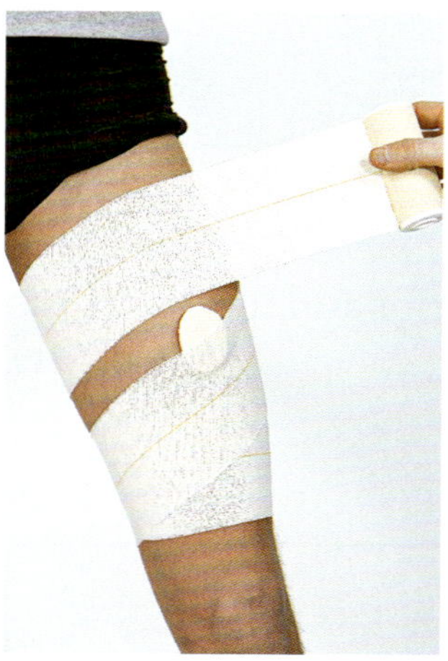

4

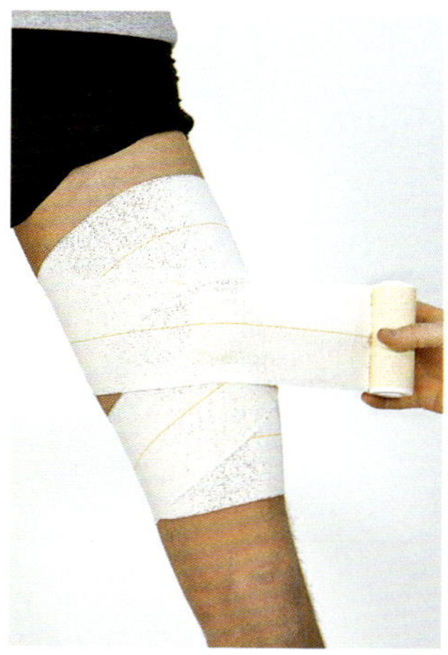

5

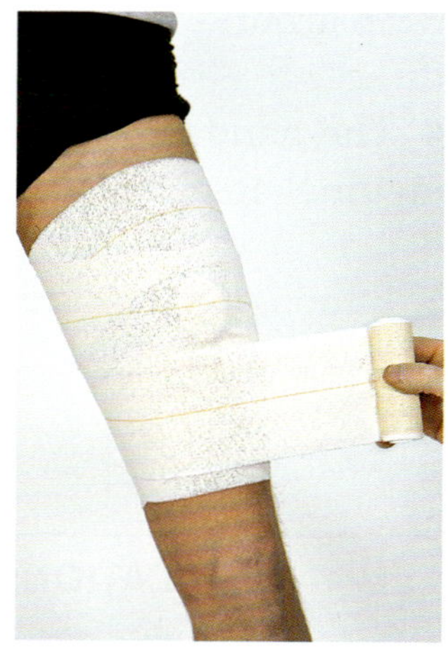

6

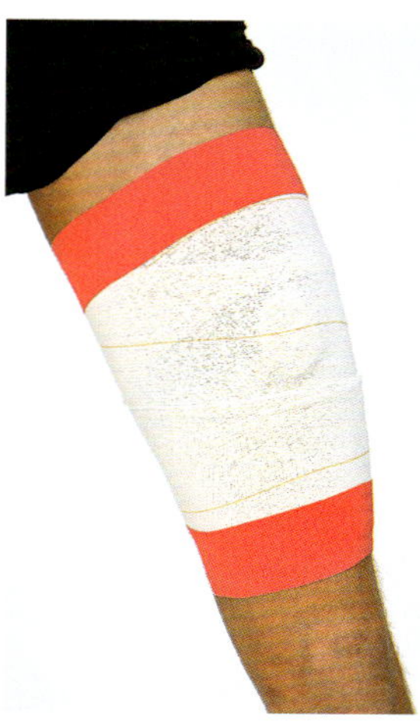

7

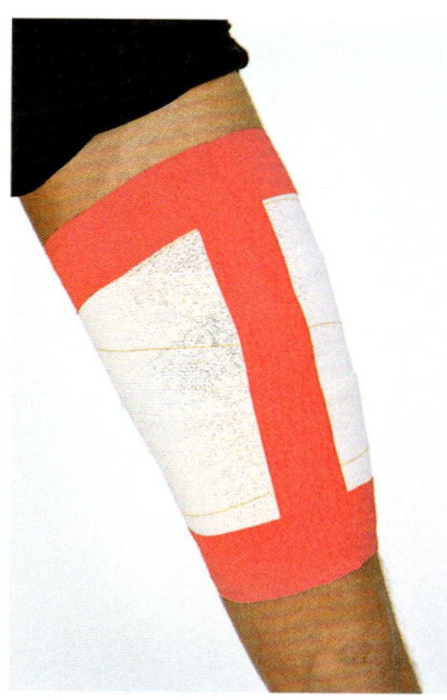

8

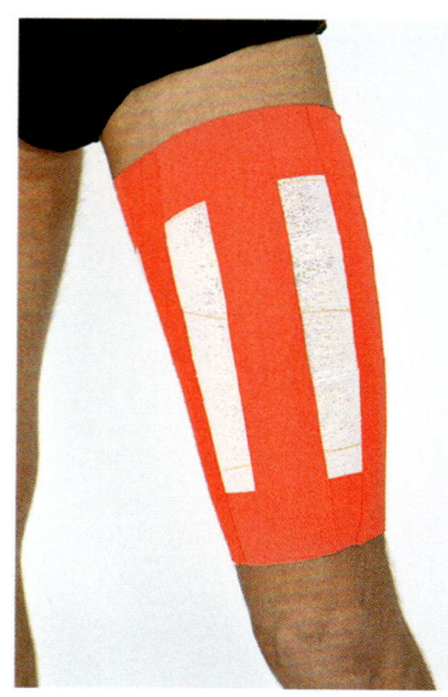

9

Muscular unloading via compressive bandaging

MATERIAL

- ✓ Cotton fabric porous elastic adhesive bandage that can be stretched lengthwise or is bi-extensible, 7.5 or 10 cm in width
- ✓ Inelastic adhesive tape
- ✓ Foam rubber compress for creating a compressive unloading pad

APPLICATION

1 Before bandaging, a foam compress must be prepared and positioned at the point of the lesion.

2 The subject stands with the weight on one leg so as to relieve the target muscle of loads. A full wrap of the bandage is applied at the distal third of the thigh.

3 With the unloading compress positioned over the point of the injury, the bandage is directed to cover the lower end of the pad, with tension at about 50% of its maximum threshold.

4 The bandage reaches the proximal third of the thigh, where a full wrap around is made.

5 The bandage descends to again cover the compress.

6 At this point, a full wrap of the bandage is applied at the distal third of the thigh, taking care to cover all free spaces.

7 Next, bandaging proceeds by preparing the proximal and distal anchoring point with two strips of inelastic adhesive tape.

8-9 Three pieces of inelastic adhesive tape are applied along the longitudinal axis of the lower limb, leaving and arriving on the distal and proximal anchoring points, respectively. The first piece of tape passes over the unloading compress; the other two run laterally and medially.

QUADRICEPS FEMORIS

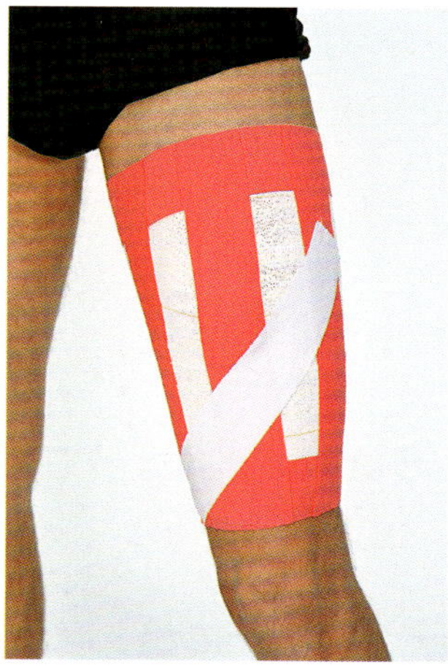

10

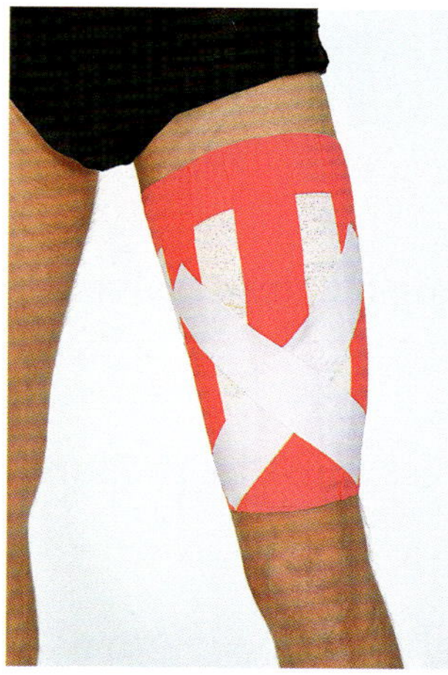

11

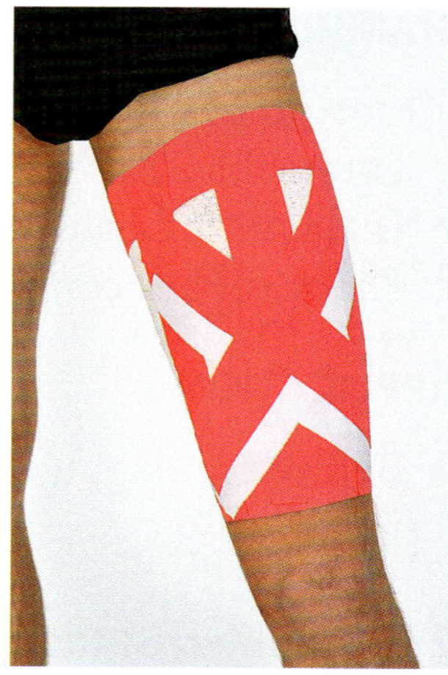

12

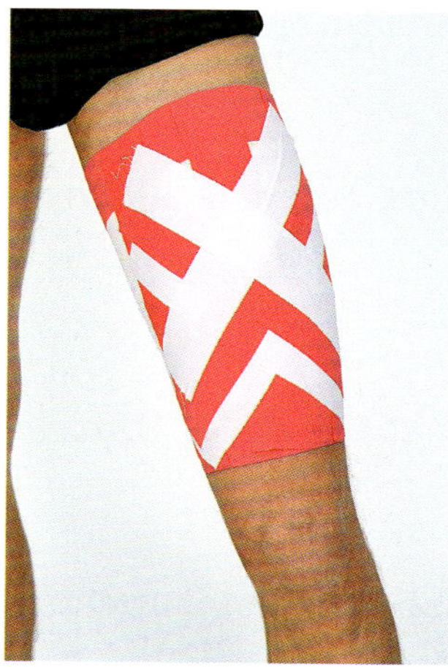

13

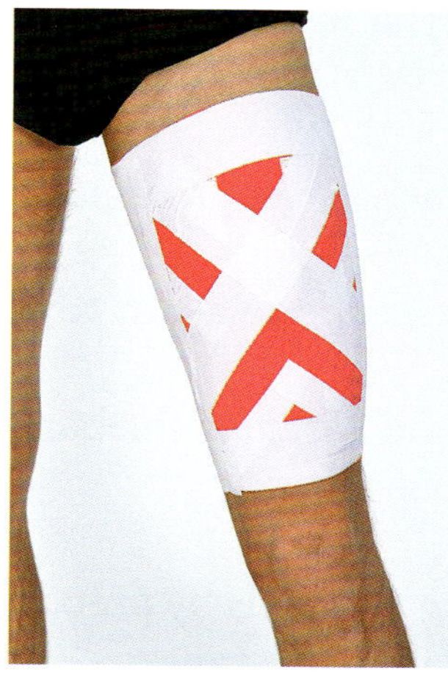

14

Muscular unloading via compressive bandaging

10-11 Beginning from the vertical anchoring points, two pieces of inelastic adhesive tape are applied, which cross at the lower end of the unloading pad to form an X.

12 Beginning as always from the vertical anchoring points, two other strips of inelastic adhesive tape are applied, crossing each other at the center of the compress to form an X, and covering the previously applied adhesive tape by 50%.

13 Again, beginning from the vertical anchoring points, two other strips of inelastic adhesive tape are applied, crossing each other at the upper edge of the compress to form an X, and covering the previously applied adhesive tape by 50%.

14 The bandaging is finished by fastening the vertical, proximal, and distal anchoring points with inelastic adhesive affixing tape.

INDICATIONS

Effects of muscular injuries such as:

- ✓ *Contractures*
- ✓ *Strains*
- ✓ *Elongations*

RECTUS FEMORIS

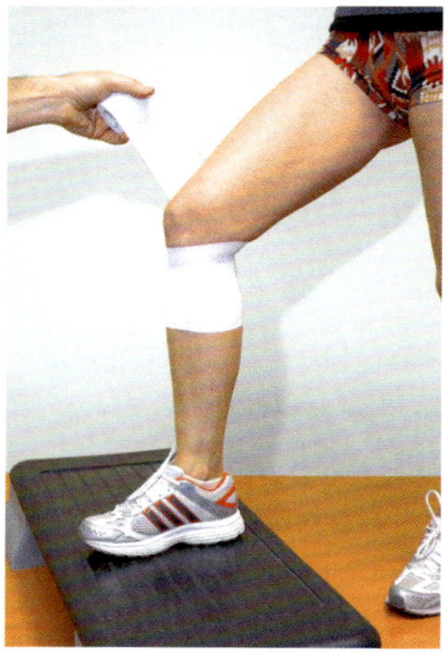

1

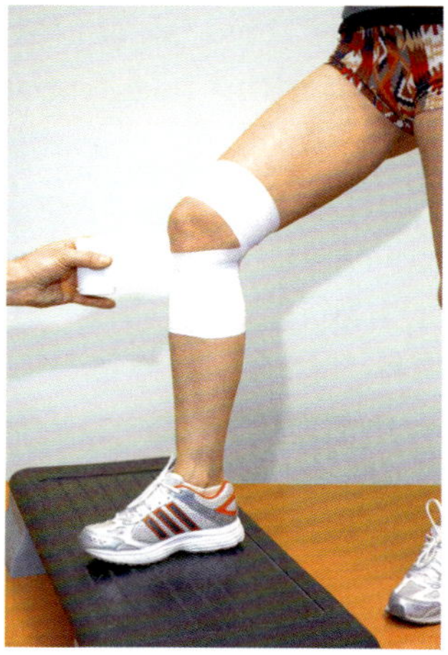

2

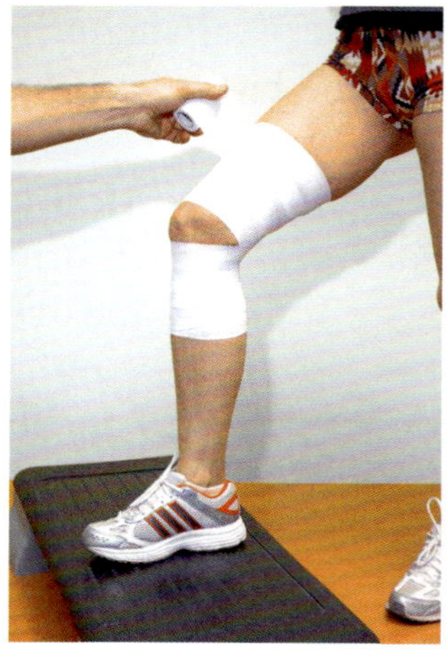

3

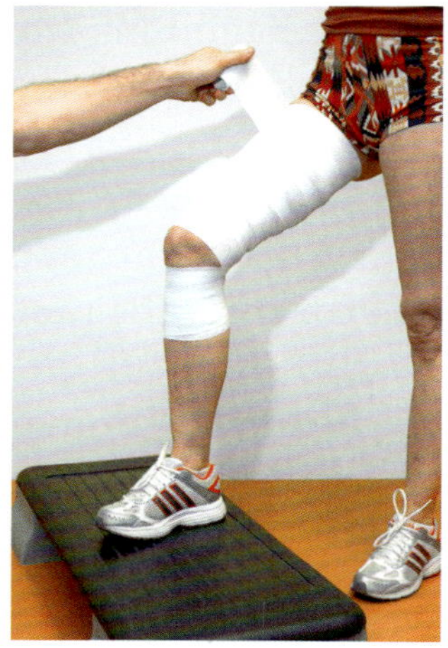

4

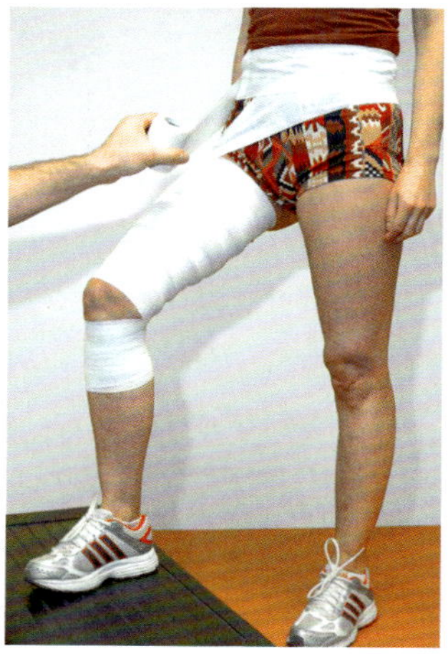

5

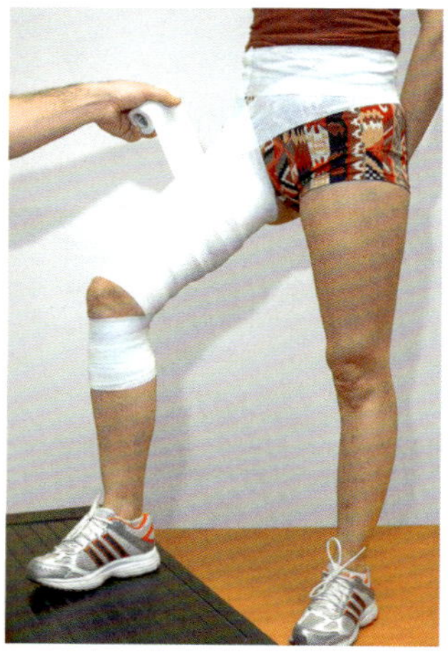

6

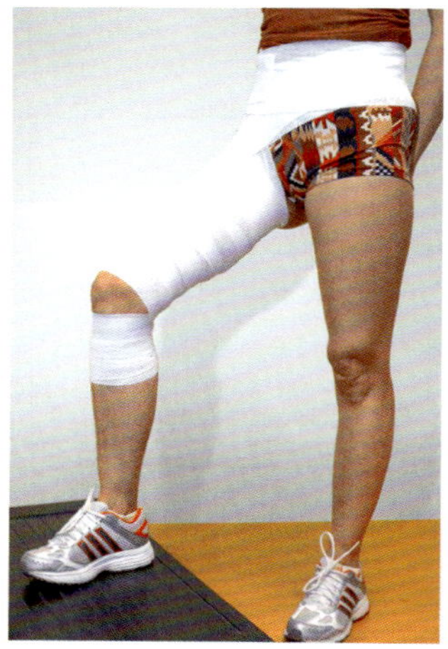

7

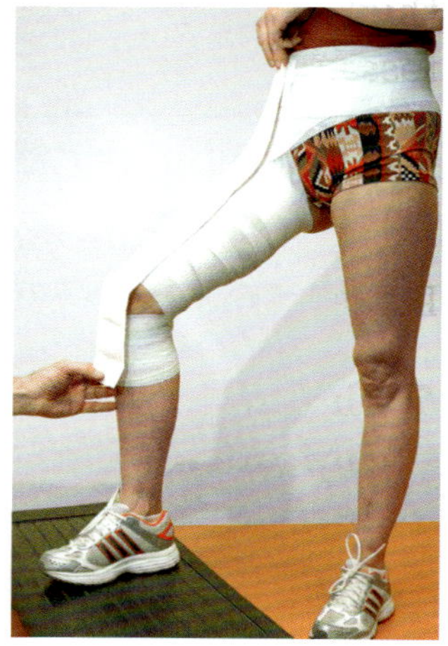

8

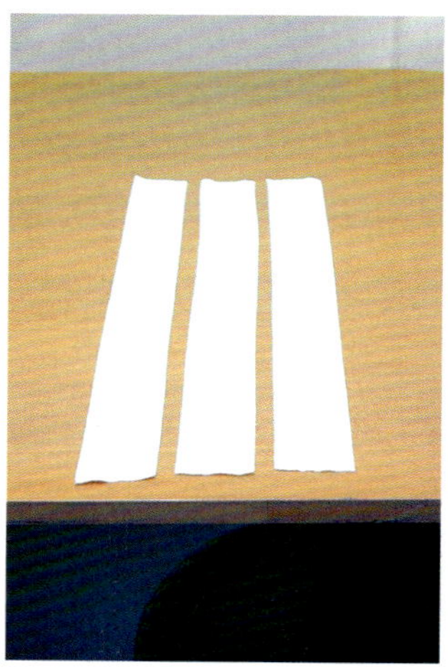

9

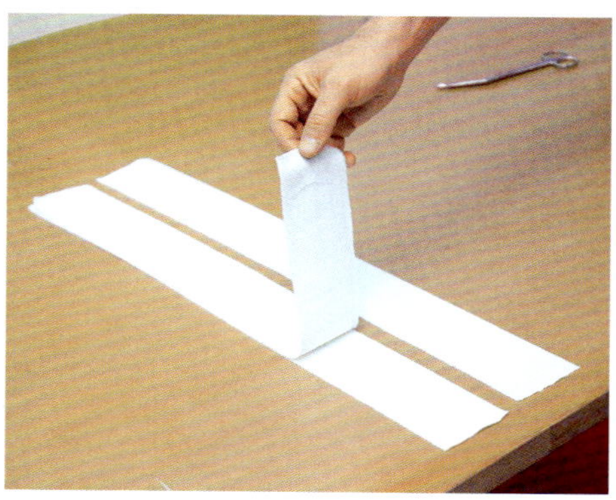

10

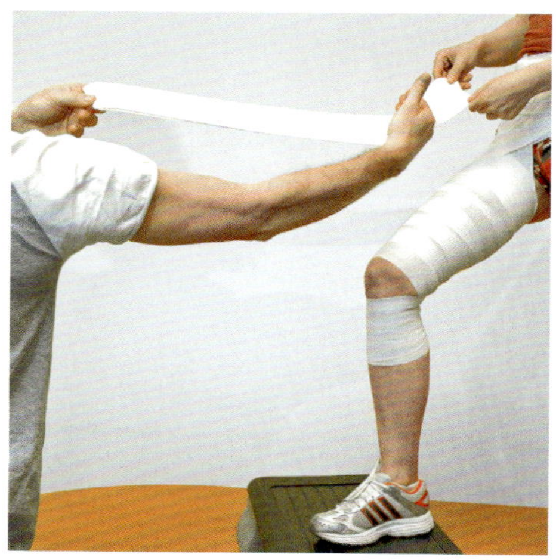

11

Unloading, support, and guidance of movement

MATERIAL

✓ Elastic cohesive bandage, 7.5 cm wide
✓ Cotton fabric porous elastic adhesive bandage that can be stretched lengthwise, 7.5 cm in width

APPLICATION

To maintain the hip and knee flexed by about 20 degrees, the foot is kept supported on a lift.

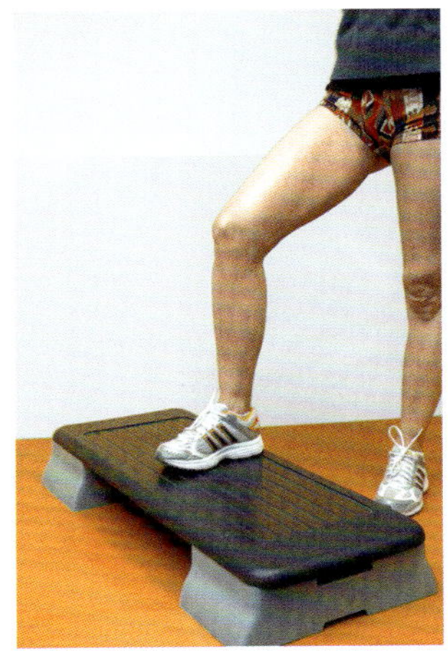

1 The subject stands up with the hip and the knee flexed by about 20 degrees. To begin, the base bandaging is prepared. Several complete wrappings are made with the cohesive bandage around the proximal third of the lower leg in the distal-proximal direction, then the bandage is moved toward the thigh making a cross behind the popliteal fossa.

2-3-4 Next, the bandage wraps around the axis of the femur with several spiral wrappings until reaching the inguinal area.

5 The bandage is directed toward the contralateral iliac crest, where it makes a complete wrapping around the pelvis before descending again toward the thigh, crossing it anteriorly.

6-7 The thigh is wrapped and the bandage is brought toward the contralateral iliac crest, where another wrapping is made around the pelvis to hold the base bandaging in place.

8 A fastener must be made out of mono-extensible elastic adhesive bandage, which runs along the tract separating the anterior superior iliac spine from the tibial crest.

9-10 Now two more strips of elastic adhesive bandage are cut to the same length, and are both overlapped over the first.

11 The fastener must be stretched using the ulnar border of the hand, passing forward and backward several times.

RECTUS FEMORIS

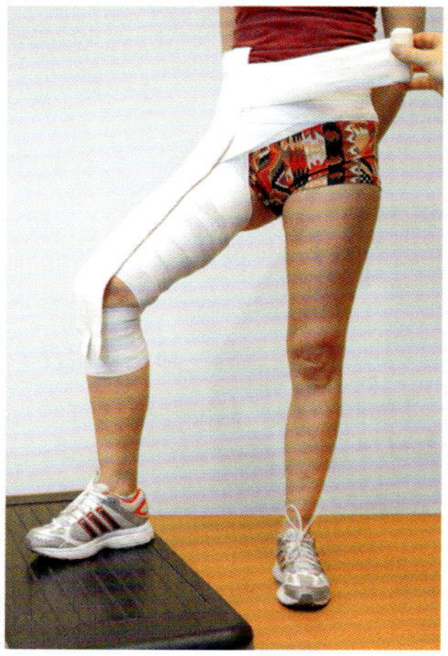

12

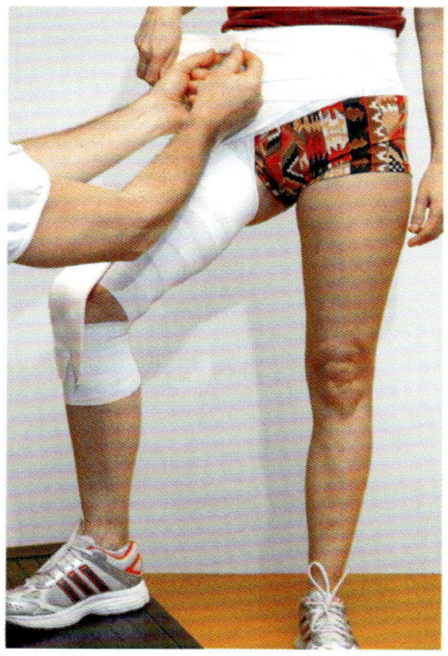

13

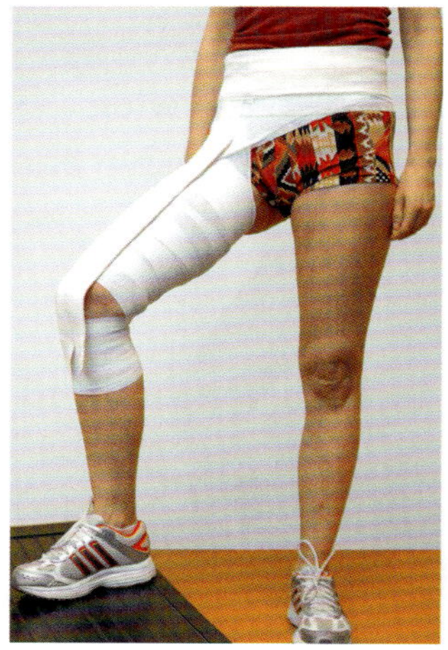

14

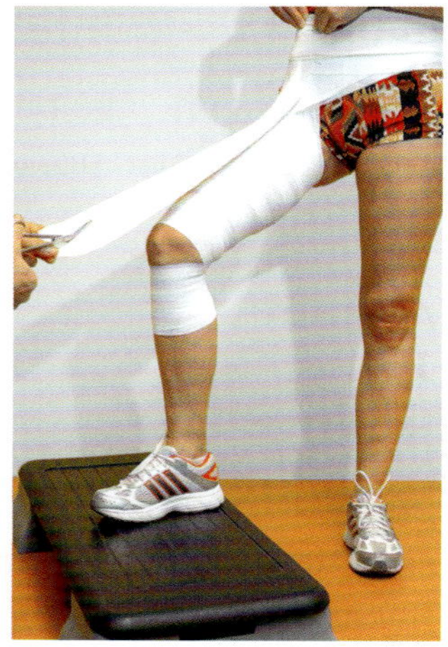

15

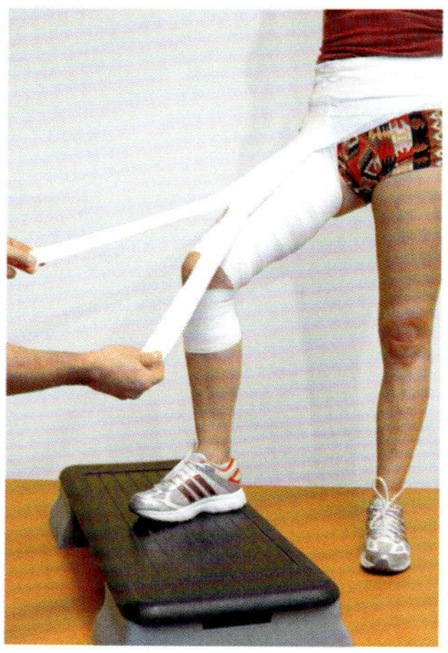

16

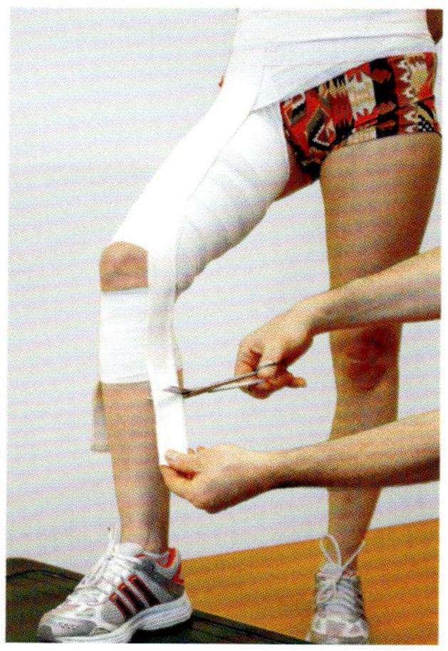

17

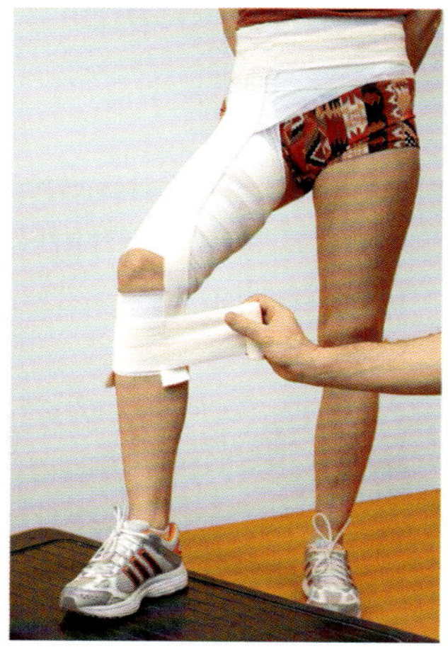

18

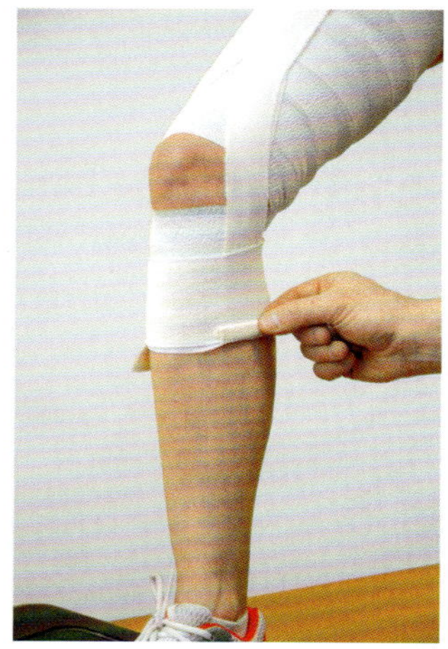

19

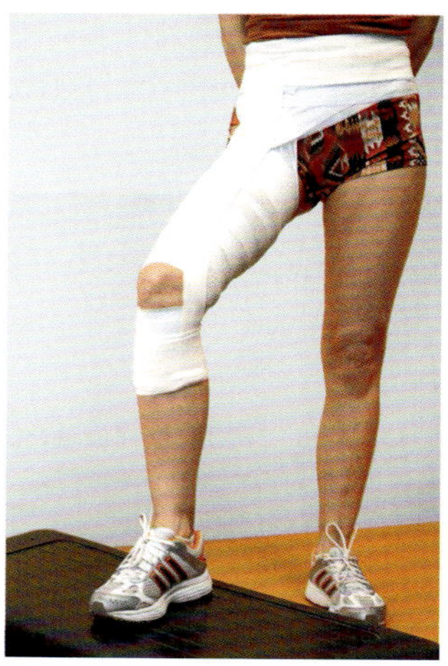

20

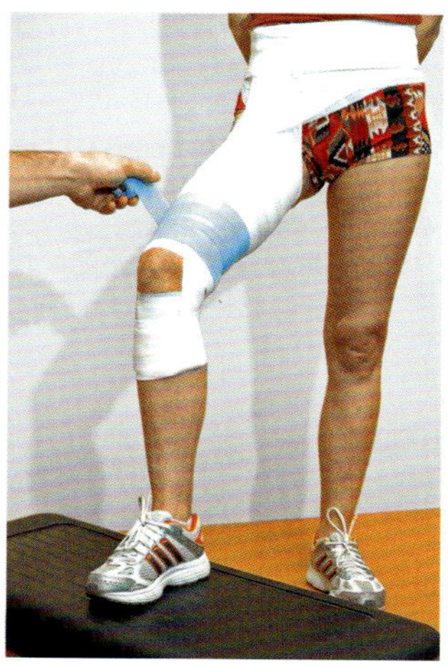

21

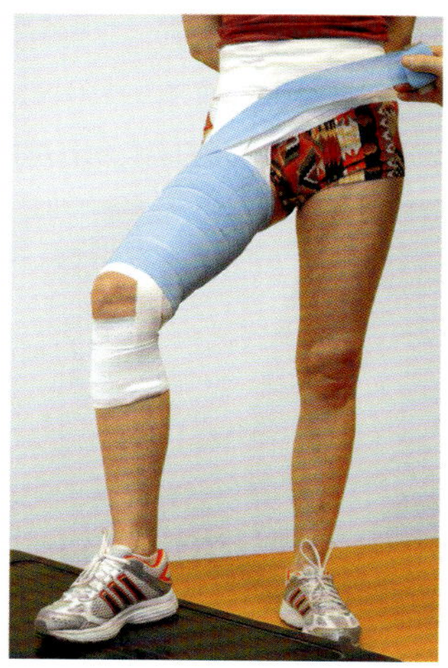

22

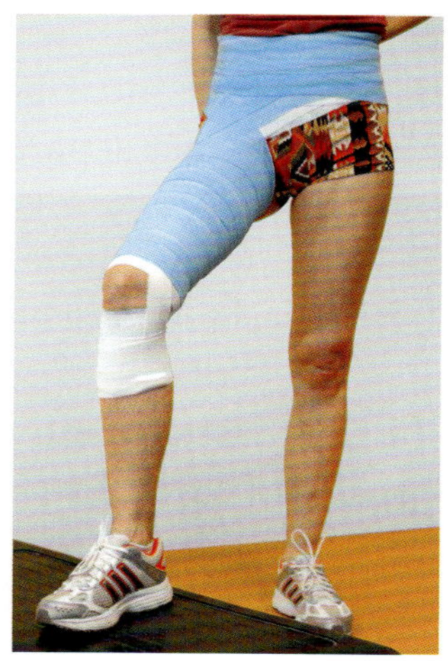

23

Unloading, support, and guidance of movement

12 Next, the reinforced elastic fastener is applied to the extension of the rectus femoris and affixed proximally with a full wrapping of the adhesive elastic bandage, covering the pelvis.

13-14 A piece of the fastener must be left free so as to be able to fold over itself and then be held in place with another wrap of the bandage around the pelvis.

15 The distal end of the reinforced elastic fastener, still free, must be cut into two parts of the same width, forming something of a Y shape.

16 The two parts of the elastic fastener must be put under tension.

17 The two pieces are applied to the lower leg, passing laterally and medially to the patella, then the excess parts are trimmed without being completely eliminated.

18 With a complete wrap of the elastic adhesive bandage, the distal parts of the Y-shaped fastener are affixed at the proximal third of the lower leg.

19-20 After the excess parts of the fastener are folded over themselves, they are held in place with another full wrap of the adhesive elastic band around the axis of the lower leg.

21-22 The bandaging is finished with a cohesive bandage applied with spiral wrapping in the distal-proximal direction, first covering the axis of the femur and then the pelvis so as to keep the base bandaging in place.

23 Bandaging is complete.

INDICATIONS

- ✓ *Posttraumatic unloading*
- ✓ *Preventative sports treatment*
- ✓ *Effects of muscular injuries*

POSTERIOR MUSCLES OF THE THIGH

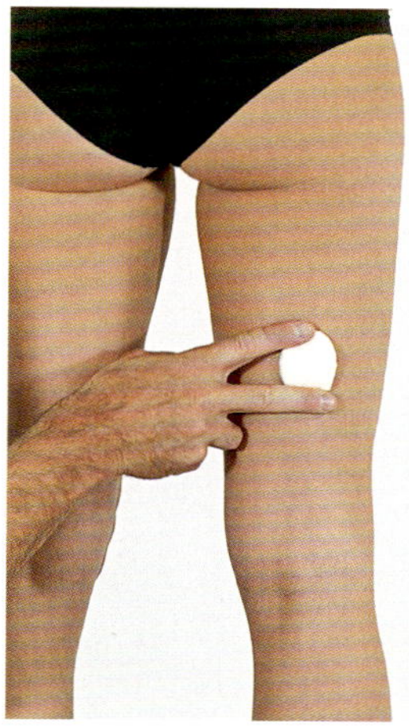
1

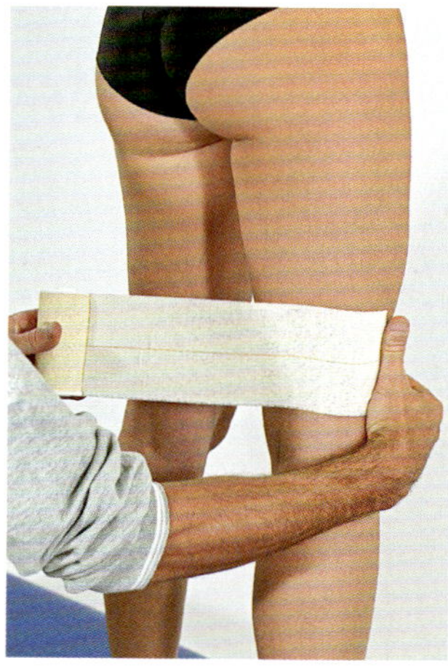
2

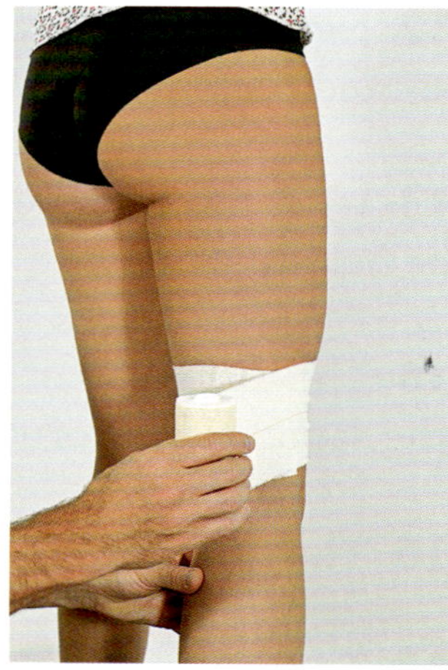
3

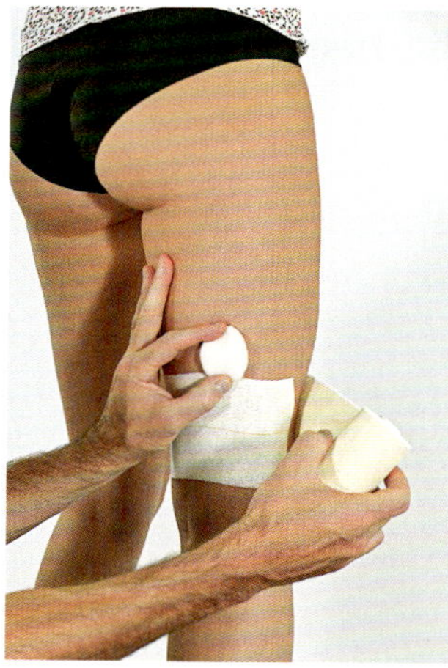
4

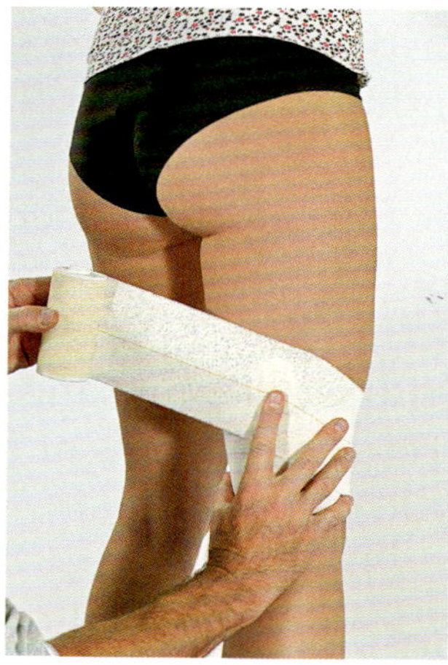
5

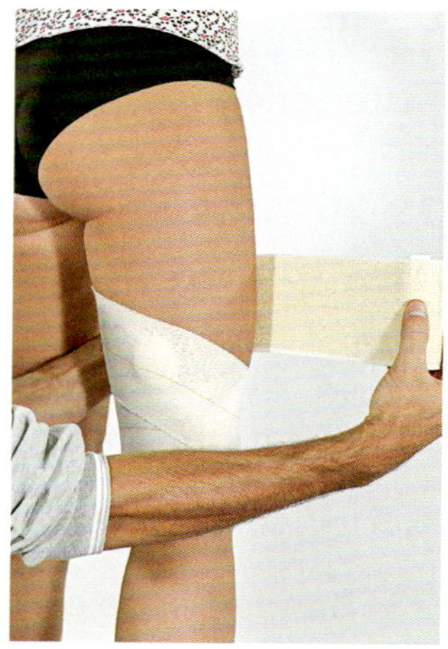
6

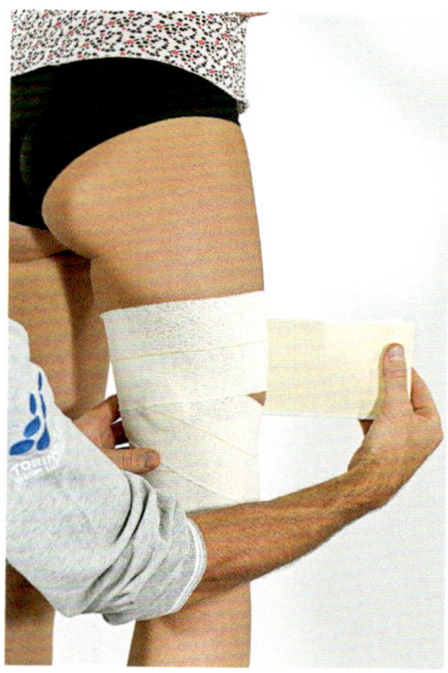
7

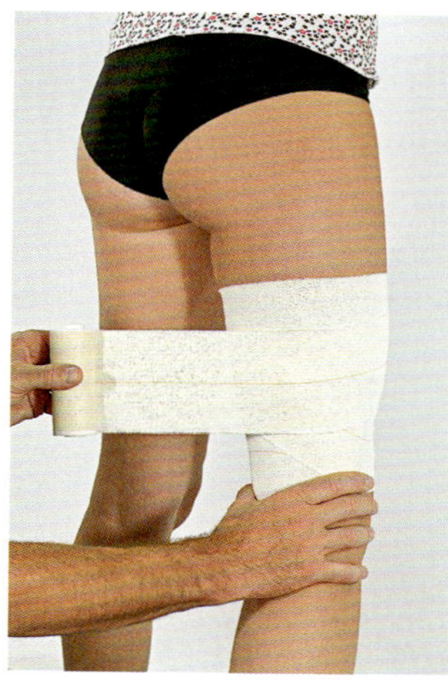
8

Muscular unloading via compressive bandaging

MATERIAL

✓ Cotton fabric porous elastic adhesive bandage that can be stretched lengthwise or is bi-extensible, 10 cm in width
✓ Foam rubber or pre-tape compress for creating a compressive unloading pad
✓ Inelastic adhesive tape

APPLICATION

1 The subject stands with the knee half-flexed and the heel supported on a 2-4 cm lift (see page 139) in order to relieve the musculoskeletal structures involved in the bandaging. Before beginning bandaging, a foam or pre-tape compress must be prepared for positioning at the point of the injury.

2-3 Below the point of the injury, a full wrap of elastic adhesive bandage is made around the thigh.

> *With regards to the unloading pad that will be subsequently positioned at the point of injury, the first wrap of the bandage must be applied at the area where its lower end will be found. In this context, the term "injury" refers to any aftereffects of muscular contracture, scars in the reparation stage, or fibrosis.*

4-5 After having placed the unloading pad at the point of the injury, it is covered with the bandage running obliquely over the thigh in the distal-proximal direction.

6-7 At this point, a complete wrap of bandage is made around the thigh, passing above the upper edge of the unloading pad.

8 The bandage is made to descend again to the thigh, such that it can cover both ends of the pad.

POSTERIOR MUSCLES OF THE THIGH

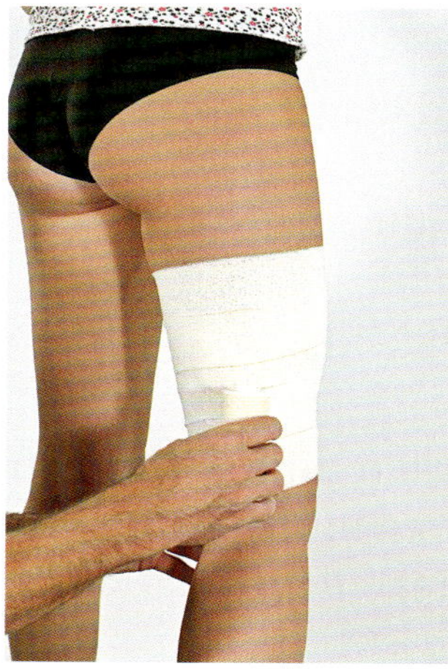
9

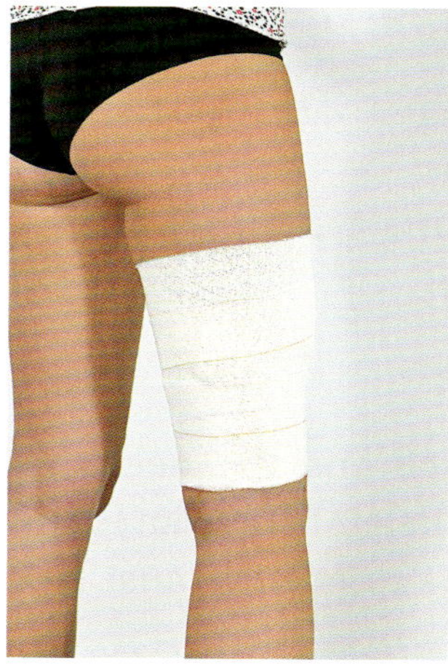
10

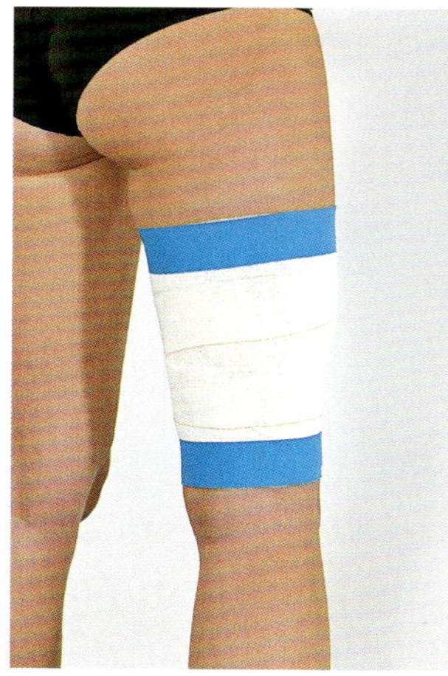
11

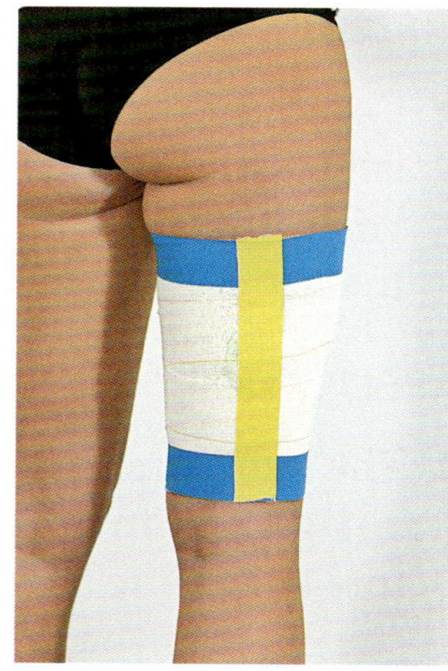
12

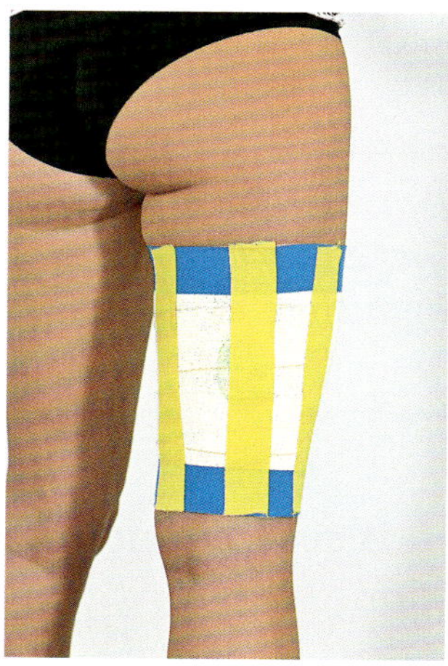
13

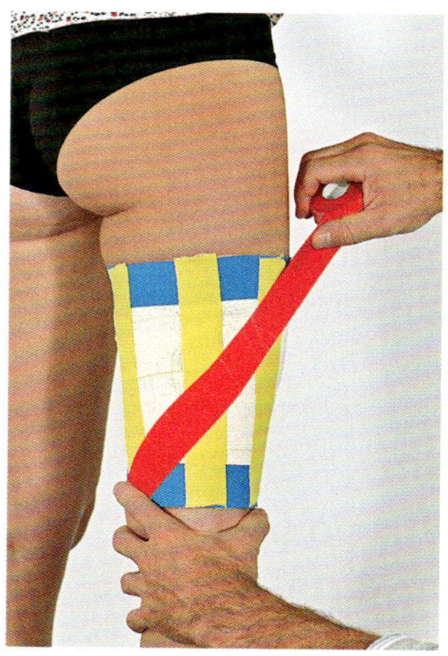
14

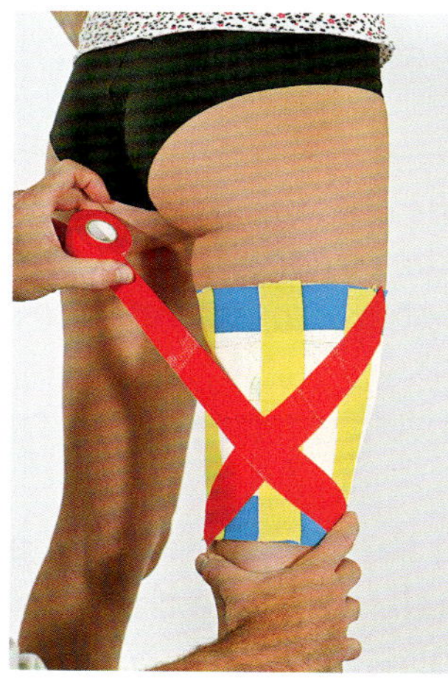
15

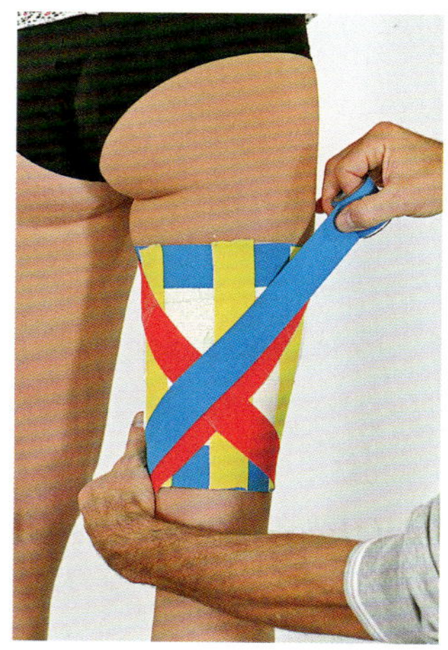
16

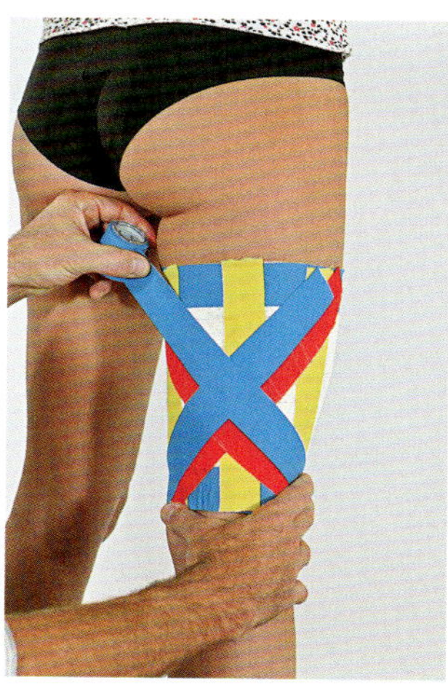
17

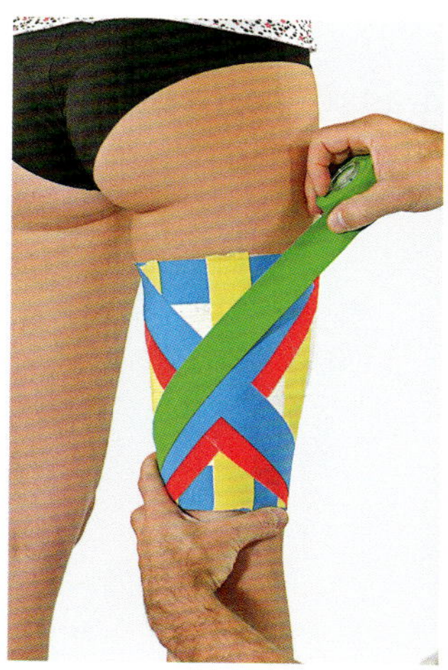
18

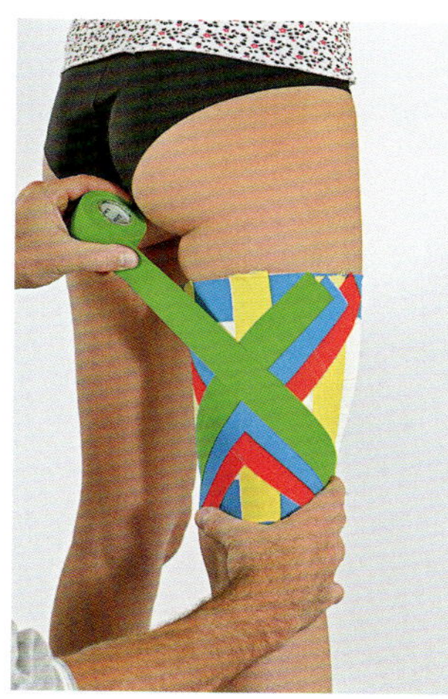
19

9-10 Next, a complete wrapping of the bandage is made to cover the lower edge of the pad.

11 The base bandaging is reinforced with strips of inelastic adhesive tape after preparing the two proximal and distal anchoring points.

12-13 Three strips are longitudinally applied to the axis of the lower limb: the first passes directly over the compress, while the other two are positioned to the sides; these pieces of tape will serve as starting and arrival points for subsequent ones.

14-15 Now bandaging proceeds, applying a bandage in X-formation beginning over the distal anchoring point and arriving at the proximal one: the first two strips cross at the lower end of the foam rubber compress.

16-17-18-19 The unloading compress must be completely covered with other tape strips applied in an X-shape and overlapping the previous ones. The tape strips must adhere perfectly to the pad.

In order to enable the aplicación of the strips of inelastic adhesive tape, it is recommended to indicate the position of the unloading pad on the bandage.

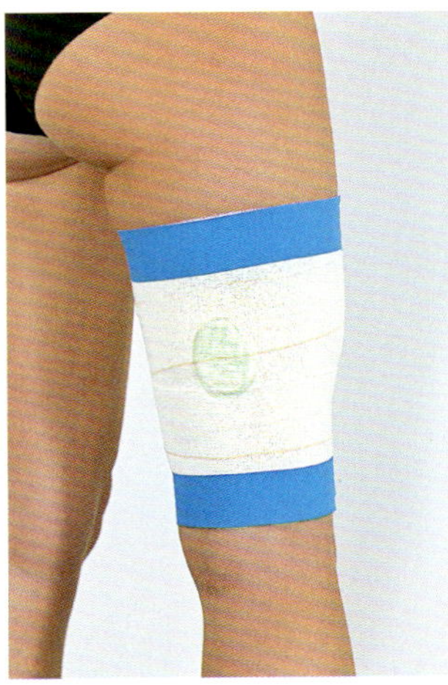

POSTERIOR MUSCLES OF THE THIGH

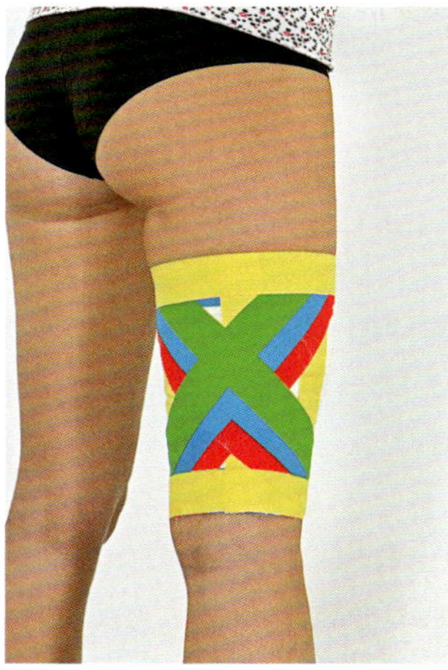

20

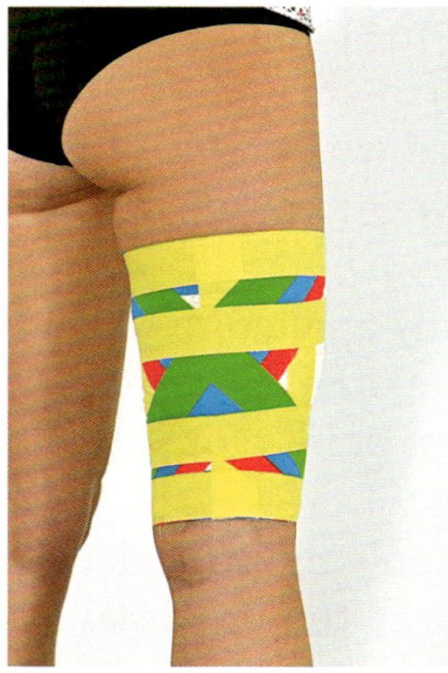

21

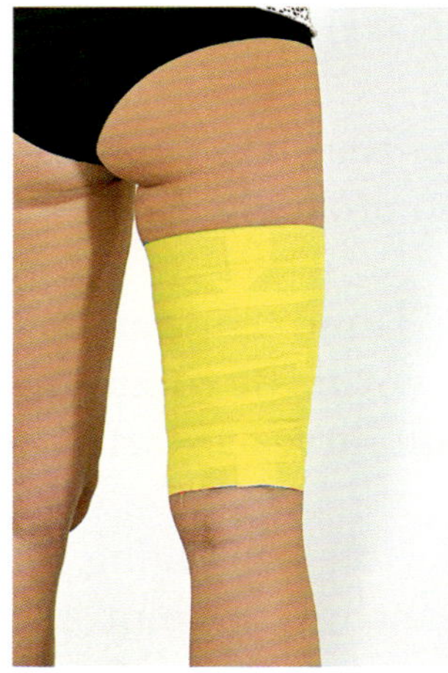

22

Muscular unloading via compressive bandaging

20-21-22 Bandaging ends with the addition of more strips applied in a semicircle perpendicular to the longitudinal axis of the thigh, until it is fully covered.

When preparing the X-shaped bandage, the strips of inelastic adhesive tape must be overlapped by 30-50%. This type of bandaging is useful for obtaining muscular unloading.

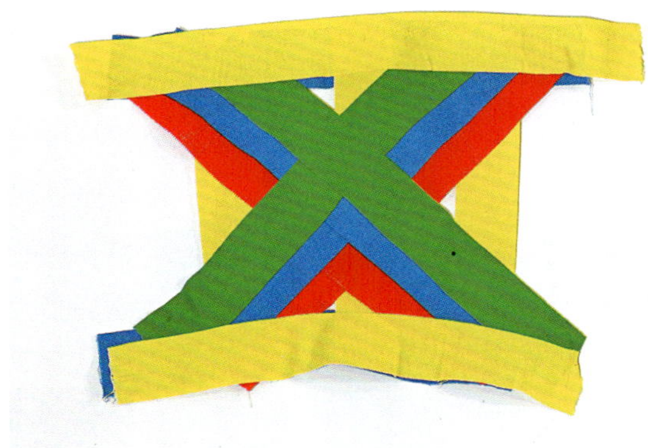

INDICATIONS

Effects of muscular injuries such as:

- ✓ *Contractures*
- ✓ *Strains*
- ✓ *Elongations*

POSTERIOR MUSCLES OF THE THIGH

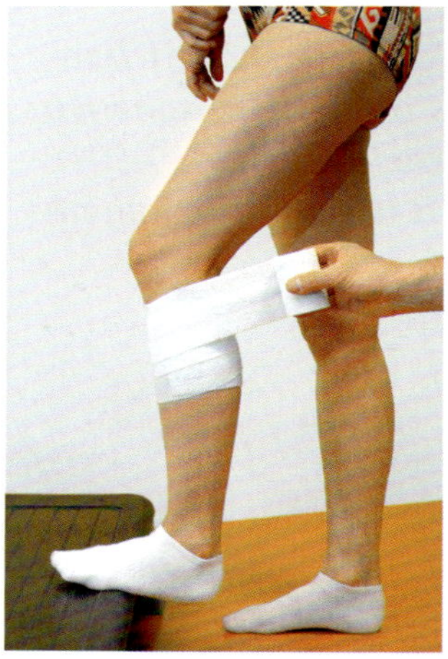

1

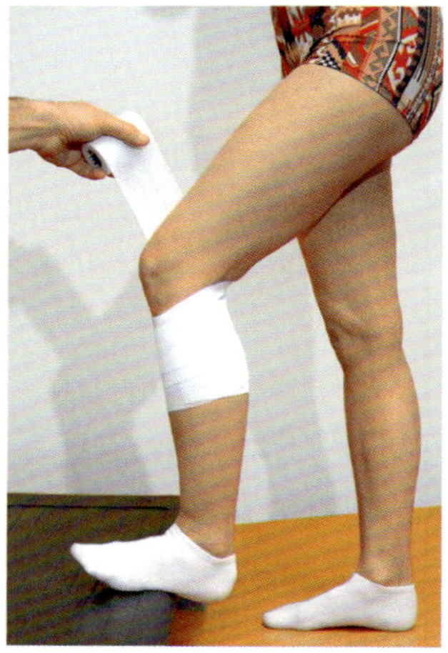

2

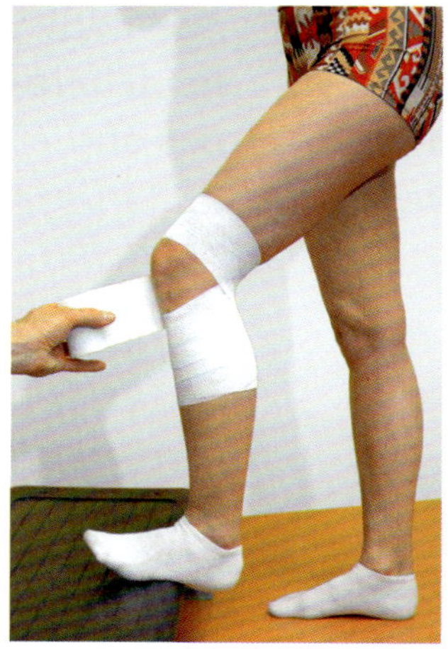

3

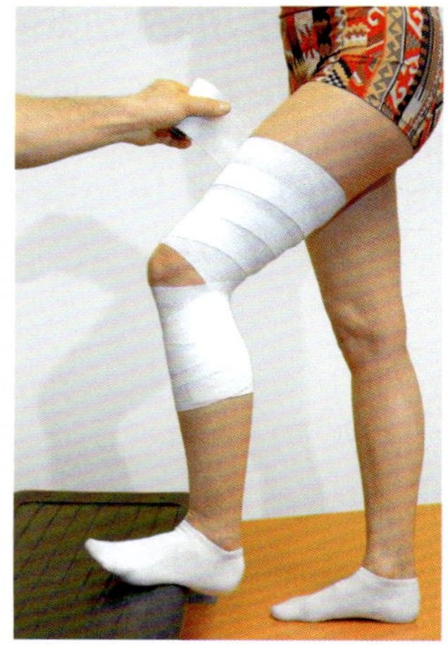

4

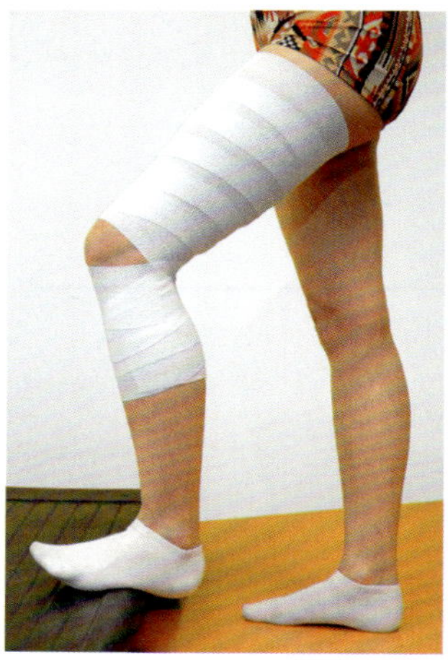

5

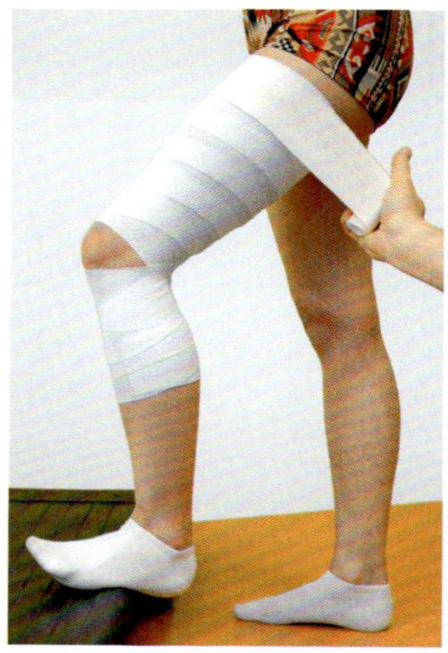

6

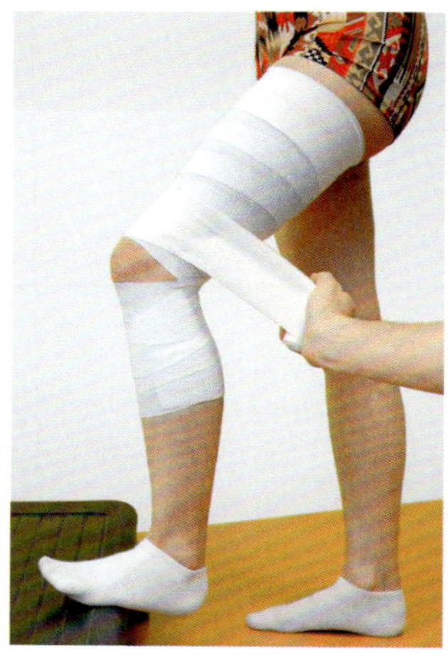

7

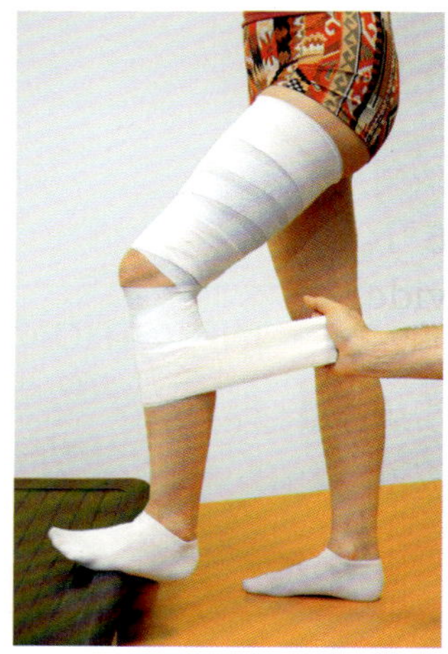

8

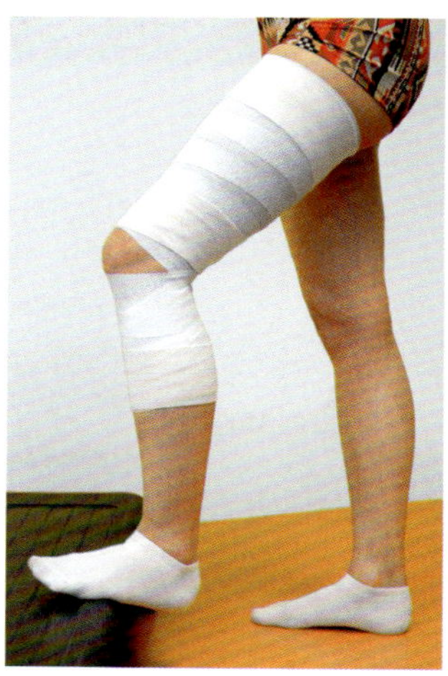

9

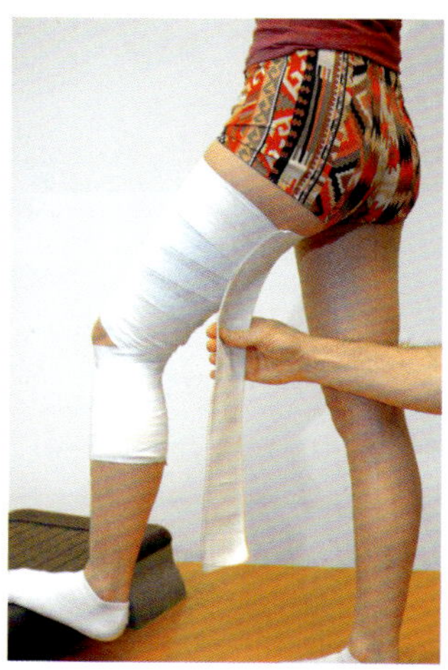

10

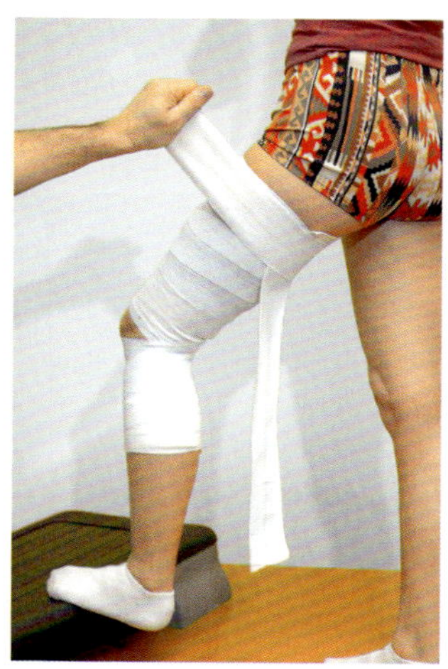

11

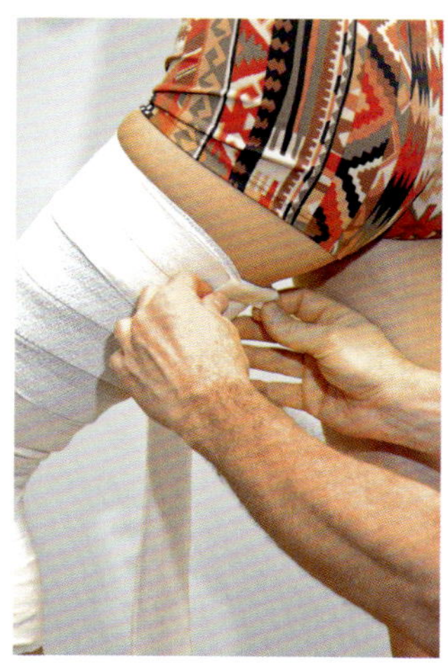

12

Unloading, support, and guidance of movement

MATERIAL

- ✓ Elastic cohesive bandage, 7.5 cm in width
- ✓ Cotton fabric porous elastic adhesive bandage that can be stretched lengthwise, 7.5 cm in width

APPLICATION

1 The subject is standing with the foot resting on a lift in order to keep the involved musculoskeletal structures relieved from load-bearing; the knee is flexed at 20 degrees and the hip at 30 degrees. In order to begin, several spiral wraps of the elastic cohesive bandage are made in the distal-proximal direction, wrapping the proximal third of the lower leg.

2-3 Passing behind the knee, the bandage is brought to the distal third of the thigh, where it makes a complete wrap, also crossing the popliteal fossa.

4-5 The bandage concludes by covering the thigh with several spiral wraps applied in the distal-proximal direction.

6 Next, an initial wrap of the mono-extensible elastic bandage is applied in order to provide the proximal anchoring point.

7 A second full wrap of bandage covers the distal third of the femur in order to provide the intermediate anchor point.

8-9 A third wrap of bandage covers the tibial axis in order to provide the distal anchoring point.

10-11 A reinforced elastic unloading fastener, made with three strips of bandage, is applied posteriorly on the proximal anchoring point, held in place with a full wrap of adhesive elastic bandage.

12 The excess part of the fastener must be folded and held in place with another full wrap of the bandage.

In order to create the reinforced elastic unloading fastener, three strips of mono-extensible elastic adhesive bandage are cut to the right measurement and placed on top of each other. The fastener, thus prepared, must be put under tension by stretching it.

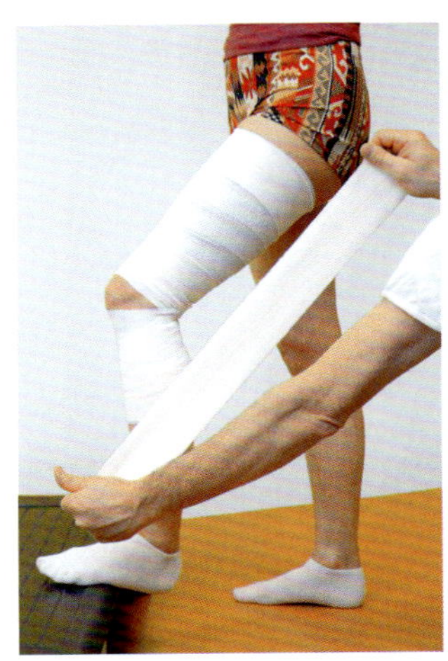

POSTERIOR MUSCLES OF THE THIGH

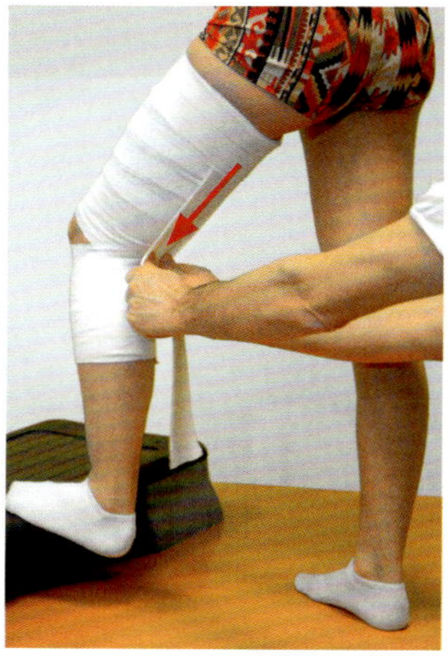

13

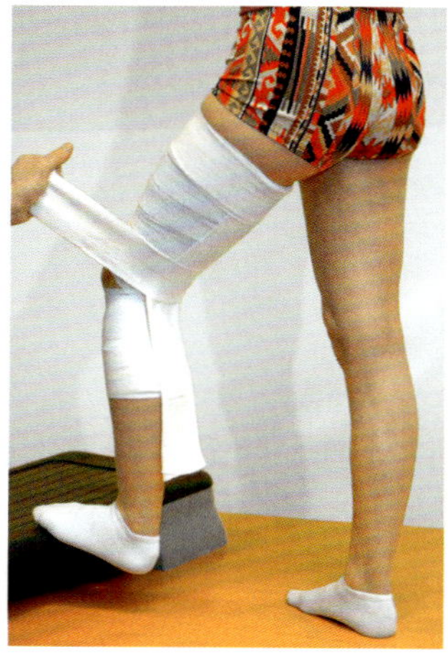

14

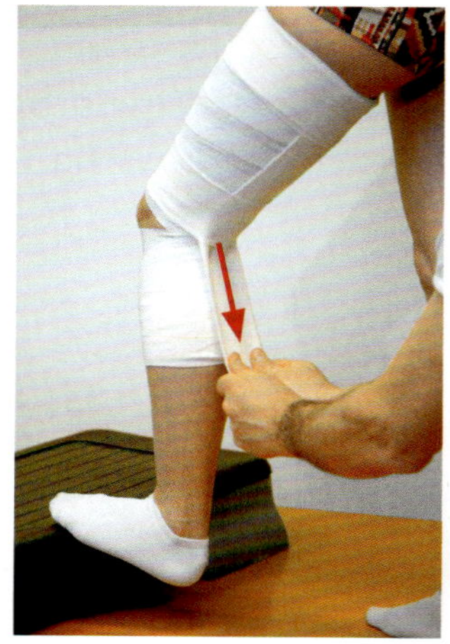

15

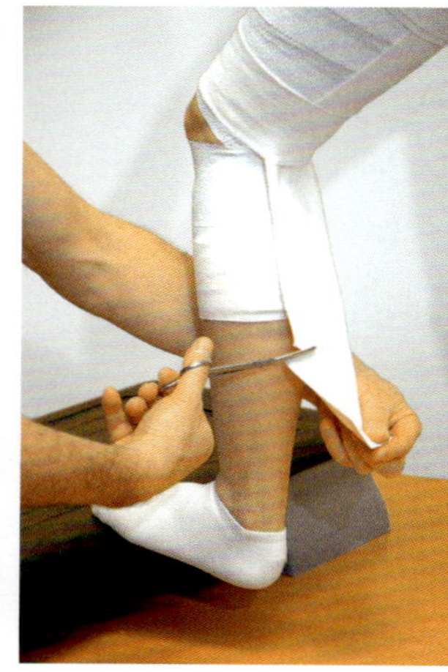

16

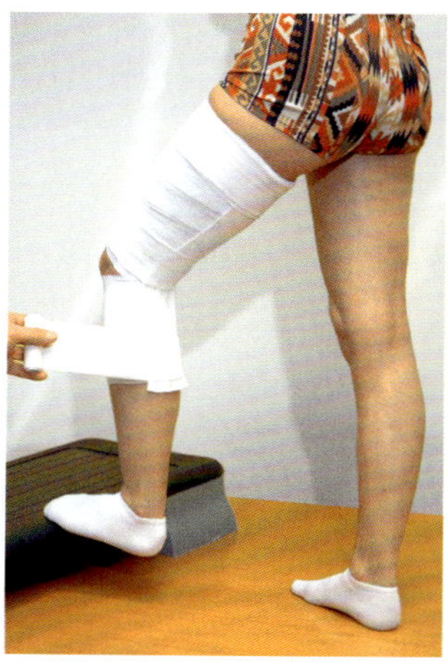

17

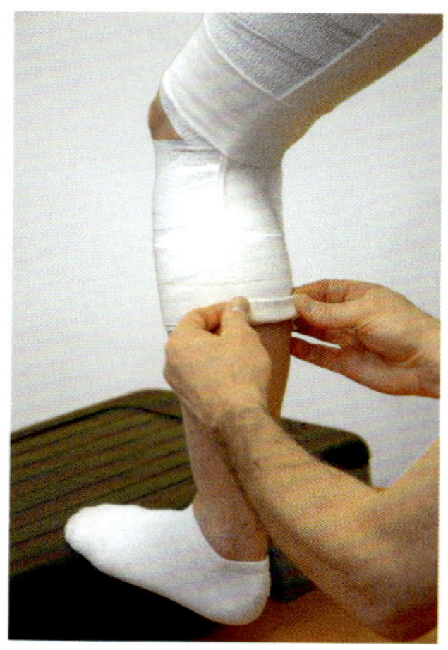

18

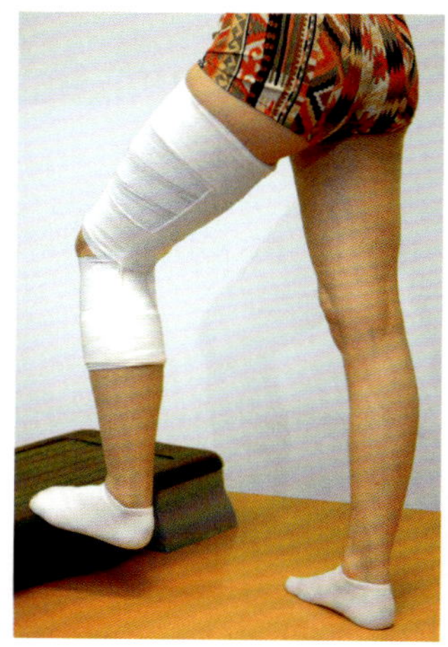

19

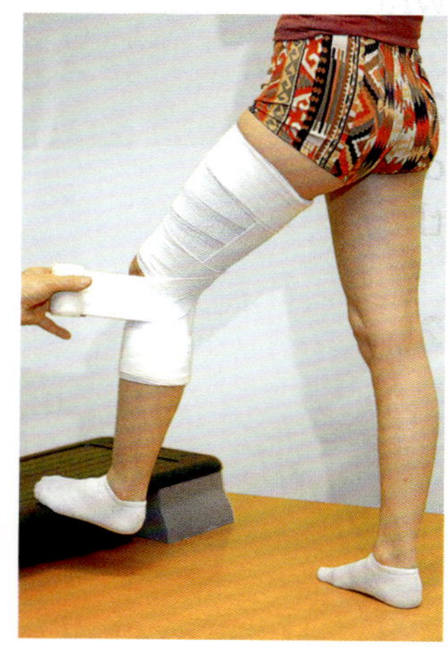

20

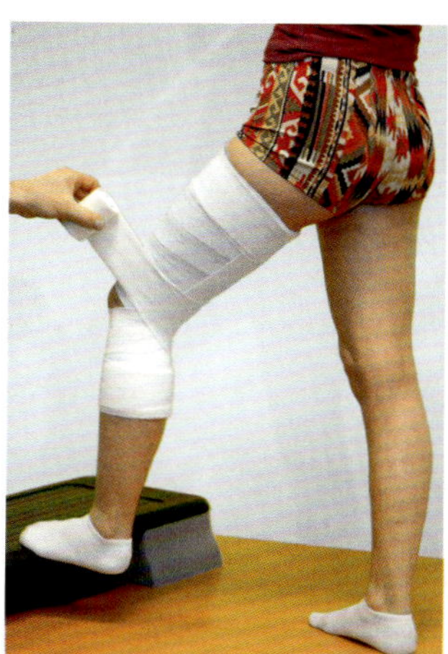

21

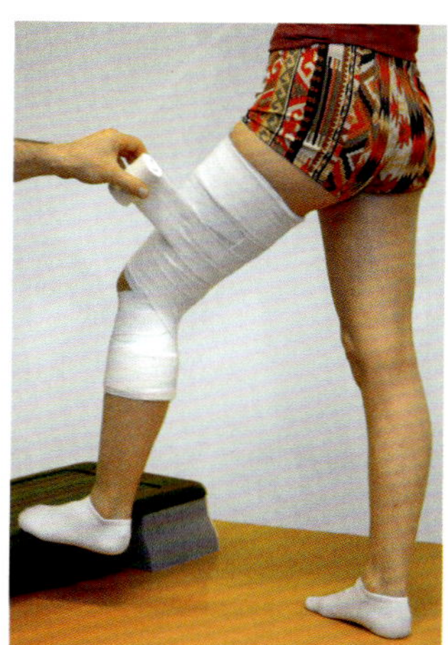

22

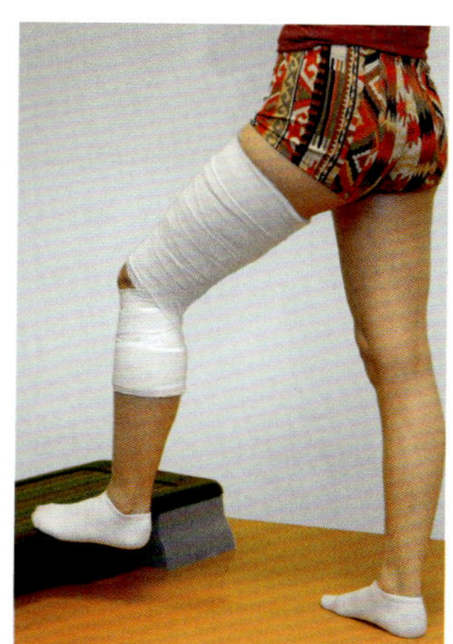

23

Unloading, support, and guidance of movement

13-14 The unloading fastener is now put under tension and affixed over the intermediate anchoring point with a complete wrap of adhesive elastic bandage.

15 The remaining bandage piece is put under tension and adhered to the distal anchoring point.

16 Bandaging proceeds by cutting the excess bandage, taking care to leave it a bit longer than the distal anchoring point.

17 With a complete wrap of the adhesive bandage around the axis of the lower leg, the fastener is also held in place distally.

18-19 The excess part of the fastener is folded over itself and held in place with another wrapping of the bandage.

20 The bandaging finishes with the application of a mono-extensible elastic adhesive bandage in the distal-proximal direction. The bandage starts from the medial region of the thigh, at the distal third, and is directed posteriorly to the knee.

21 Once a full wrap is completed around the proximal third of the lower leg, the bandage crosses the popliteal fossa and runs toward the thigh.

22 The thigh is covered with several spiral wraps applied in the distal-proximal direction.

23 Bandaging is complete.

INDICATIONS

- ✓ *Posttraumatic conditions*
- ✓ *Preventative sports treatment*
- ✓ *Effects of muscular injuries*

POSTERIOR MUSCLES AND JOINT OF THE KNEE

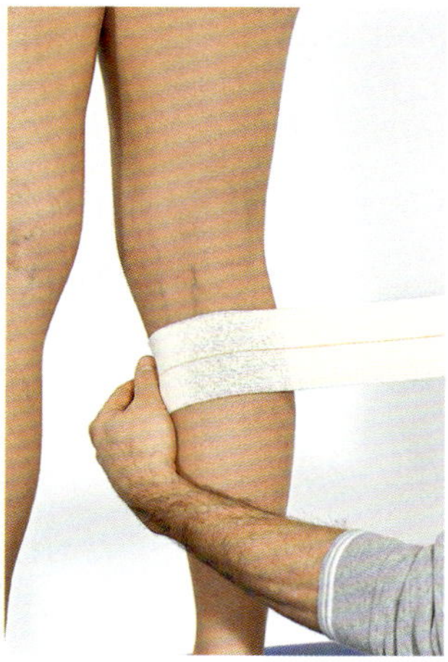

1

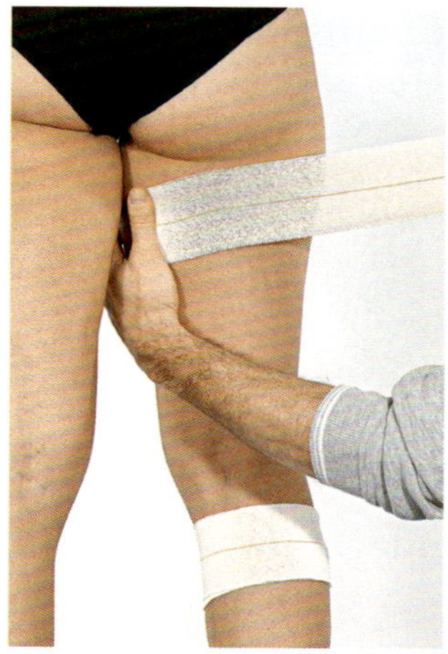

2

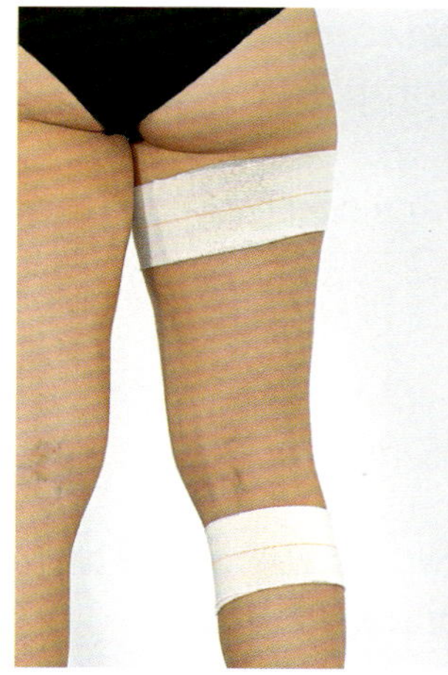

3

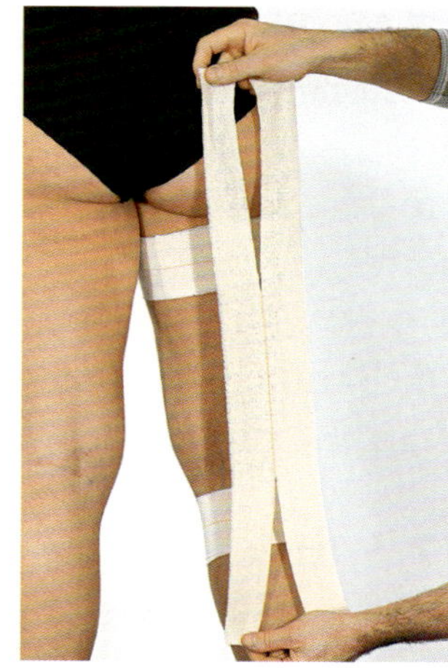

4

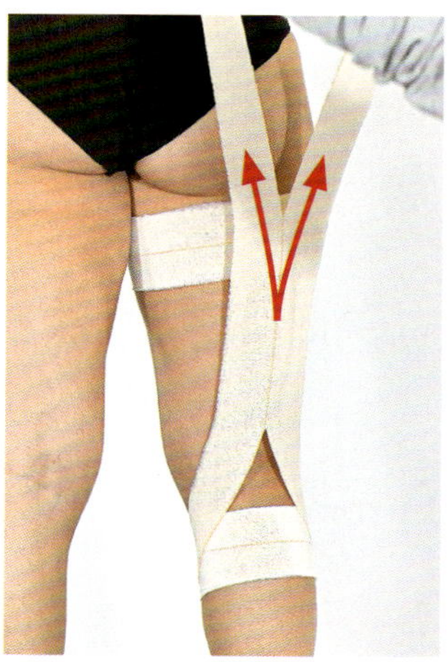

5

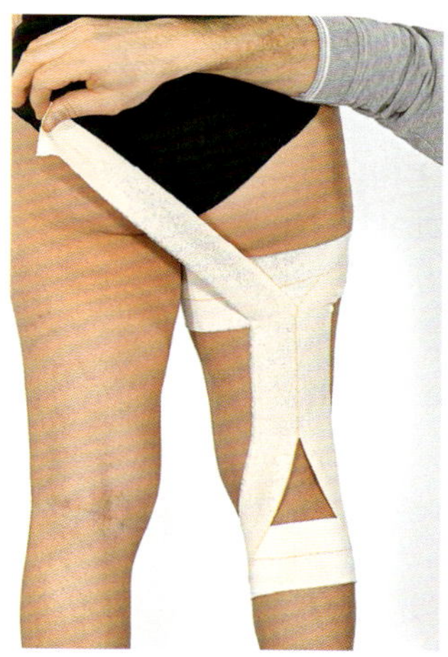

6

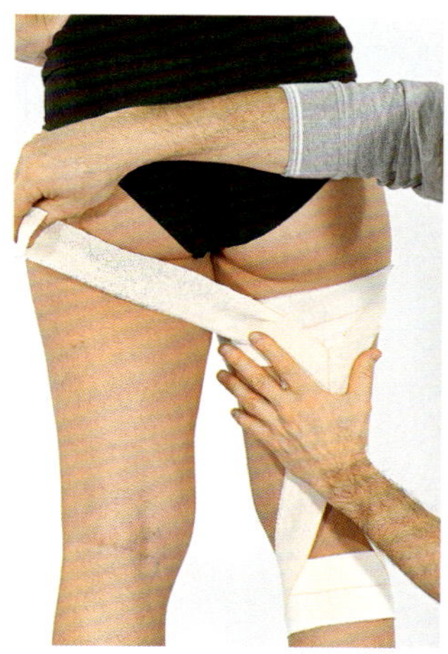

7

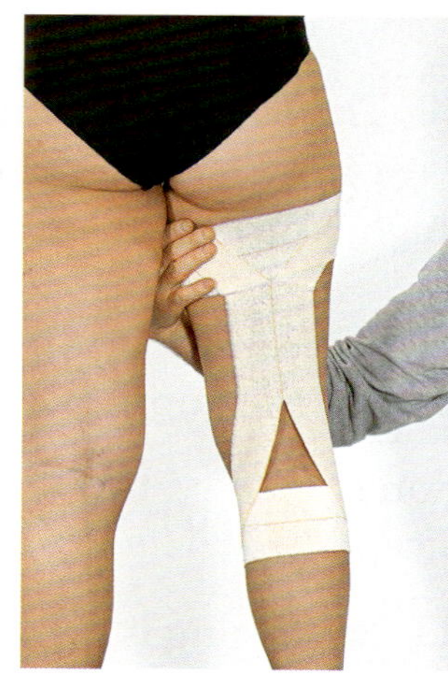

8

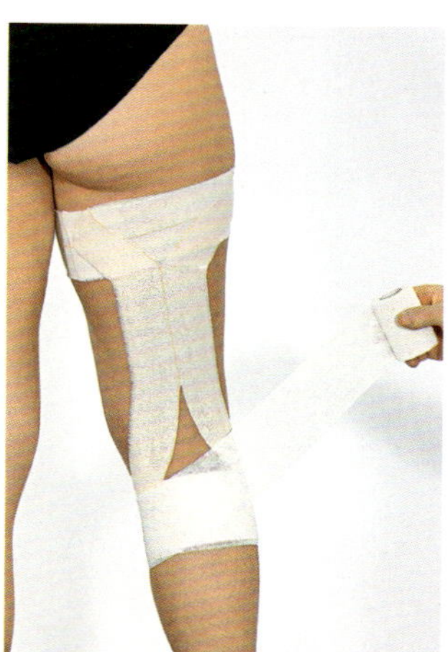

9

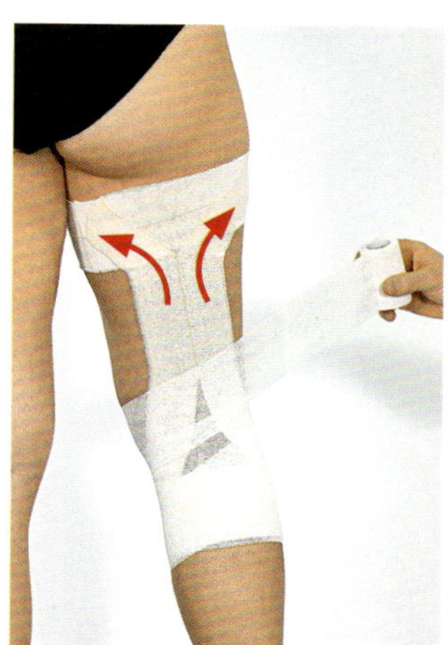

10

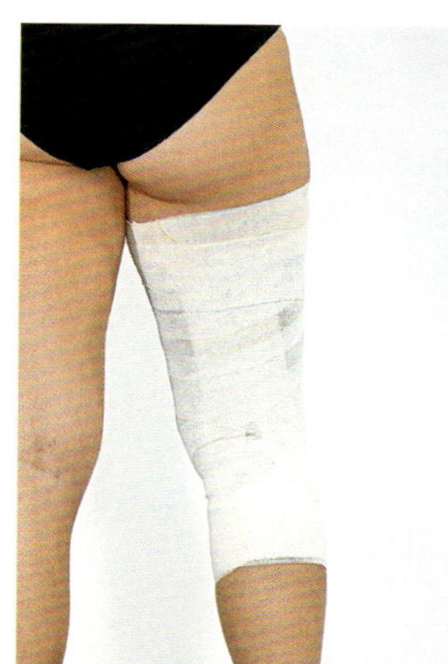

11

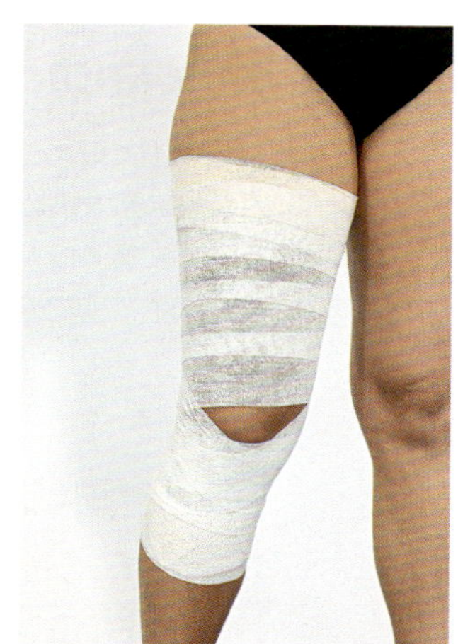

12

Muscular unloading with bandage in X-shape, taking on of the satellite joint

MATERIAL

✓ Cotton fabric porous elastic adhesive bandage that can be stretched lengthwise, 7.5 or 10 cm in width
✓ Elastic cohesive bandage to cover base bandaging

APPLICATION

1 The subject stands with the lower limb in slight flexion of the knee and the heel supported on a lift. The distal anchoring point is prepared at the proximal third of the lower leg with the application of a full wrap of adhesive elastic bandage.

The heel of the lower limb to be treated must be held on a 2-4 cm lift in order to put the involved musculoskeletal structures in a situation of load relief.

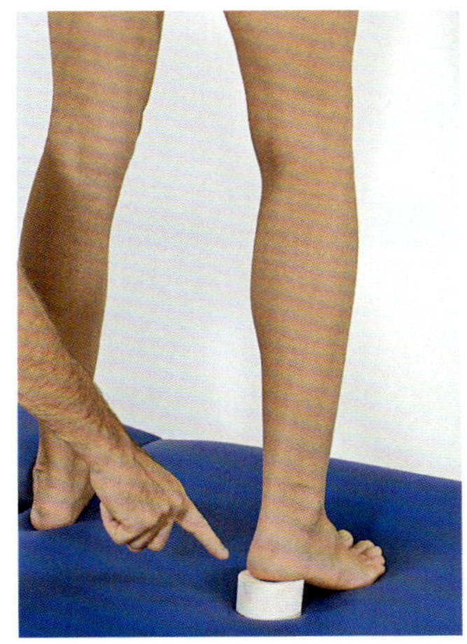

2-3 The proximal anchoring point is applied at the proximal third of the thigh.

4 A bandage of ideal length for this process is longitudinally cut from both ends in order to form an X.

5 The parts of one end are applied on the distal anchoring point, following the skin projection of the tendons of the semimembranosus and semitendinosus medially and that of the biceps femoris laterally. The bandage is then placed in tension in the distal-proximal direction, longitudinally to the muscle fibers.

6-7-8 The parts of the other end of the bandage are held in place at the proximal anchoring point, taking care that they are well adhered.

9-10 The bandaging finishes with a cohesive bandage applied with spiral wrapping in the distal-proximal direction, so as to keep the adhesive bandaging in place and reinforce the base application.

11-12 Bandaging is complete.

INDICATIONS

✓ *Injuries of the posterior muscles of the thigh*

KNEE JOINT

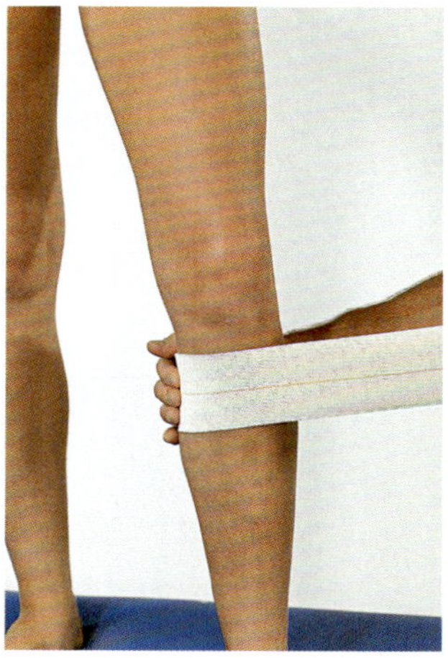

1

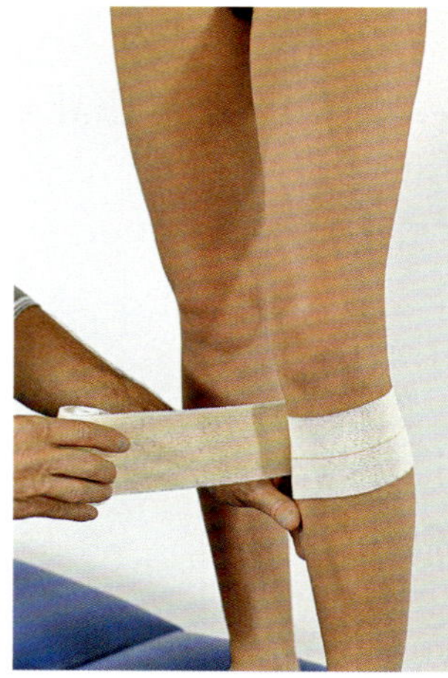

2

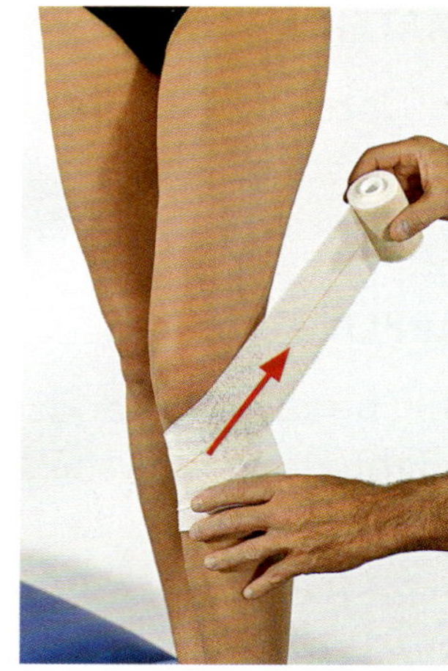

3

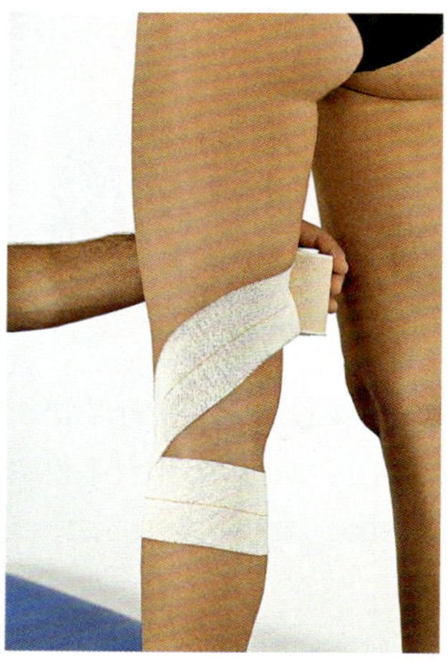

4

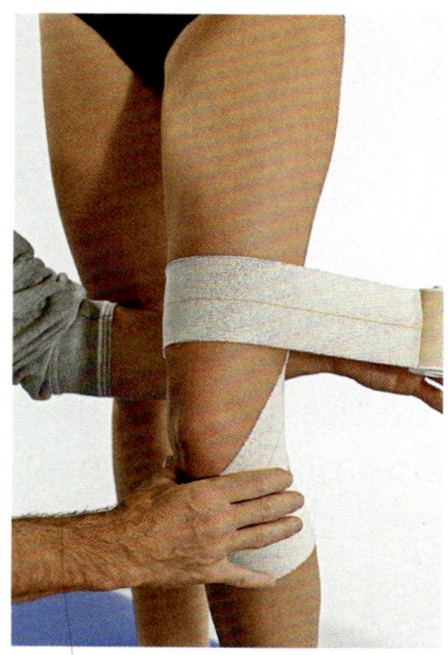

5

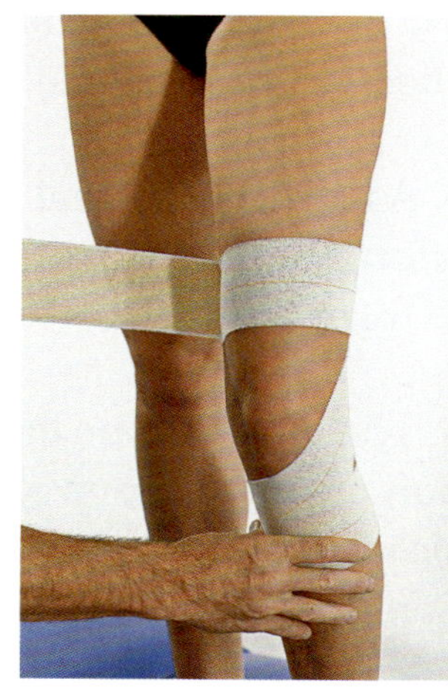

6

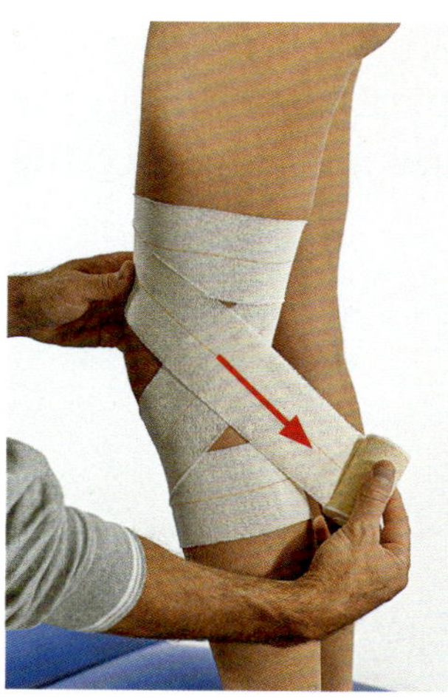

7

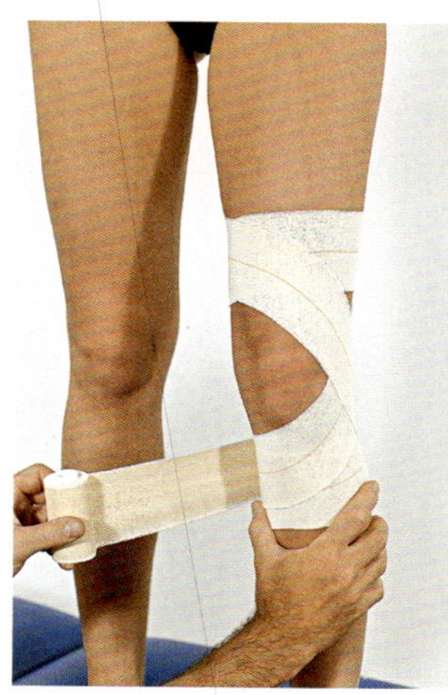

8

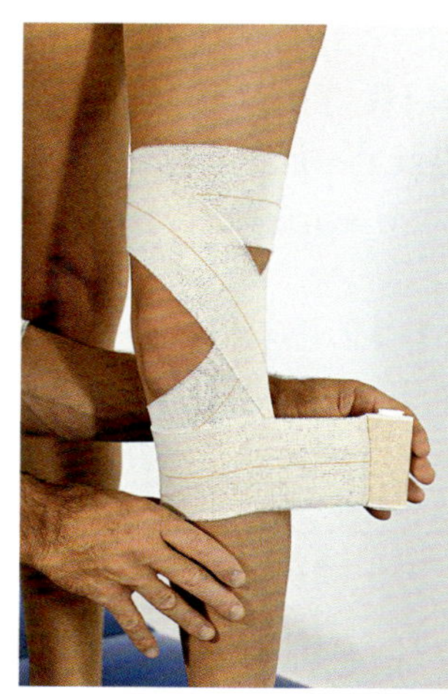

9

Base bandaging

MATERIAL

✓ Cotton fabric porous elastic adhesive bandage that can be stretched lengthwise, 7.5 cm in width

APPLICATION

1-2 The subject is standing with the lower limb to be treated in slight semi-flexion. To begin, a full wrap of bandage is done at the proximal third of the lower leg near the knee joint.

> *In order to improve the unloading of the musculotendinous structures, a 2-4 cm wide lift may be positioned under the heel (see page 139).*

3 The bandage is obliquely pulled to laterally border on the lower end of the patella, going on to cover the skin projection of the lateral collateral ligament.

4 Posteriorly, the bandage goes directly over the distal third of the thigh, leaving the popliteal fossa free.

5-6 Next, a complete wrap of the bandage is made around the thigh.

7 The bandage is obliquely pulled to laterally border on the upper end of the patella, then cross the previous bandage's path at the skin projection of the lateral collateral ligament.

8-9 A full wrap of bandage is made at the proximal third of the lower leg, without covering the popliteal fossa.

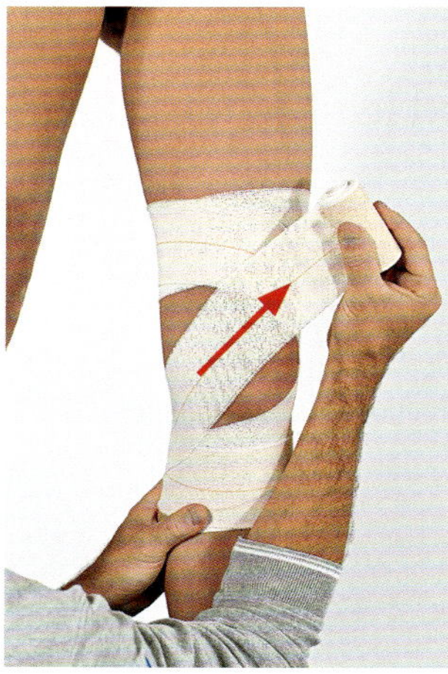
10

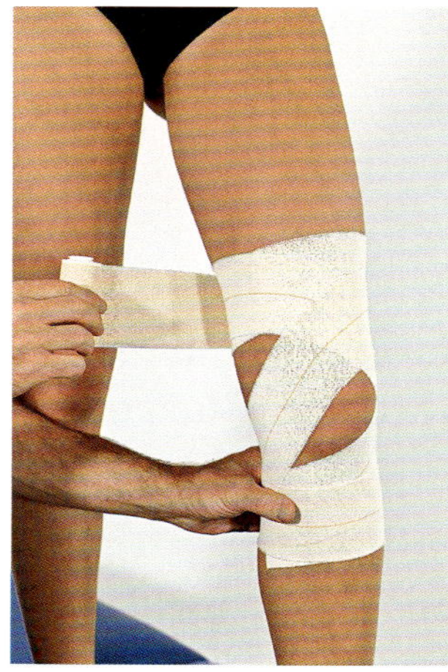
11

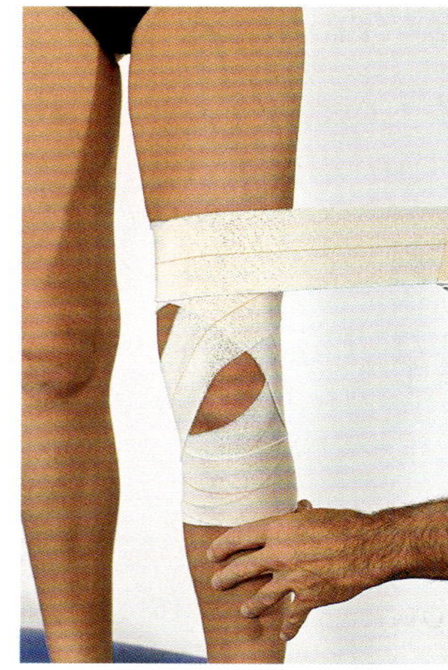
12

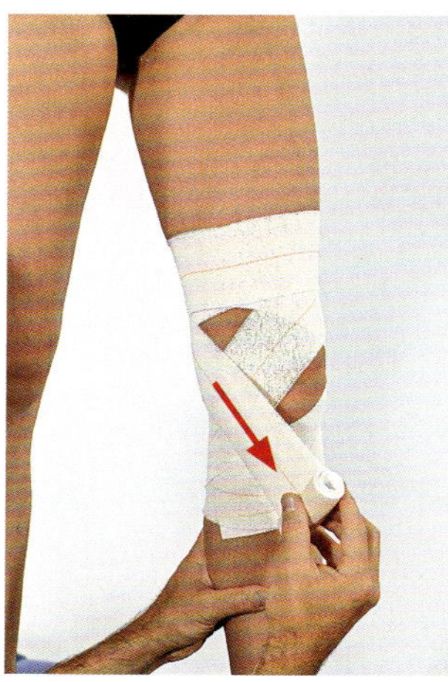
13

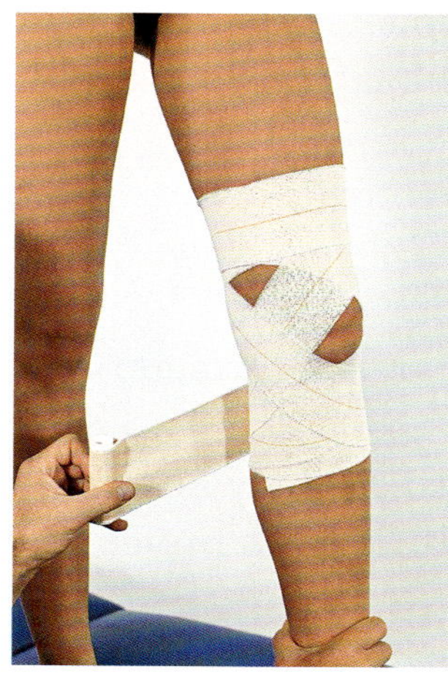
14

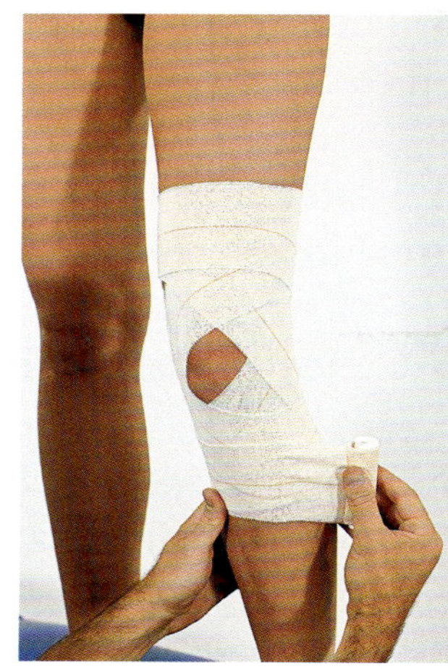
15

Base bandaging

10 The bandage is obliquely pulled to medially border on the upper end of the patella, passing over the medial collateral ligament.

11-12 At this point, a full wrap of bandage is applied around the distal third of the thigh, covering the previous wrap of bandage.

13 The bandage is obliquely pulled to medially border on the lower end of the patella, passing over the skin projection of the medial collateral ligament.

14-15 To finish, another full wrap of the bandage is made around the proximal third of the lower leg, securing the bandaging.

INDICATIONS

- ✓ *Support for sprain trauma*
- ✓ *Bilateral injuries of the collateral ligaments*
- ✓ *Mono-compartmental injuries of the collateral ligaments*
- ✓ *Retention of posttraumatic capsuloligamentous instability*

KNEE JOINT

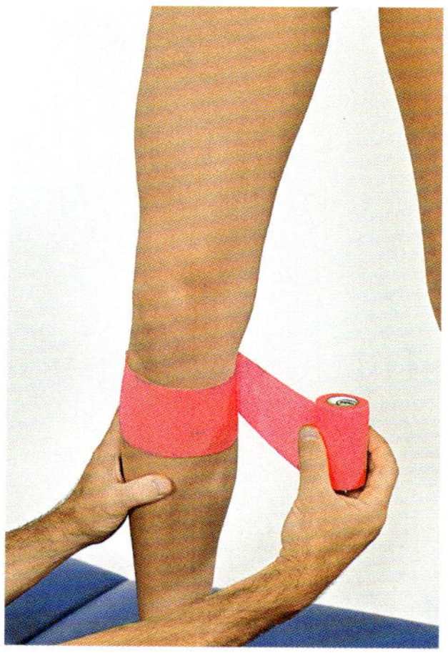
1

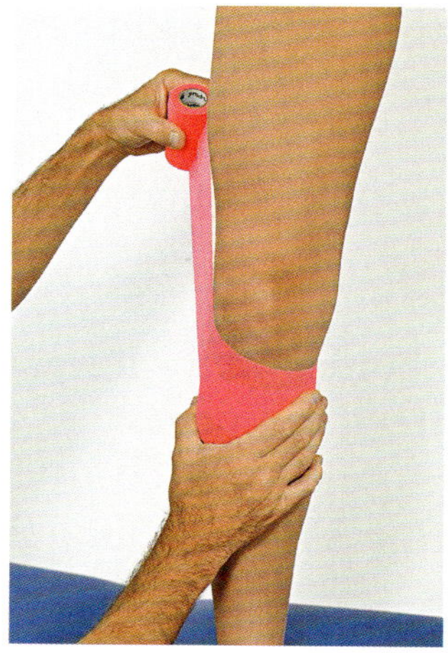
2

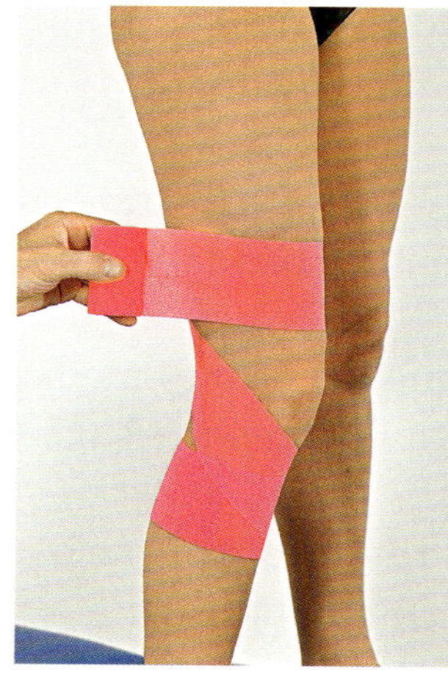
3

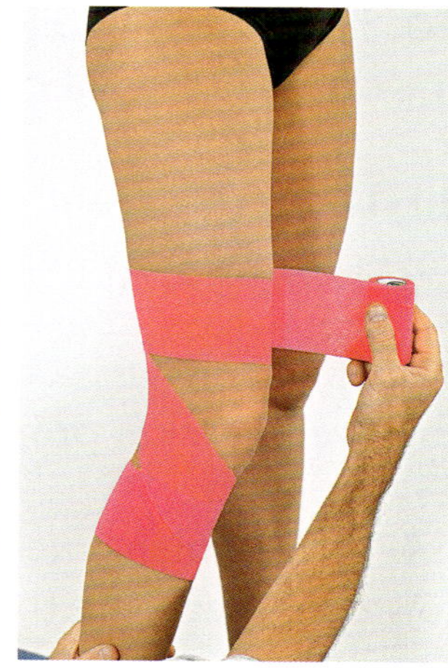
4

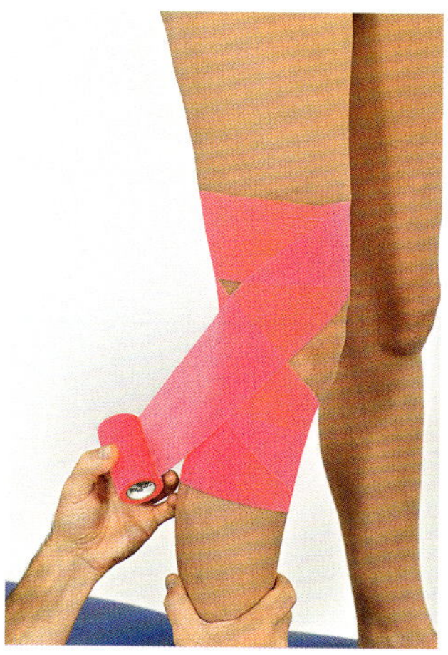
5

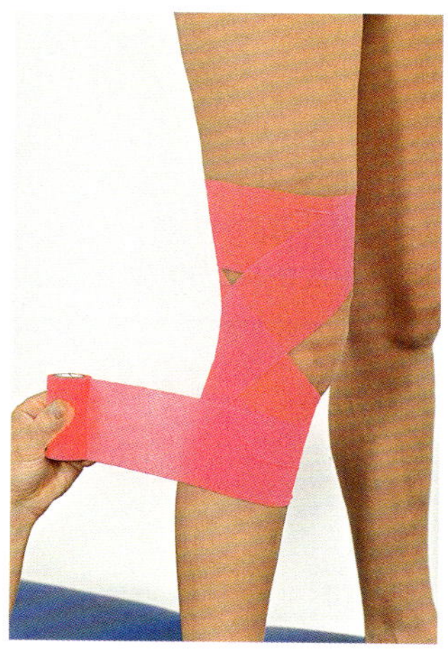
6

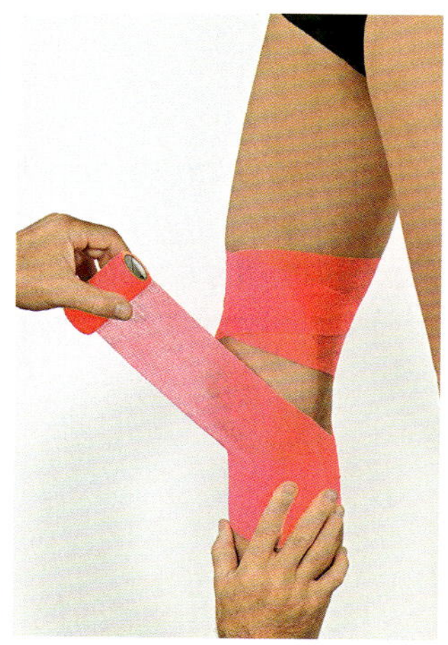
7

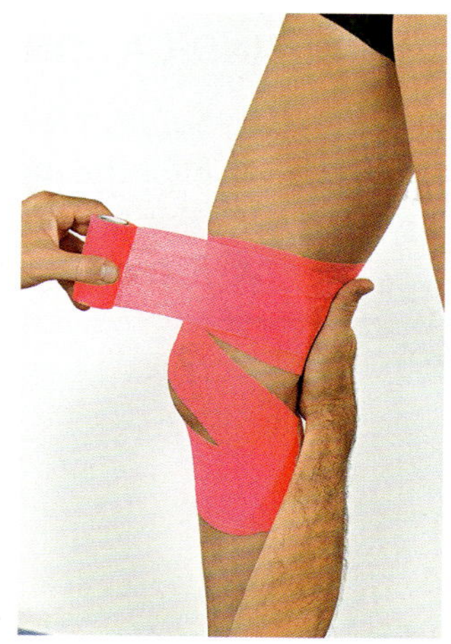
8

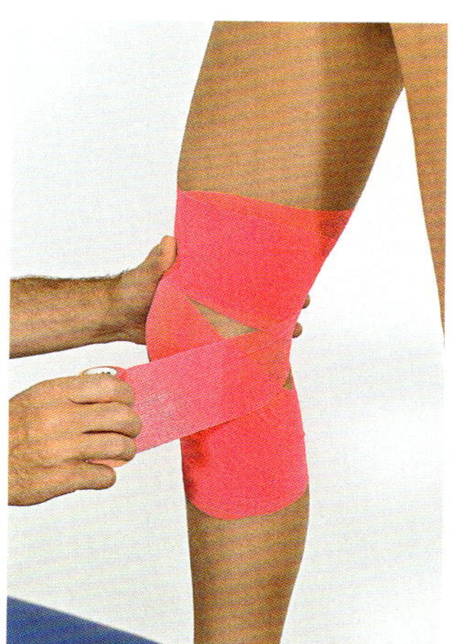
9

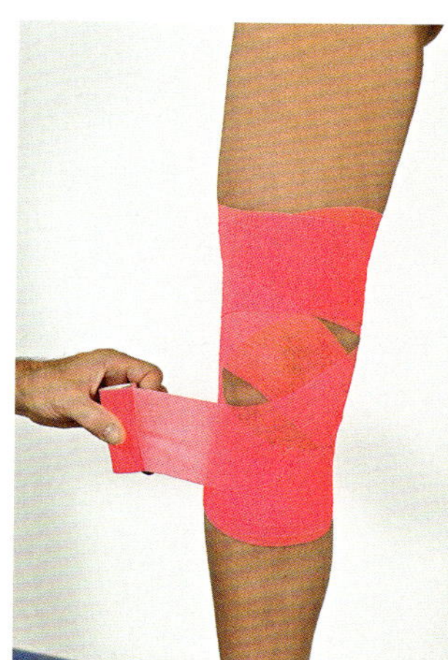
10

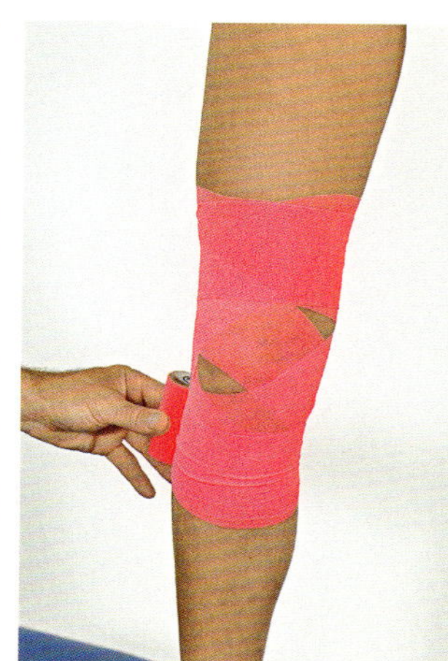
11

Base bandaging with cohesive bandage

MATERIAL

✓ Elastic cohesive bandage, 7.5 cm in width

APPLICATION

1 To begin, a full wrap of bandage is made at the proximal third of the lower leg.

2 The bandage is pulled distal to proximal and, bordering on the lower end of the patella, is passed over the skin projection of the lateral collateral ligament of the knee.

3 The bandage is then directed between the medial and distal thirds of the thigh, passing posteriorly and leaving the popliteal fossa free.

4 Next, a complete wrap of the bandage is made around the thigh.

5 Bordering on the upper end of the patella, the bandage is brought in the anterior-posterior and proximal-distal directions to cross the previous path on the skin projection of the lateral collateral ligament of the knee.

6 The bandage is directed posteriorly and makes a full wrap at the proximal third of the lower leg without covering the popliteal fossa.

7 At the skin projection of the medial collateral ligament of the knee, the bandage is pulled in a posterior-anterior and distal-proximal direction until reaching the distal third of the thigh after having covered the upper end of the patella.

8 Proceed with a full wrap of the bandage around the thigh, passing over the bandaging that has already been placed.

9 At the skin projection of the medial collateral ligament of the knee, the bandage is pulled in a posterior-anterior and proximal-distal direction until reaching the proximal third of the lower leg after having covered the lower end of the patella.

10-11 To finish, a full wrap of bandage is applied at the proximal third of the lower leg, without covering the popliteal fossa. The bandaging concludes with the application of the proximal and distal anchoring points.

KNEE JOINT

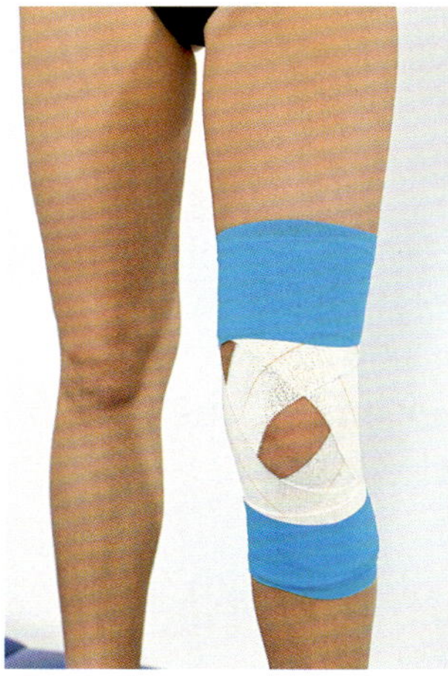

1

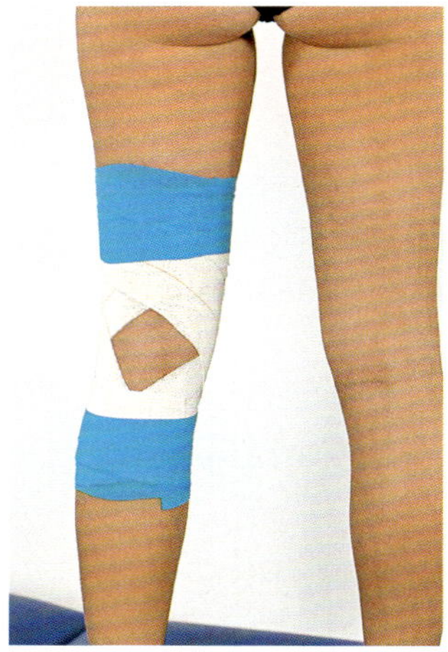

2

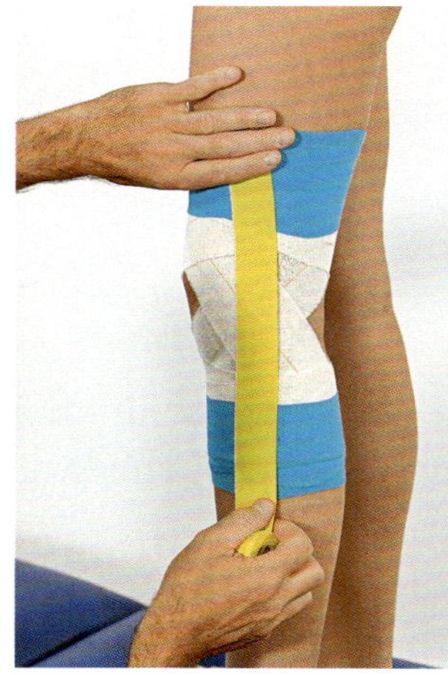

3

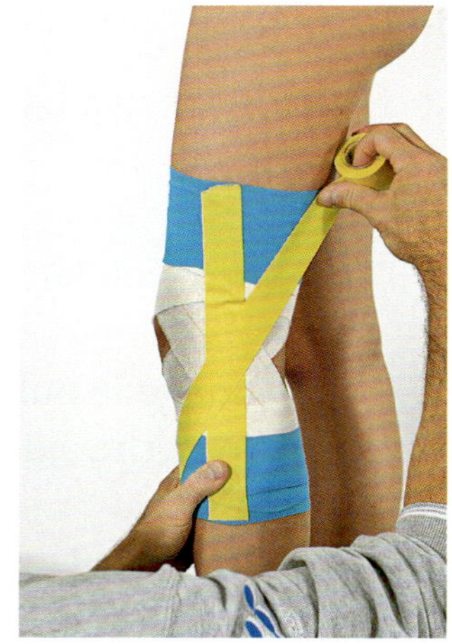

4

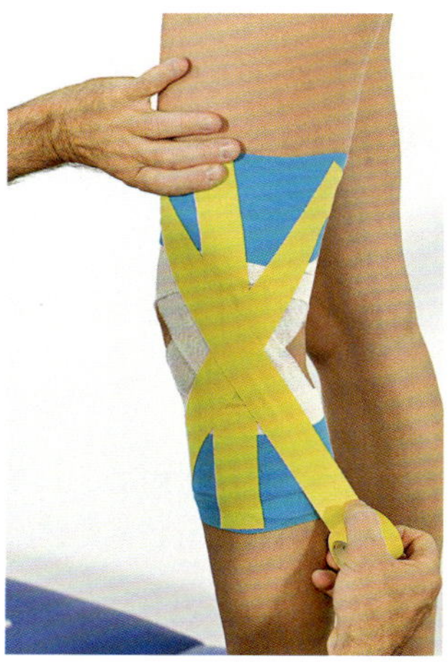

5

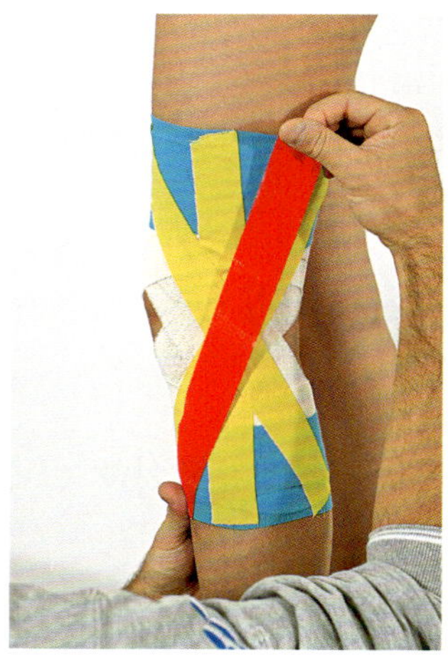

6

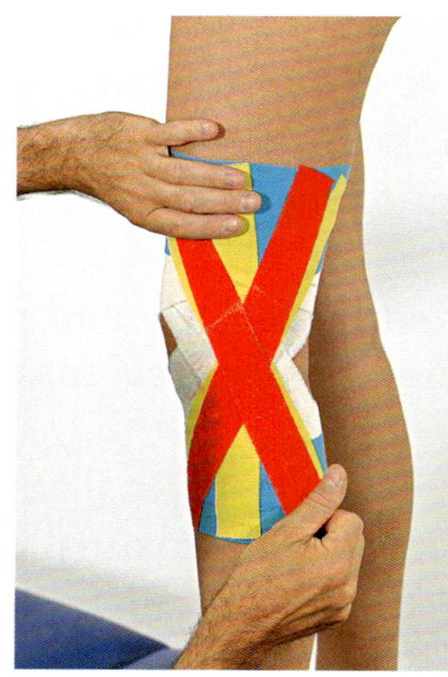

7

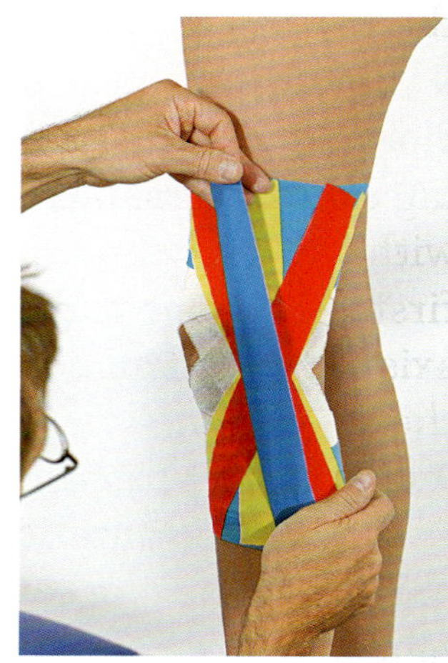

8

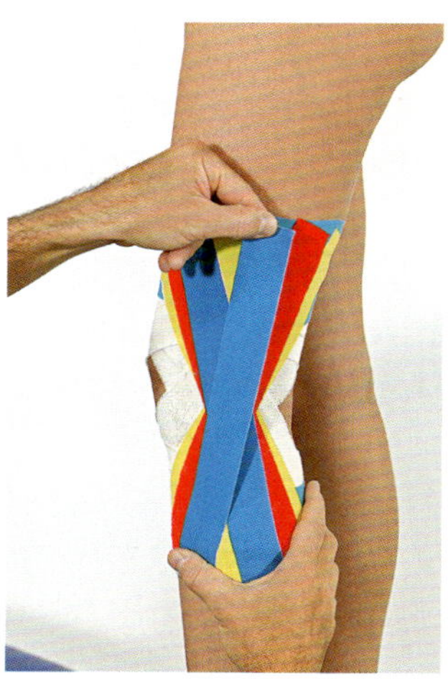

9

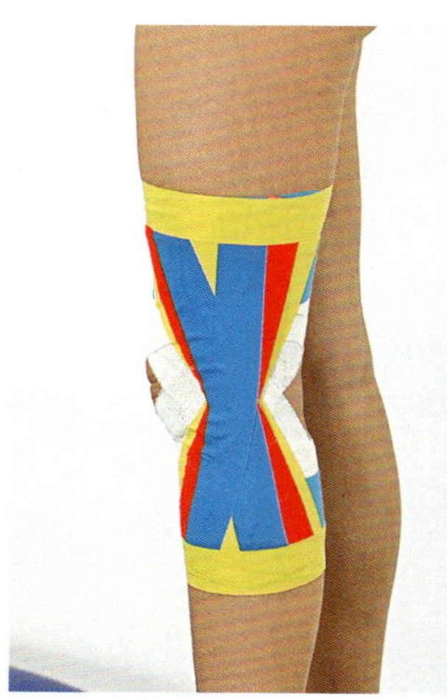

10

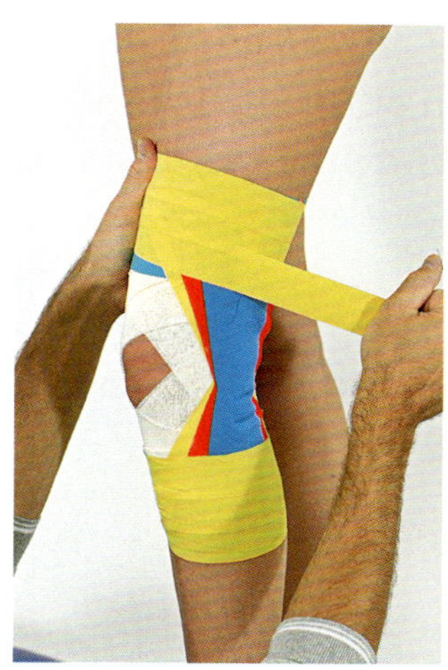

11

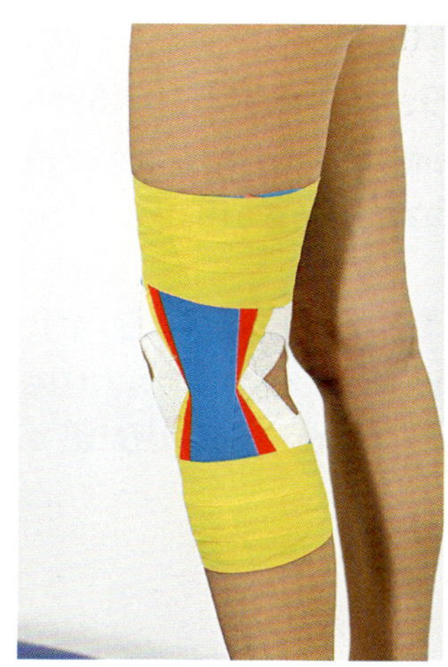

12

Stabilization of the collateral ligament on the base bandaging

MATERIAL

- ✓ 7.5 cm wide cotton fabric porous elastic adhesive bandage that can be stretched lengthwise to create base bandaging
- ✓ Elastic adhesive tape for affixing the base bandaging
- ✓ Inelastic adhesive tape

APPLICATION

1-2 After having done base bandaging (see pages 140-143), it is finished with two wraps of elastic adhesive tape applied at the proximal and distal anchoring points. Note how the bandage leaves both the patella and the popliteal fossa open.

3 Bandaging for stabilization and unloading of the lateral collateral ligament is done with the use of inelastic adhesive tape. The first strip is applied longitudinally to the axis of the lower limb, having it pass over the projection of the lateral collateral ligament.

When preparing the X-shaped bandage, the strips of inelastic adhesive tape must be overlapped by 75%. The bandaging is held in place with pieces of tape applied in a semicircle.

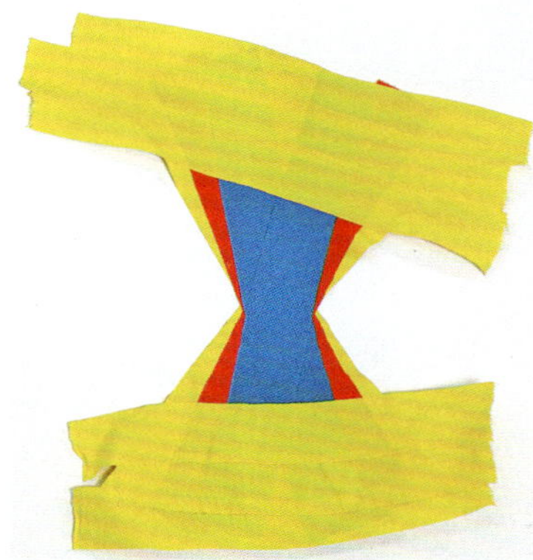

4-5-6-7-8-9 In order to stabilize and contain the point of injury, another six strips of inelastic adhesive tape are crossed two-by-two at the skin projection of the lateral collateral ligament, with an overlap of 75%.

10-11-12 The bandaging is set in place and completed by applying several strips of inelastic adhesive tape in a semicircle, starting from the proximal and distal anchoring points in order to cover the reinforcement fasteners and thus increase the stabilization force of the bandaging.

This type of bandaging may be used in cases of injuries of the medial collateral ligament by applying the reinforcement fasteners in the medial area.

INDICATIONS

- ✓ *Mono-compartmental injuries of the collateral ligaments*
- ✓ *Sprain trauma*

KNEE JOINT

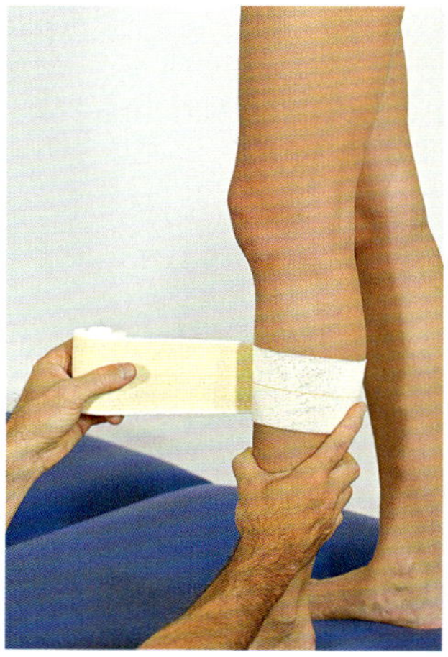
1

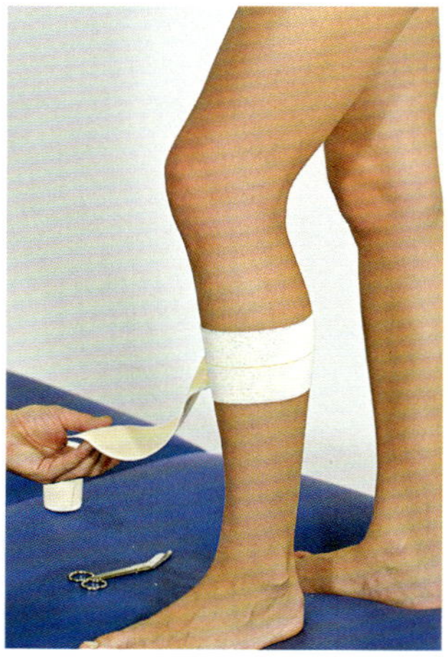
2

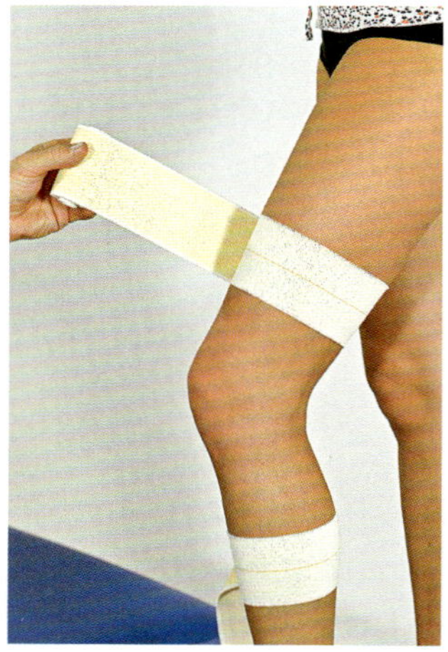
3

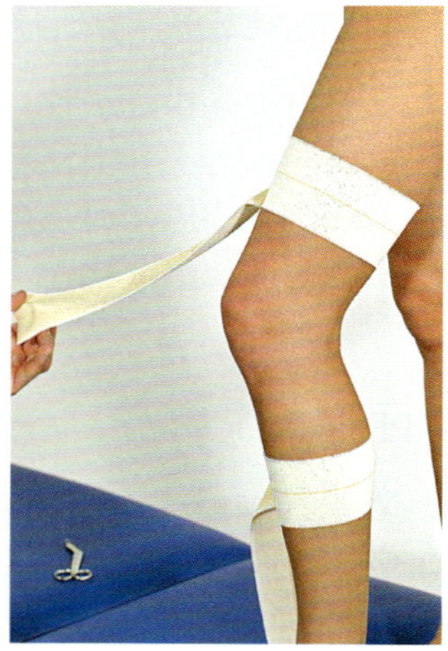
4

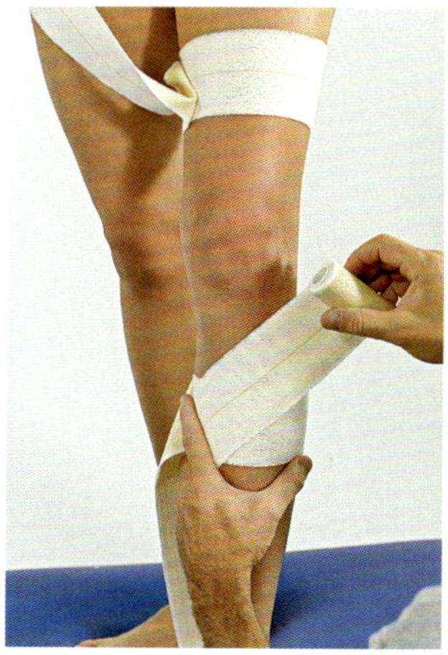
5

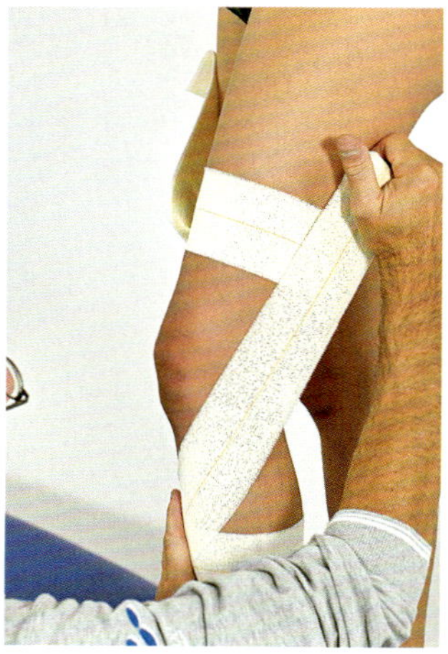
6

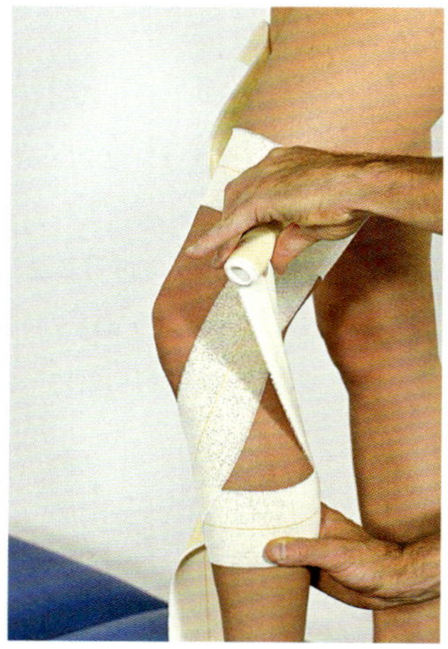
7

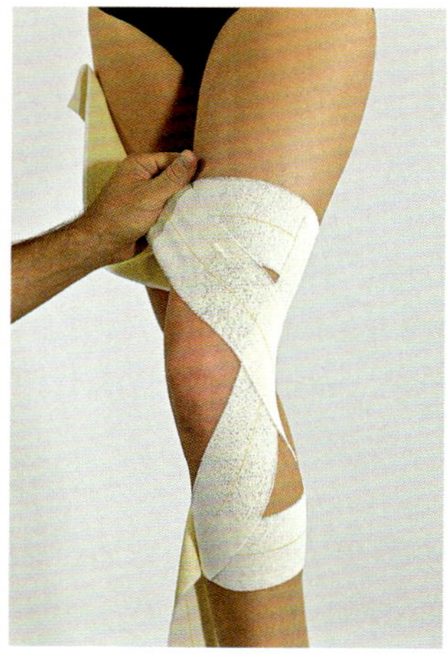
8

Unloading and stabilization with reinforcement of the collateral ligaments

MATERIAL

- ✓ Cotton fabric porous elastic adhesive bandage that can be stretched lengthwise, 7.5 cm in width
- ✓ Inelastic adhesive tape

APPLICATION

1-2-3-4 The subject, standing, keeps the lower limb to be treated in semi-flexion, outward rotation of the lower leg, and slight valgus of the knee. The proximal and distal anchoring points are applied at the middle third of the thigh and the middle third of the lower leg, respectively. To make these, a complete wrap of bandage is made around the limb, and then a piece of necessary length is left free to cover and secure the distal anchoring point.

> *In order to improve the unloading of the musculotendinous structures, a 2-4 cm high lift may be positioned under the heel (see page 139).*

5-6-7-8 Shown here is bandaging for injuries of the lateral collateral ligament. Two strips of adhesive elastic bandage are crossed over the skin projection of the lateral collateral ligament. The first bandage is applied from the distal anchoring point on the lower leg to the proximal anchoring point on the thigh in the anterior-lateral direction; the second is applied in the posterior-lateral direction. The tension of the two stabilizing bandages is between 70% and 80% of the total elastic capacity of the bandage. The direction of the two bands thus also has the function of countering the torsional forces between tibia and femur.

> *This type of bandaging may be used in cases of injuries of the medial collateral ligament by applying the reinforcement fasteners in the medial area.*

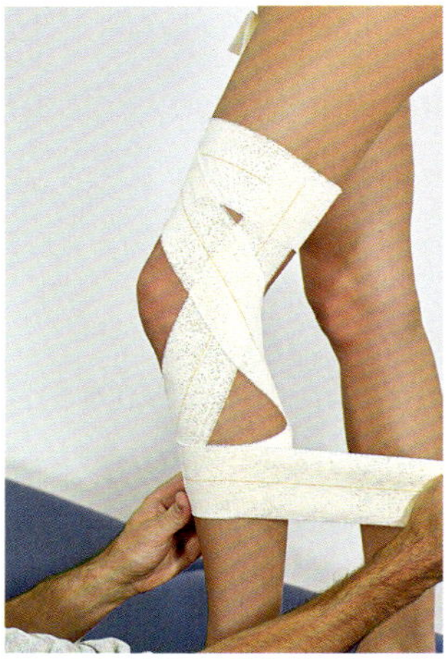
9

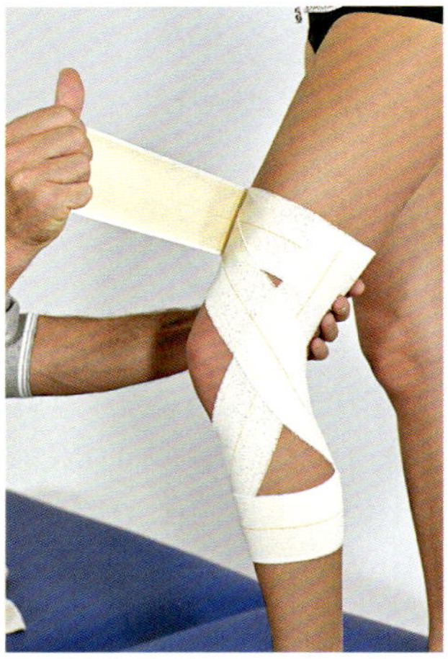
10

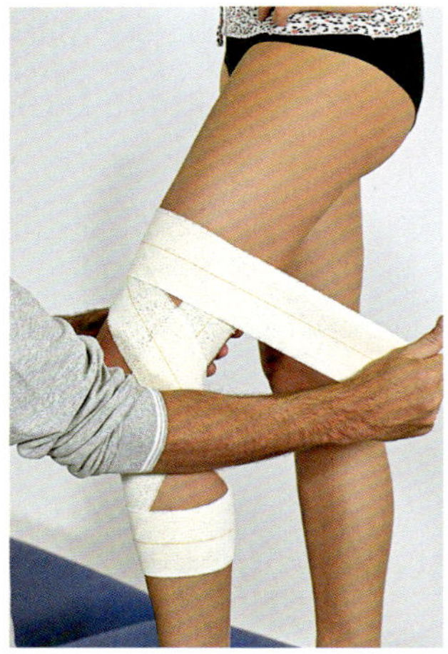
11

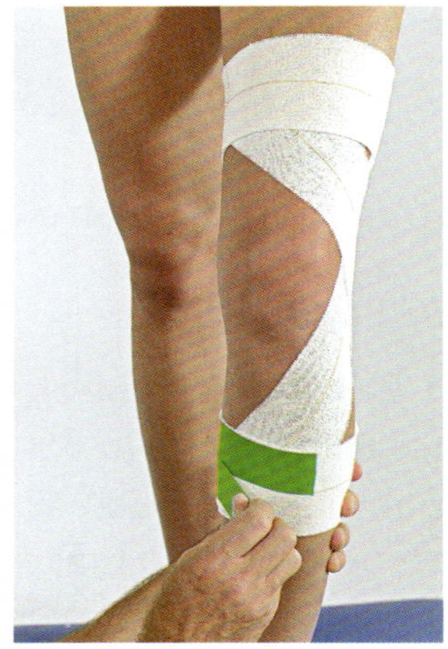
12

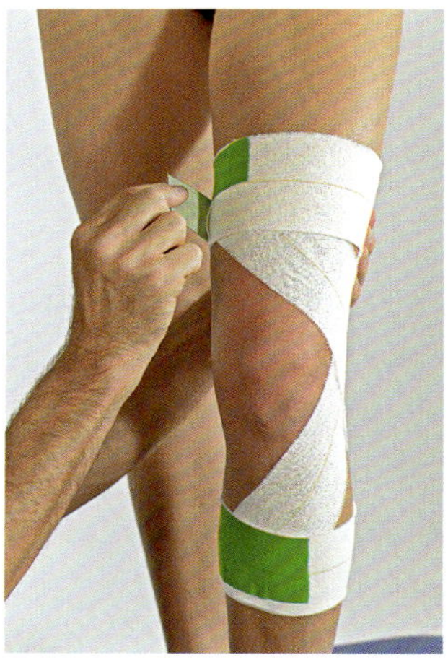
13

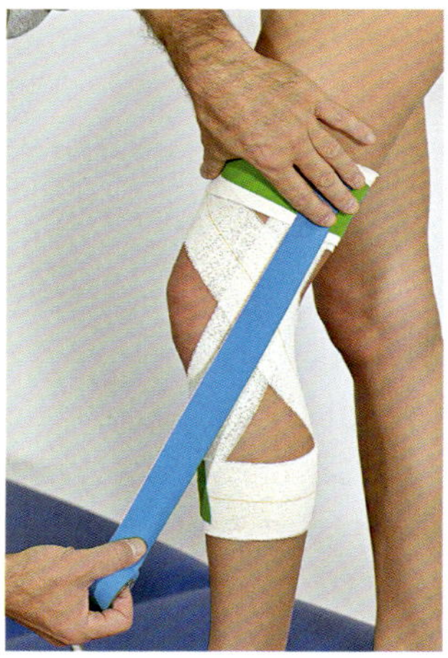
14

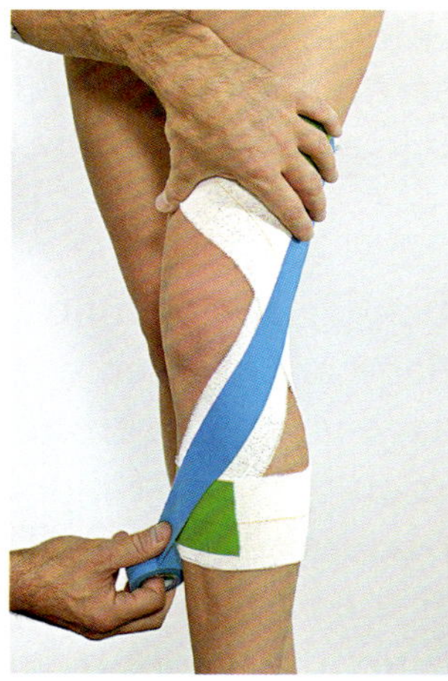
15

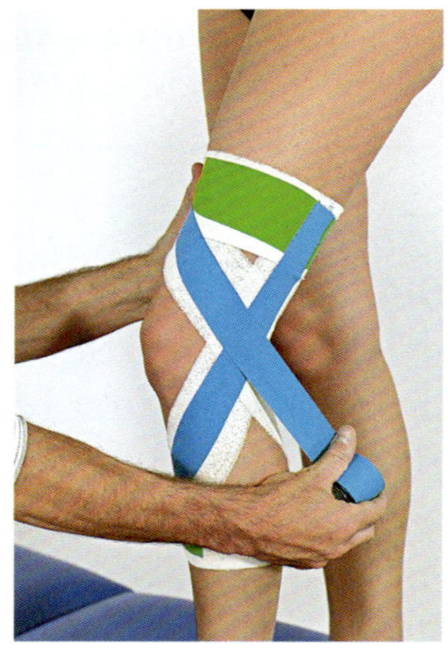
16

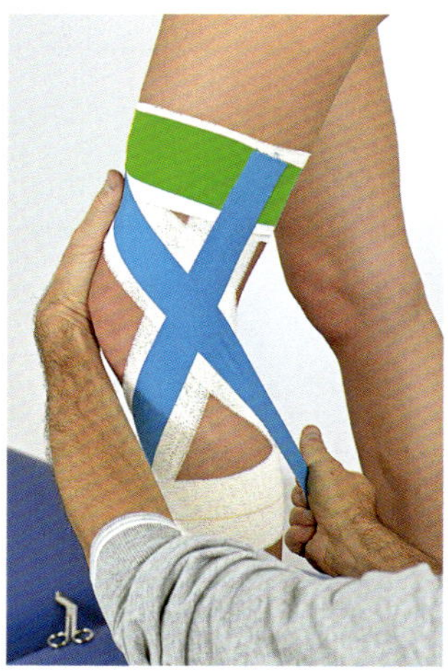
17

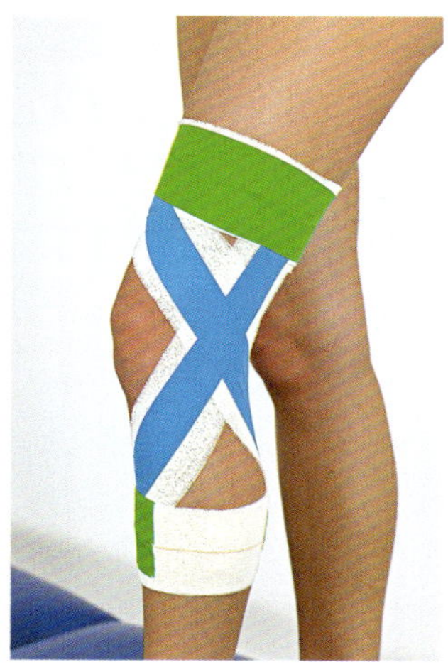
18

Unloading and stabilization with reinforcement of the collateral ligaments

9-10-11 The distal and proximal anchoring points are then secured, and the pieces of bandage previously left free are adhered to the lower leg and thigh.

12-13 The anchoring points are reinforced with inelastic adhesive tape applied in a semicircle.

14-15-16-17 Bandaging proceeds with the application of two strips of inelastic adhesive tape crossed over the projection of the lateral collateral ligament. The strips are adhered over the previously applied adhesive elastic bandages, always having them cross over the skin projection of the lateral collateral ligament.

18 Bandaging finishes with the securing of the anchoring points.

INDICATIONS

- ✓ *Mono-compartmental injuries of the collateral ligaments*
- ✓ *Bilateral injuries of the collateral ligaments*

KNEE JOINT

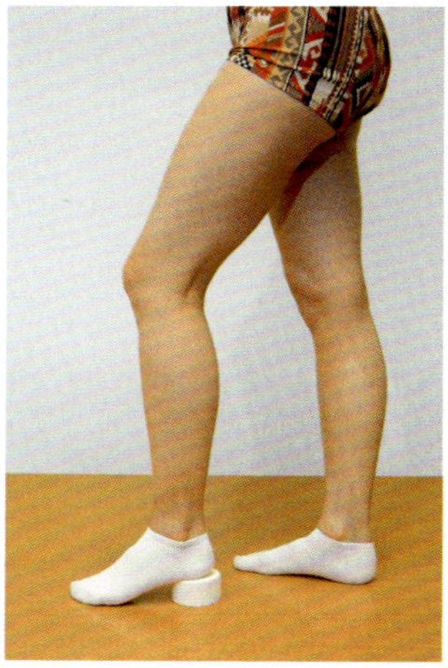

1

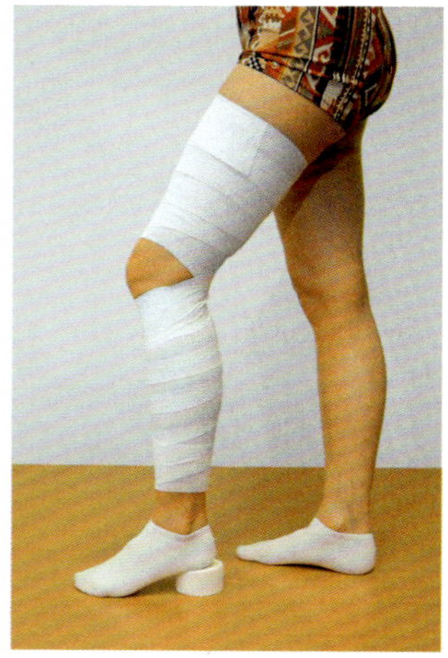

2

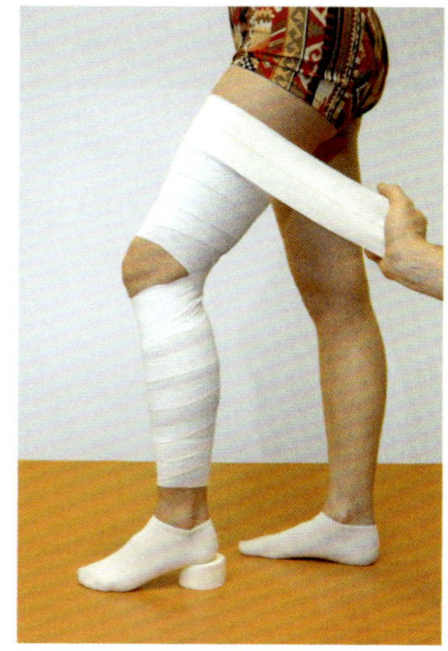

3

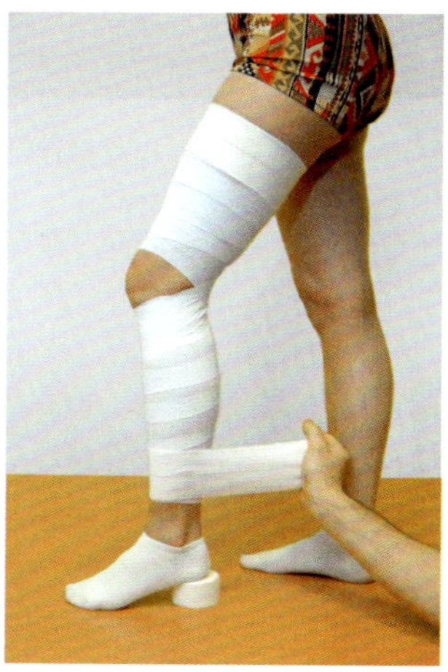

4

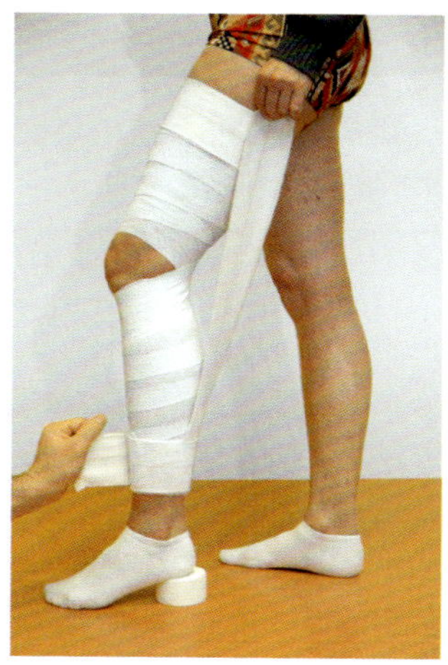

5

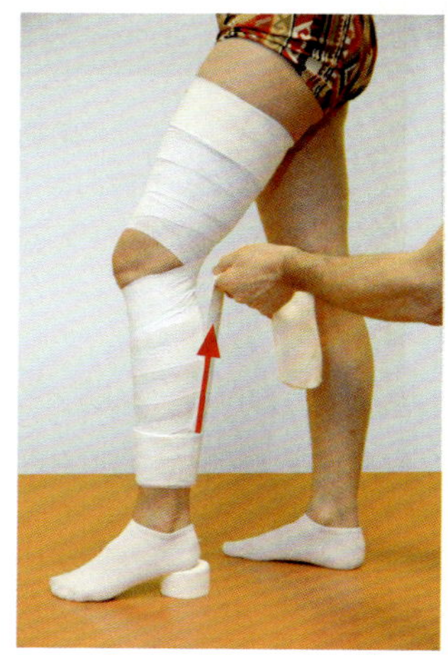

6

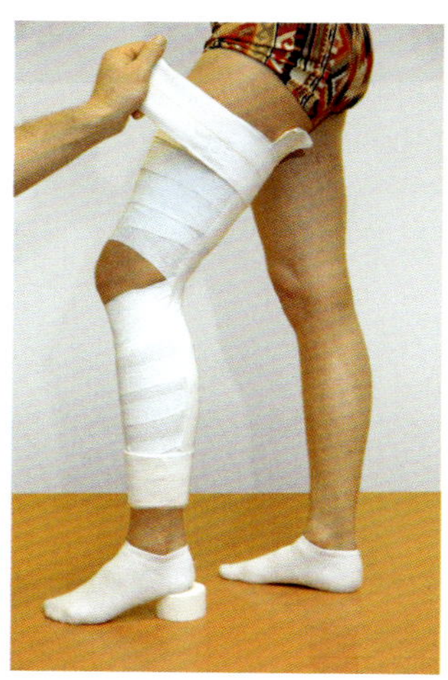

7

Limitation of extension, support for collateral ligaments

MATERIAL

✓ Elastic cohesive bandage, 7.5 cm in width
✓ Cotton fabric porous elastic adhesive bandage which can be stretched lengthwise, 7.5 cm in width

APPLICATION

1 The subject stands upright, with the limb to be treated unloaded and the knee flexed by about 30 degrees.

In order to improve the unloading of the musculotendinous structures, a 2-4 cm high lift may be positioned under the heel, or the bandaging may be applied with the subject lying on the table in a supine position. A reinforced fastener must be made in order to support the ligaments, overlapping two strips of adequate length.

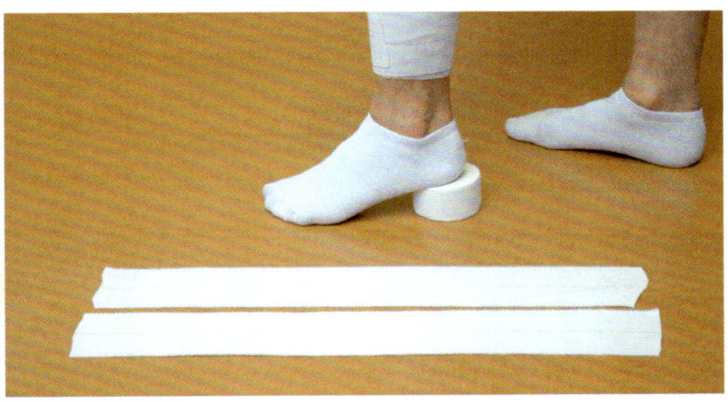

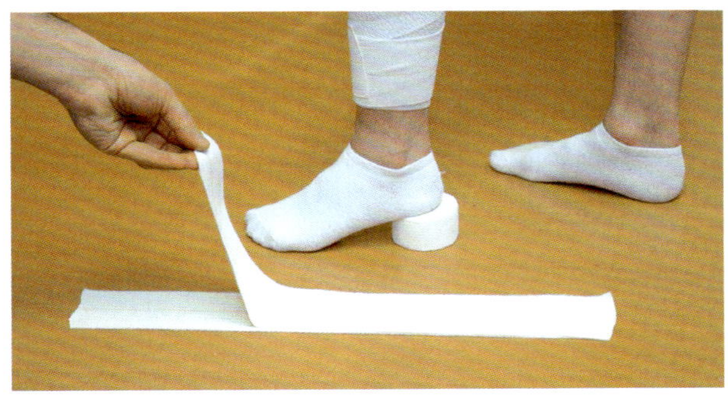

2 Base bandaging is done with the cohesive bandage, covering the entire lower limb with several spiral wraps in the distal-proximal direction and crossing behind the popliteal fossa (see pages 134-135).

3 A wrap of mono-extensible adhesive elastic bandage is applied in order to provide the proximal anchoring point.

4 An adhesive elastic bandage is used for the distal anchoring point as well, applied with a full wrap at the distal third of the lower leg.

5 A reinforced fastener is prepared by overlapping two strips, and is applied posteriorly to the axis of the lower limb beginning from the distal anchoring point, where it is secured with a full wrap of bandage.

6 Once the fastener is placed under tension, it is adhered posteriorly to the lower leg.

7 The tension-bearing fastener must also adhere to the posterior surface of the thigh, and must then be secured with a wrap of adhesive elastic bandage.

KNEE JOINT

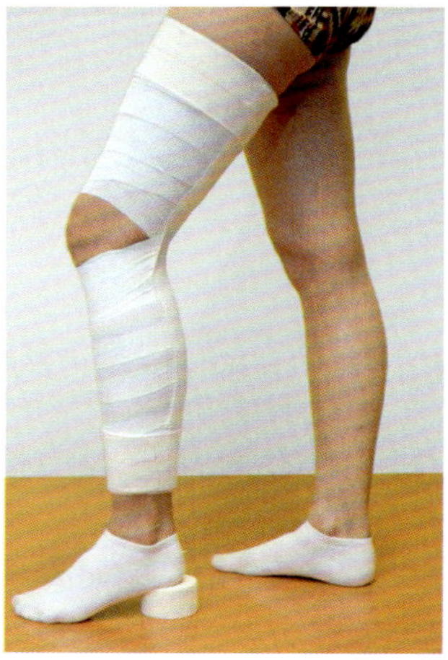

8

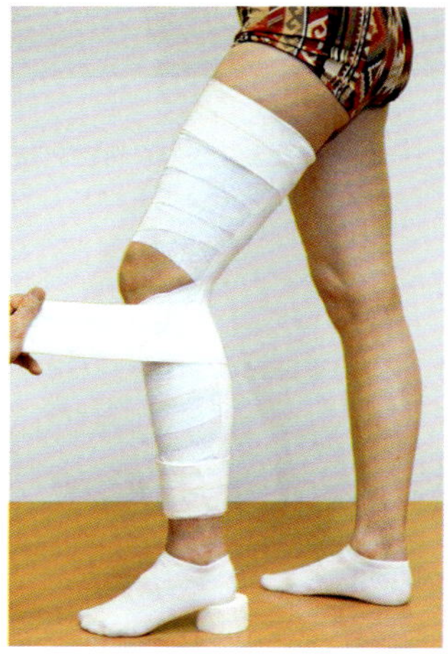

9

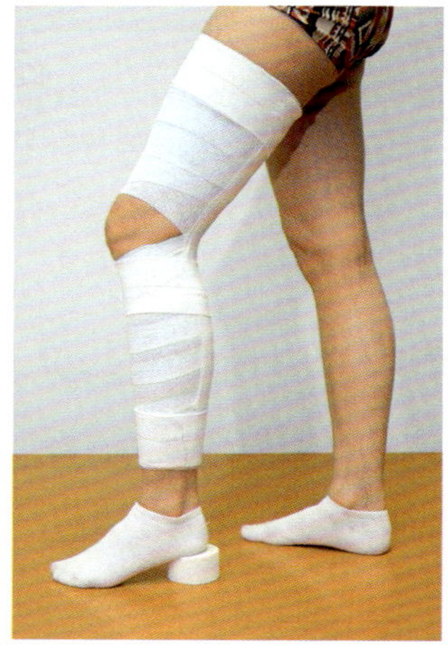

10

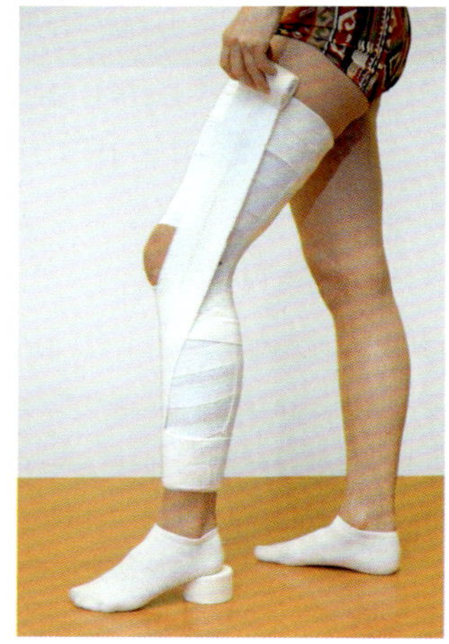

11

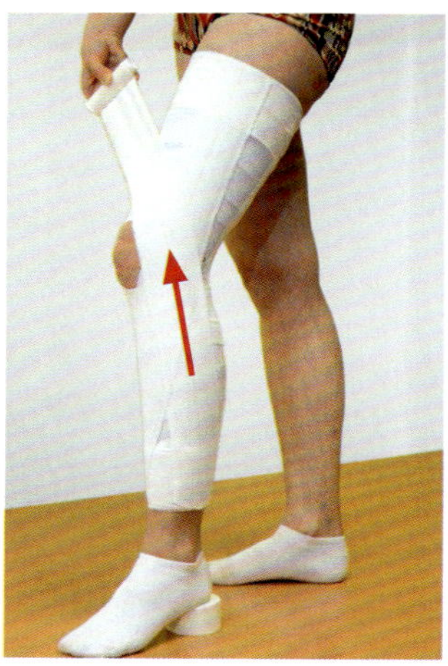

12

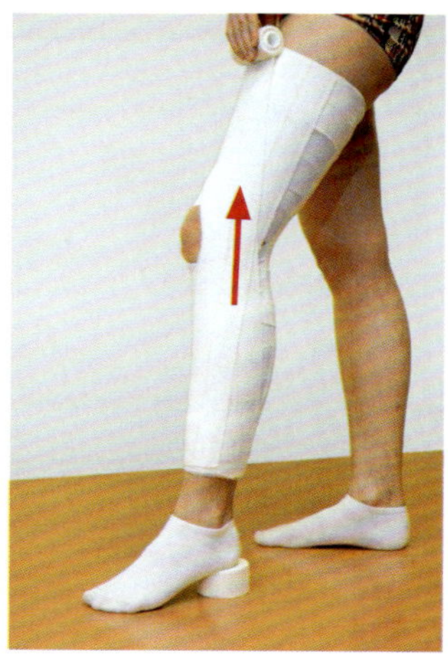

13

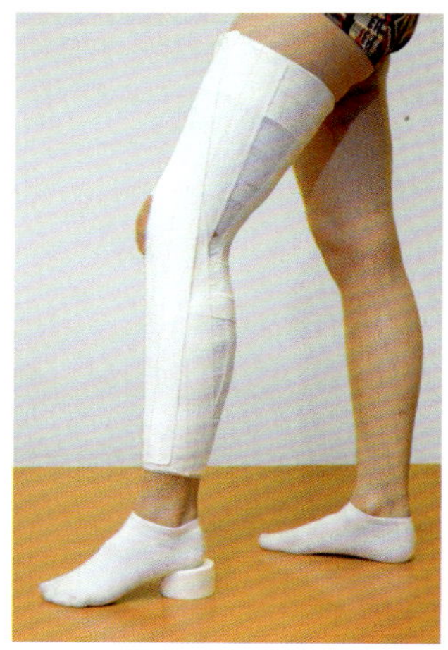

14

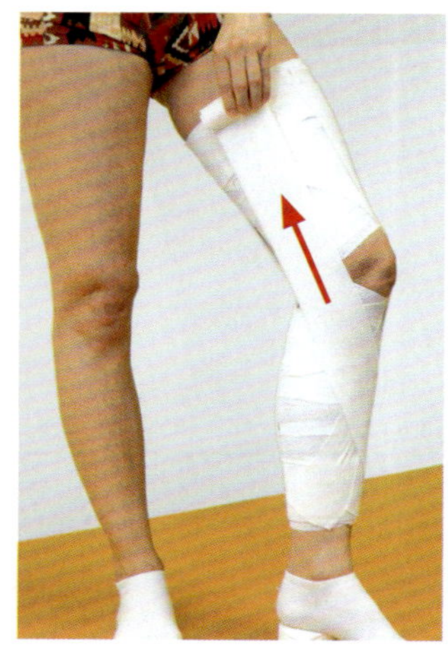

15

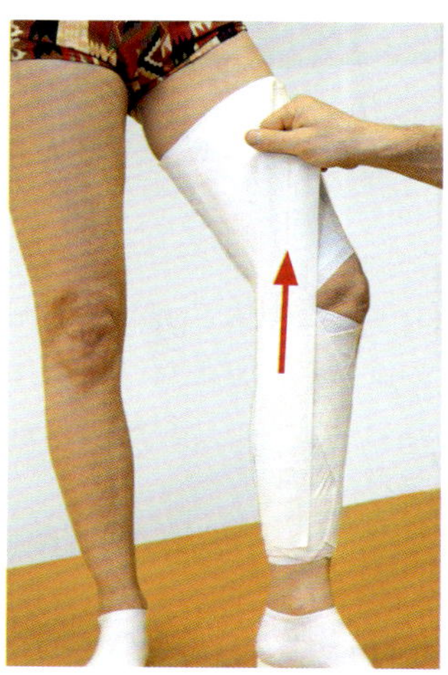

16

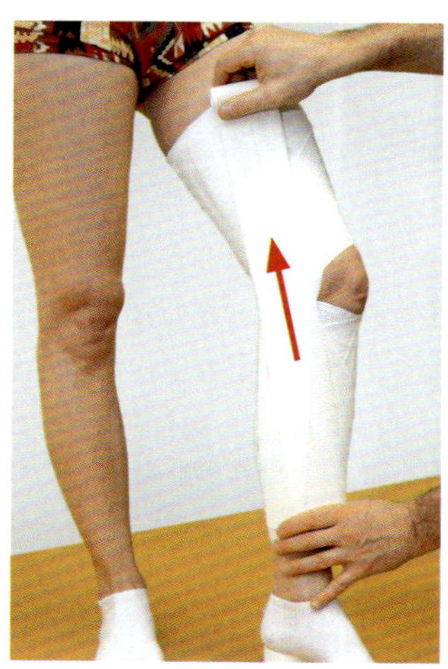

17

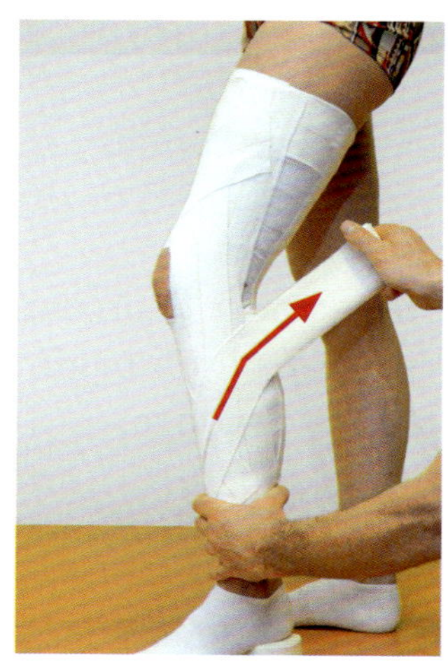

18

Limitation of extension, support for collateral ligaments

8 The excess part of the fastener is folded over itself and held in place with another wrapping of the bandage.

9-10 The posterior elastic fastener must also be secured with a wrap of adhesive bandage at the proximal third of the lower leg.

11 Three strips of adhesive elastic bandage are applied to the bandaging in order to exert a distal-proximal traction. The first strip is applied starting from the distal anchoring point on the medial surface of the lower leg, then is brought in the contralateral direction in order to go on to cover the skin projection of the lateral collateral ligament, and is finally secured over the proximal anchoring point on the lateral surface of the thigh.

12 The second strip is applied, starting from the distal anchoring point on the lateral surface of the lower leg, then brought in the contralateral direction in order to go on to cover the skin projection of the lateral collateral ligament, and is finally secured over the proximal anchoring point on the medial surface of the thigh.

13-14 The third strip is applied, starting from the distal anchoring point in an intermediate area between the beginning points of the two preceding strips, then brought to cover the skin projection of the lateral collateral ligament, and is finally secured over the proximal anchoring point between the first and second strips.

15 Next, the same procedure is repeated to cover the medial collateral ligament with three strips of bandage. The first strip is applied starting from the distal anchoring point on the lateral surface of the lower leg, then brought in the contralateral direction in order to go on to cover the skin projection of the medial collateral ligament, and is finally secured over the proximal anchoring point on the medial surface of the thigh.

16 The second strip is applied, starting from the distal anchoring point on the medial surface of the lower leg, then brought in the contralateral direction in order to go on to cover the skin projection of the medial collateral ligament, and is finally secured over the proximal anchoring point on the lateral surface of the thigh.

17 The third strip is applied, starting from the distal anchoring point in an intermediate area between the beginning points of the two preceding strips, then brought to cover the skin projection of the medial collateral ligament, and finally secured over the proximal anchoring point between the first and second strips.

18 Next, several strips of adhesive elastic bandage are applied in order to counter outward and inward rotation. The first bandage starts from the distal anchoring point on the medial surface of the lower leg and is directed proximally over its lateral surface. A complete wrap of bandage is made at the proximal third of the lower leg.

KNEE JOINT

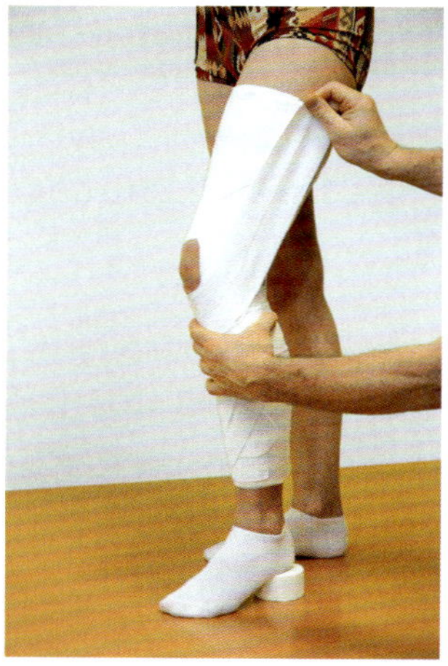
19

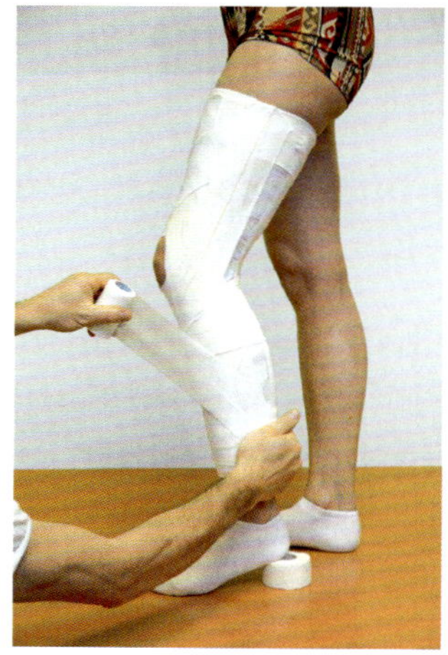
20

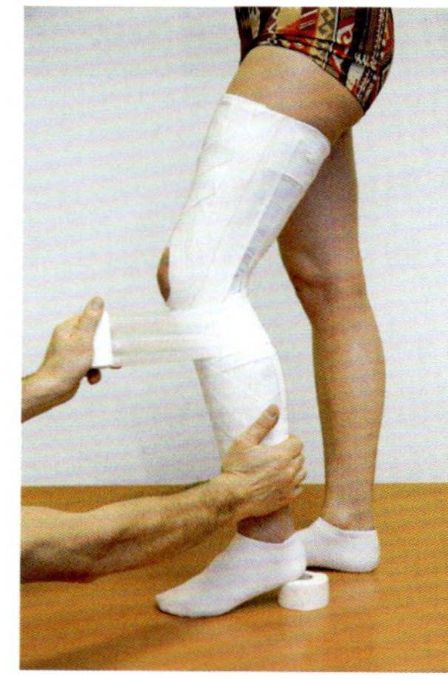
21

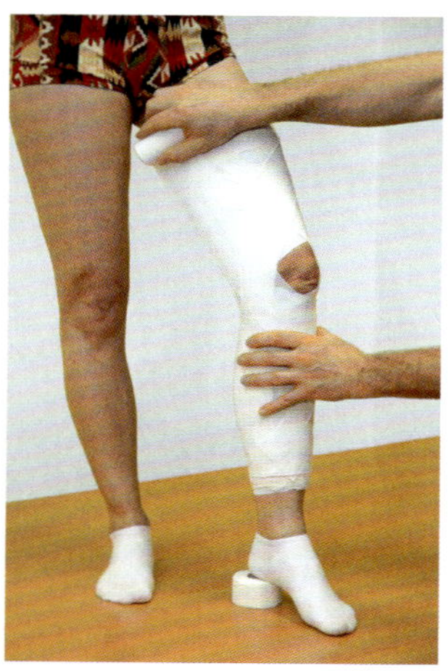
22

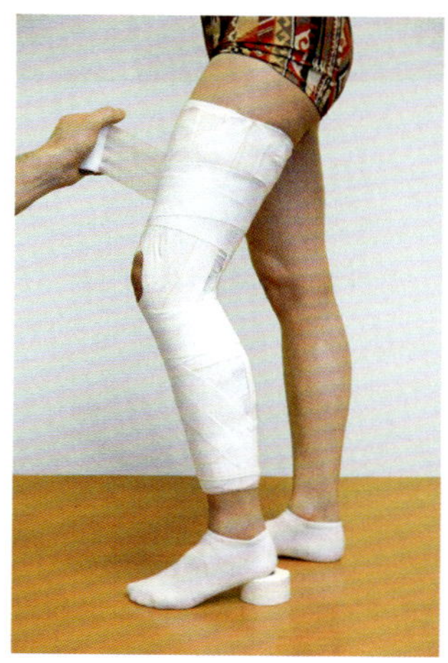
23

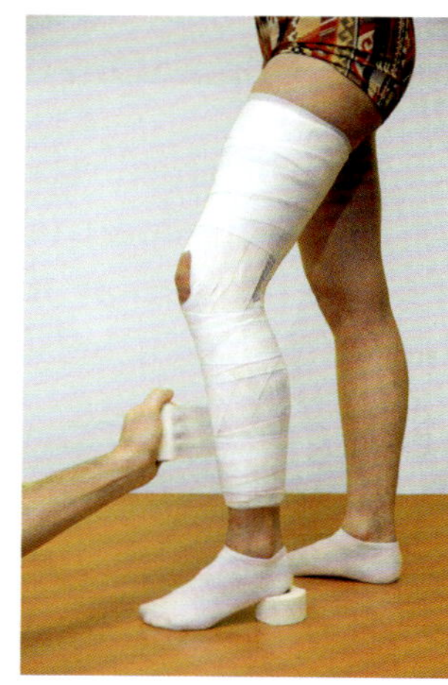
24

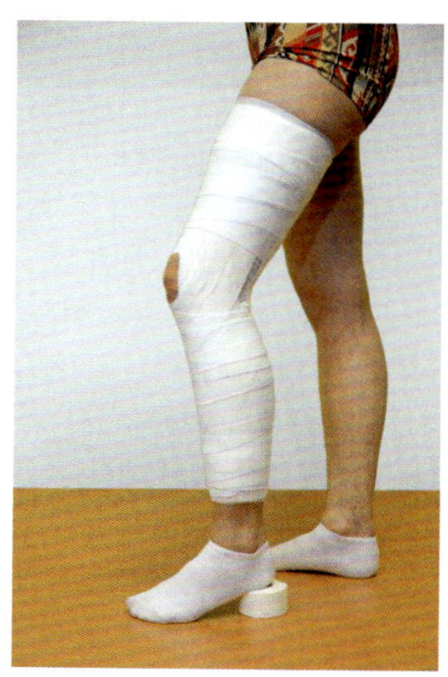
25

Limitation of extension, support for collateral ligaments

19 The bandage is made to run along the lateral surface of the thigh and is then secured over the proximal anchoring point.

20 The second bandage starts from the distal anchoring point on the lateral surface of the lower leg and is directed proximally over its medial surface.

21 A complete wrap of bandage is made at the proximal third of the lower leg.

22 The bandage is made to run along the medial surface of the thigh and is then secured over the proximal anchoring point.

23 The bandaging is secured with several spiral wraps, covering the thigh.

24 The wraps of bandage must be applied around the axis of the lower leg as well.

25 Bandaging is complete.

INDICATIONS

✓ *Posttraumatic capsuloligamentous injuries*
✓ *Pulling of ligaments following sprain*
✓ *Preventative sports treatment*

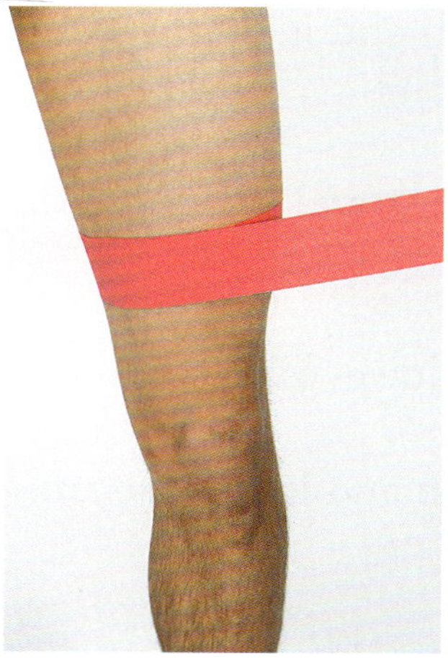
1

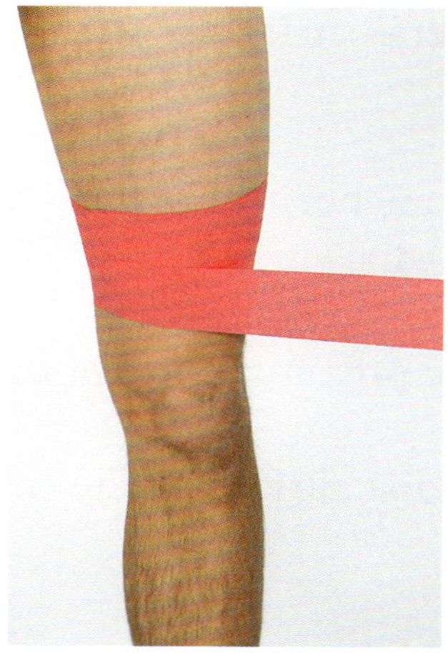
2

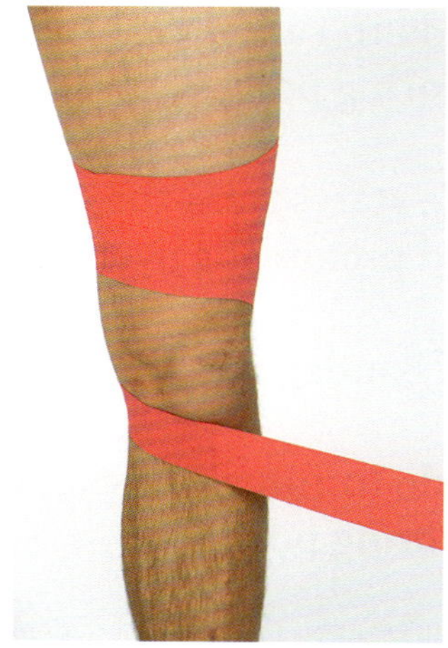
3

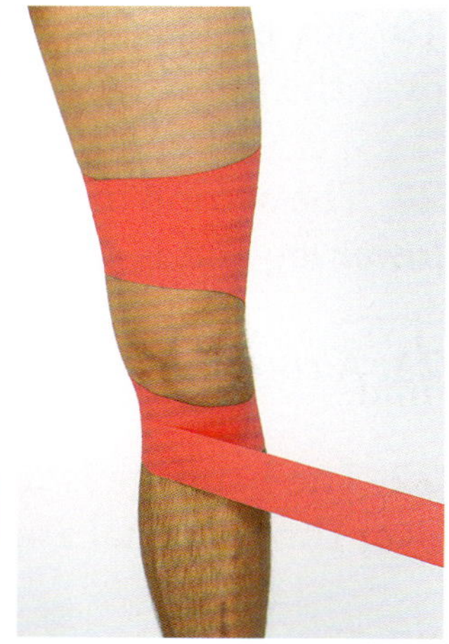
4

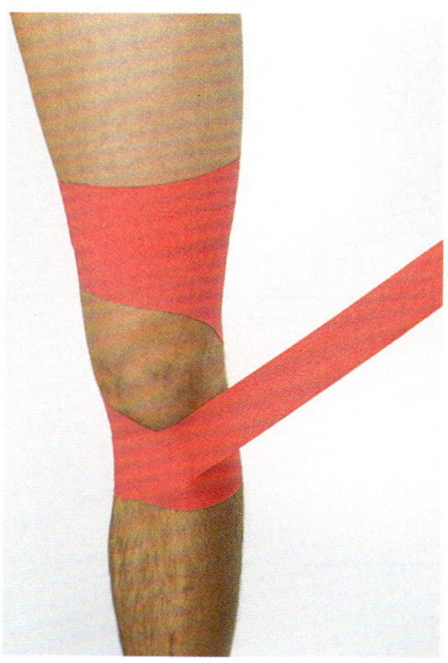
5

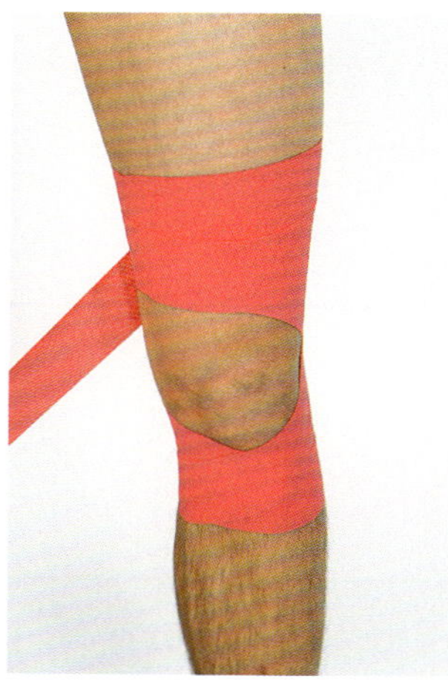
6

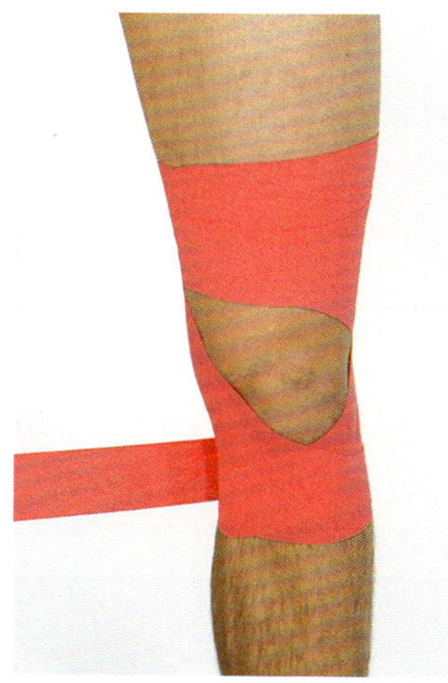
7

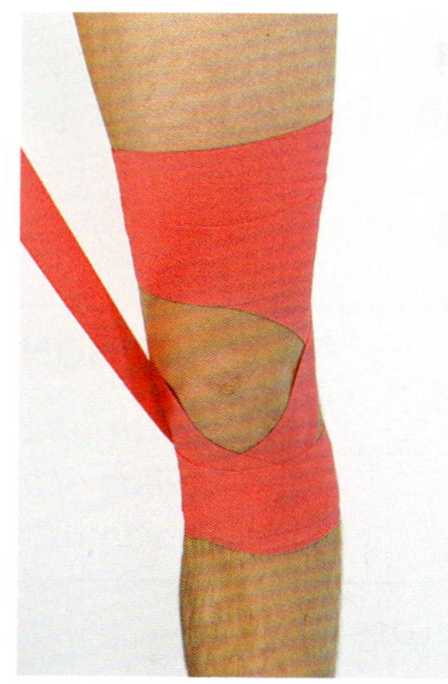
8

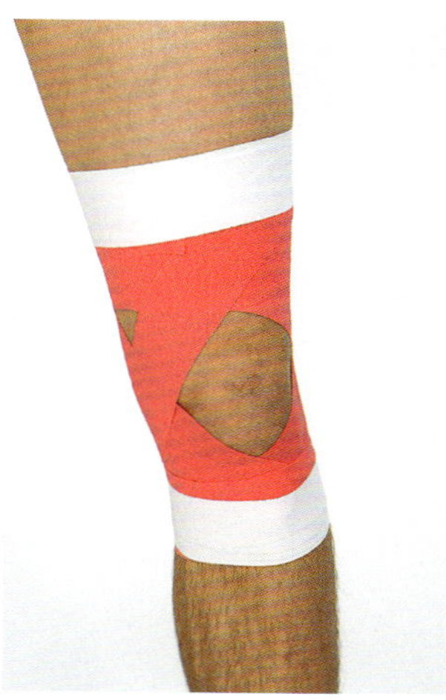
9

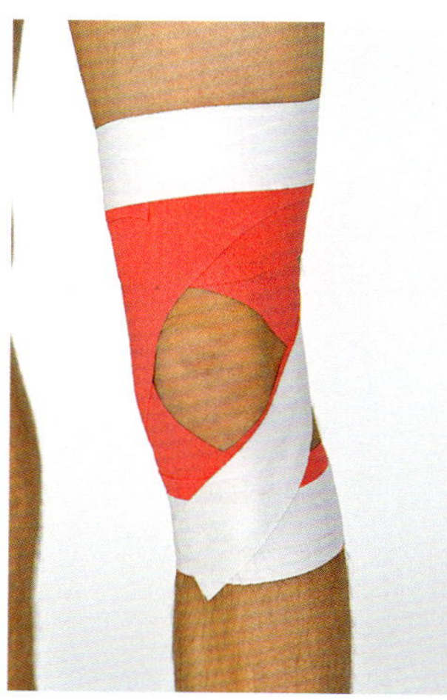
10

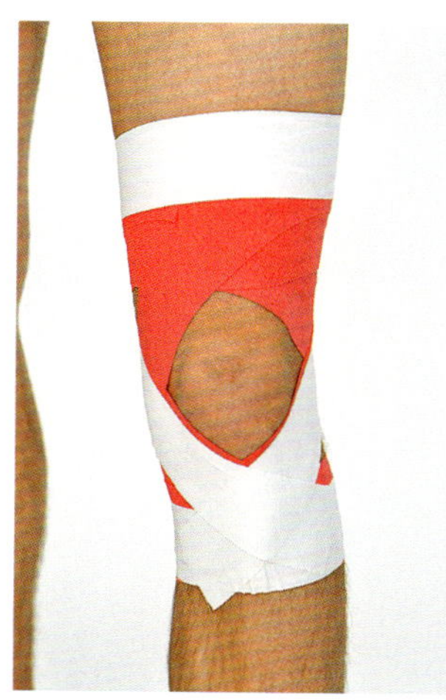
11

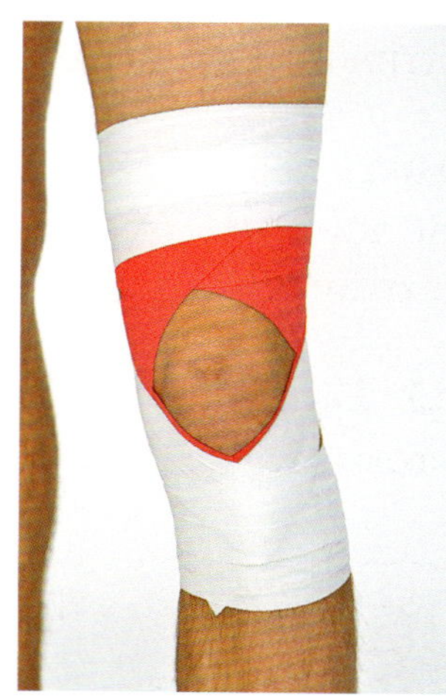
12

Support of the anterior cruciate ligament

MATERIAL

✓ Elastic adhesive tape, extensible lengthwise, 5/7.5 cm in width
✓ Inelastic adhesive tape

APPLICATION

1 The subject is standing up. A complete wrap of elastic adhesive bandage is made at the middle third of the thigh.

2 Several wraps of bandage are made in a proximal-distal direction, covering the previous bandage by 50%.

3 The bandage obliquely goes down, passing over the skin projection of the lateral collateral ligament.

4 Next, a complete wrapping of the bandage is made, bordering on the lower edge of the patella.

5 The bandage is made to cross the previous path over the skin projection of the lateral collateral ligament.

6-7 A full wrap of bandage is made around the axis of the thigh; the bandage is brought obliquely to cover the skin projection of the medial collateral ligament.

8 The bandage borders on the upper edge of the patella, and passes medially to the knee to cross the previous path over the skin projection of the medial collateral ligament.

9 Finishing the base bandaging with a full wrap of elastic adhesive tape around the distal third of the thigh, the distal and proximal anchoring points are prepared using several strips of inelastic adhesive bandage applied in a semicircle.

10-11 Beginning from the anterior area of the distal anchoring point, two strips of inelastic adhesive bandage are applied that cross at the tibial crest and end posteriorly over the proximal anchoring point. One strip passes laterally to the patella, the other medially.

12 The bandaging is secured with several full wraps of inelastic adhesive bandage at the proximal and distal anchoring points.

INDICATIONS

✓ *Limitation of anterior slippage of the tibia with posterior-anterior instability due to injury of the anterior cruciate ligament*

KNEE JOINT

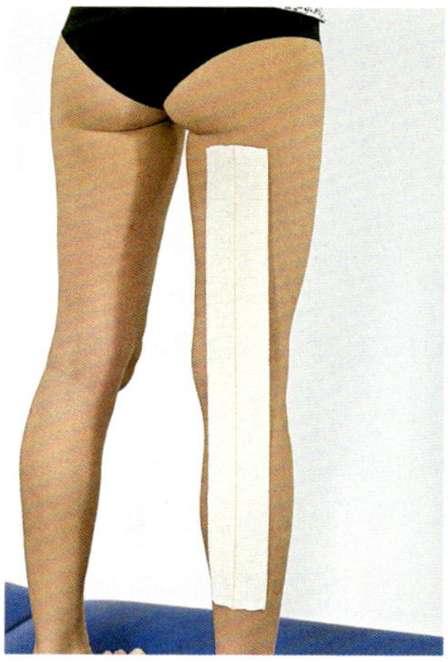
1

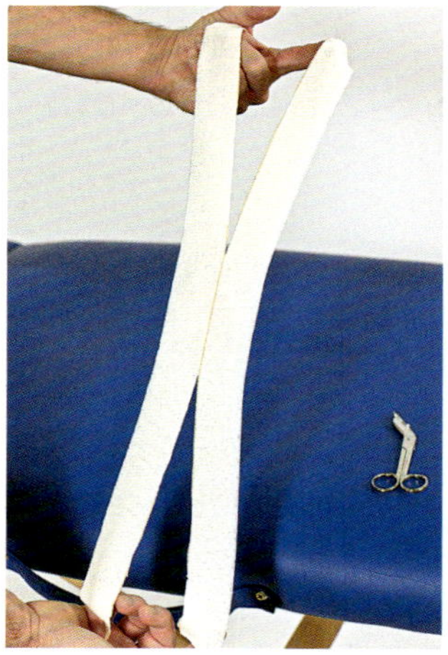
2

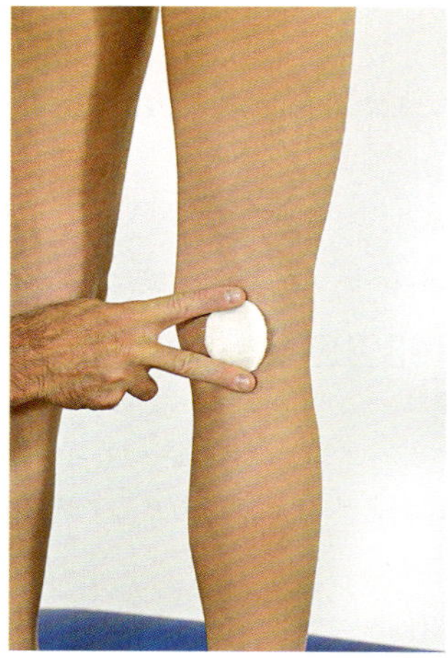
3

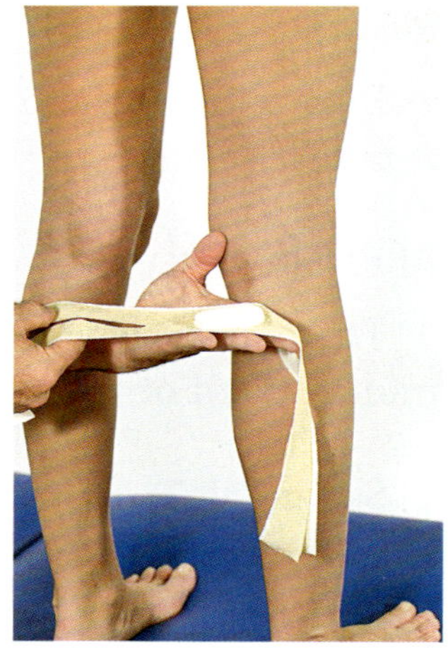
4

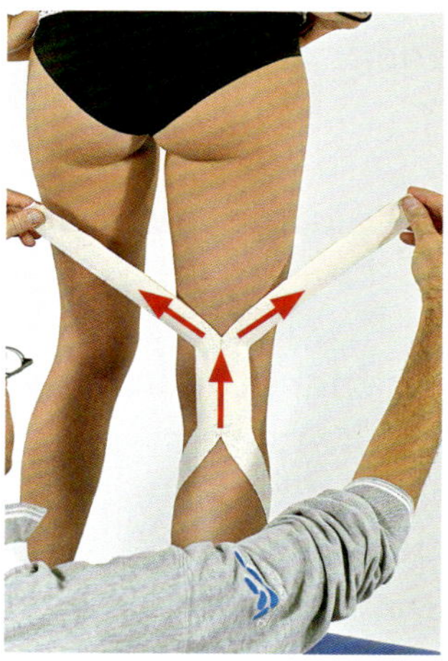
5

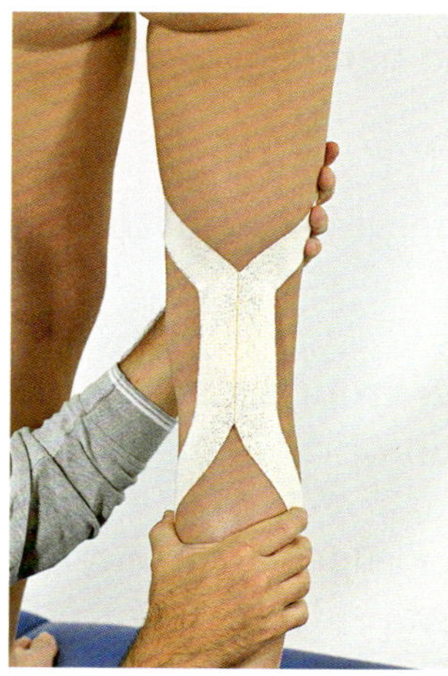
6

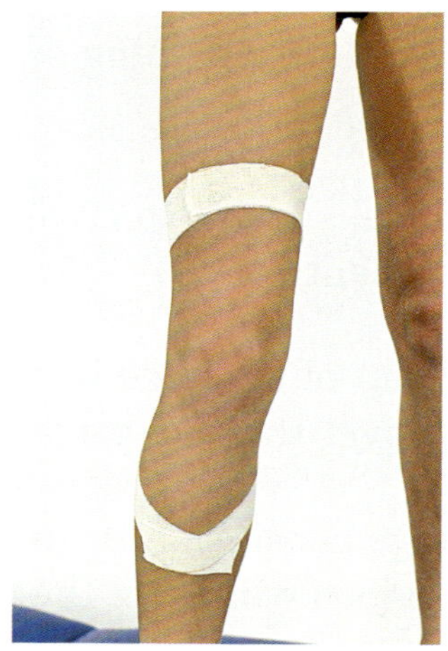
7

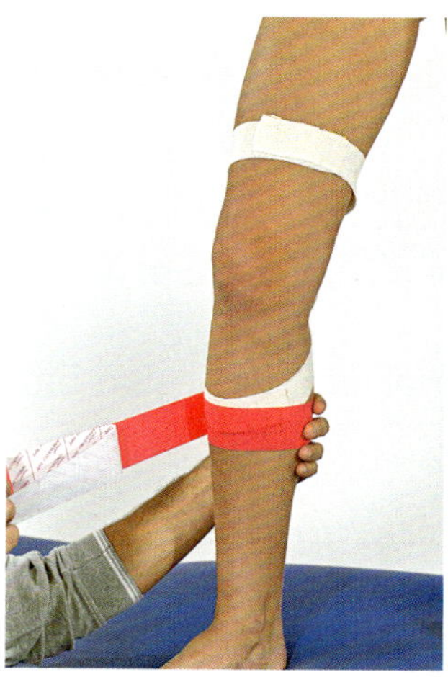
8

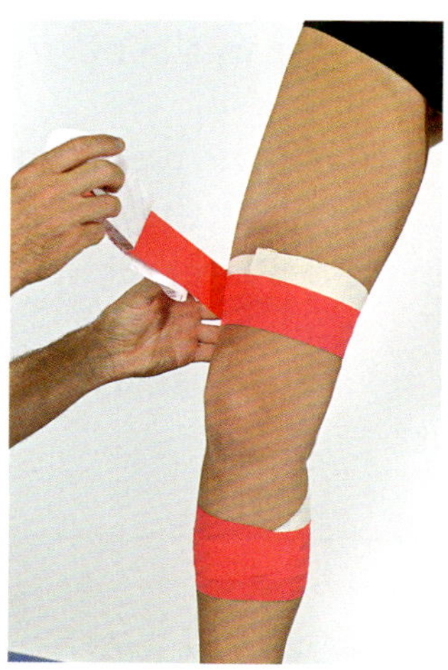
9

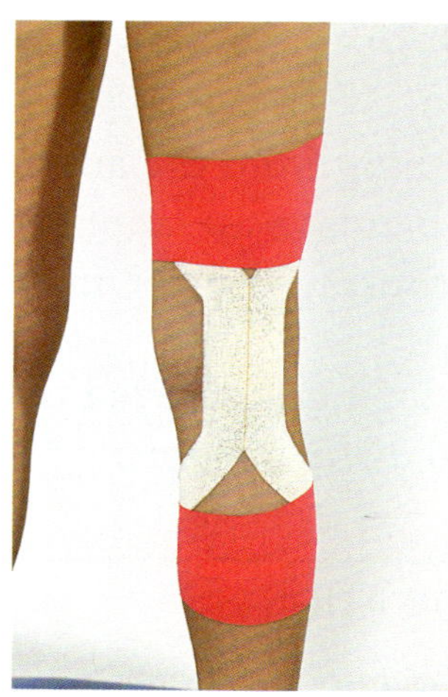
10

Limitation of extension

MATERIAL

✓ Cotton fabric porous elastic adhesive bandage which can be stretched lengthwise, 7.5 cm in width
✓ Pre-tape compress for creating a skin protective pad
✓ Elastic adhesive tape for securing anchoring points

APPLICATION

1-2 To begin, a bandage of the appropriate length is cut longitudinally from both ends, taking care to leave about 10 cm of uncut bandage in the central area.

3 A pre-tape compress is prepared for protection of the structures at risk in the popliteal area.

4 The compress is applied to the center of the bandage.

5-6-7 The subject is standing with the lower limb to be treated in semi-flexion. The central area of the bandage with the pre-tape pad is applied to the popliteal fossa while the distal pieces of bandage are adhered on the middle third of the lower leg; the two proximal pieces are put under tension and adhered at the middle third of the thigh.

In order to improve the unloading of the musculotendinous structures, a 2-4 cm high lift may be positioned under the heel (see page 139).

8-9-10 The bandaging finishes by applying several wraps of elastic adhesive tape over the distal and proximal anchoring points.

INDICATIONS

✓ *Hyperextension of the knee*
✓ *Recurvatum of the knee*
✓ *Pain from overpressure on the anterior tibial plateau*

KNEE JOINT

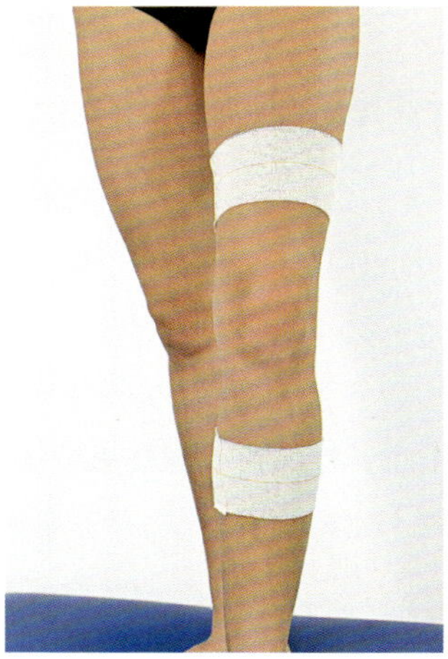

1

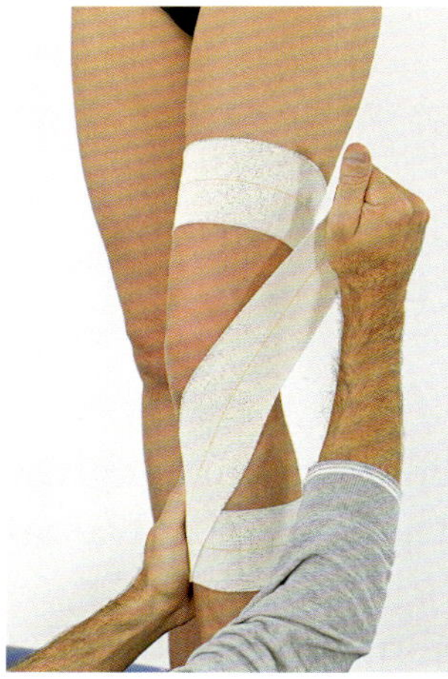

2

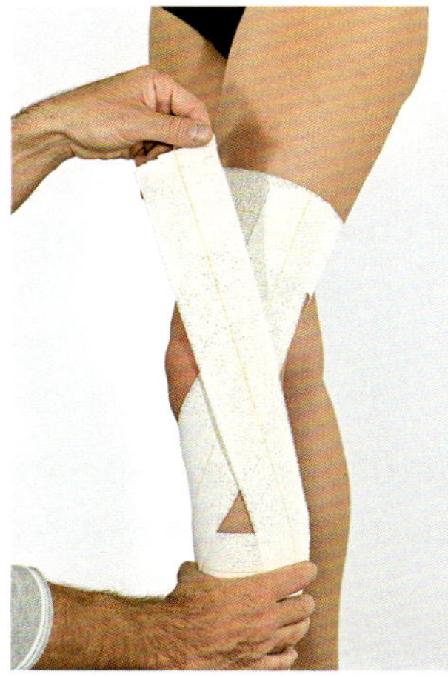

3

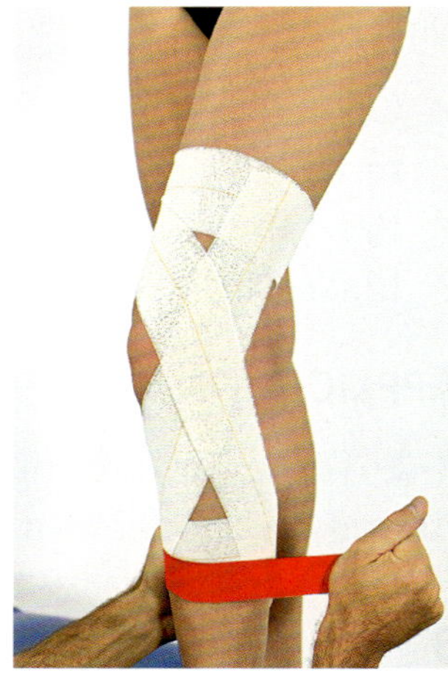

4

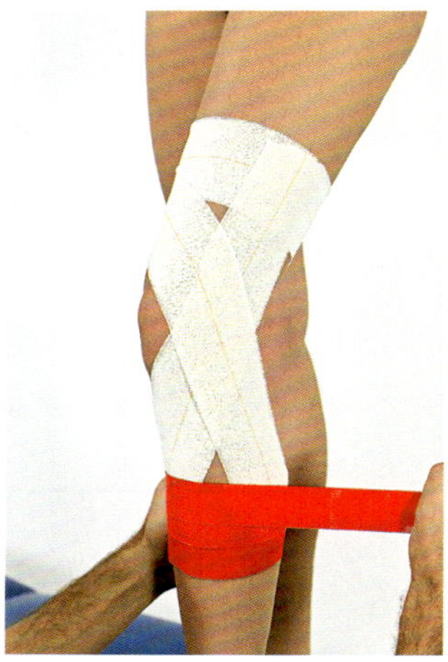

5

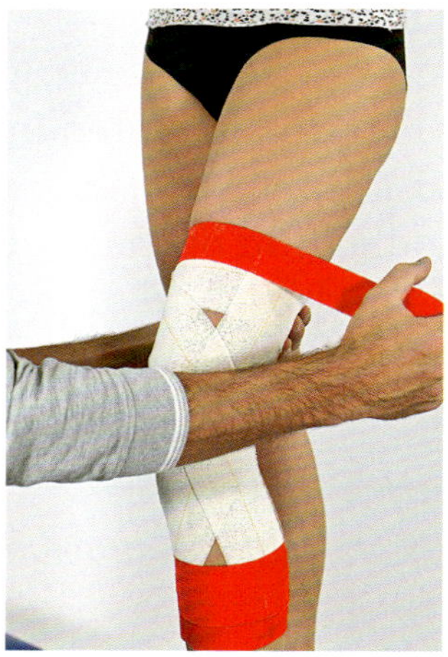

6

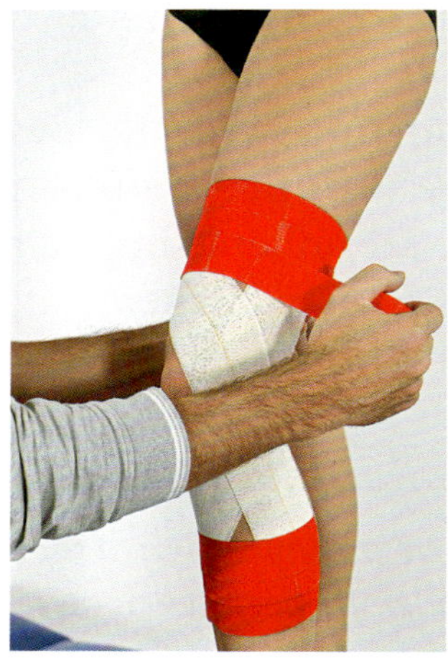

7

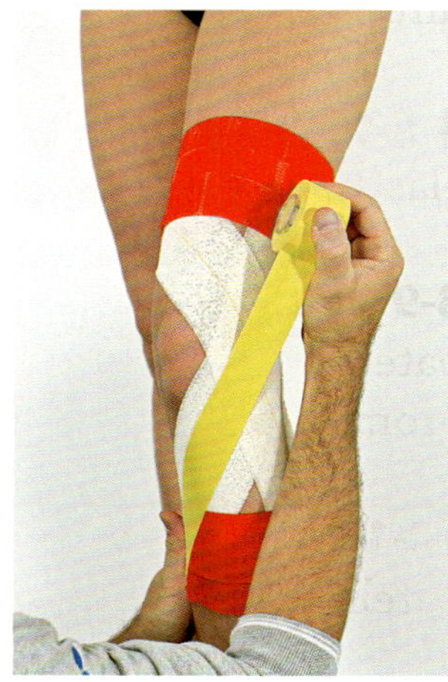

8

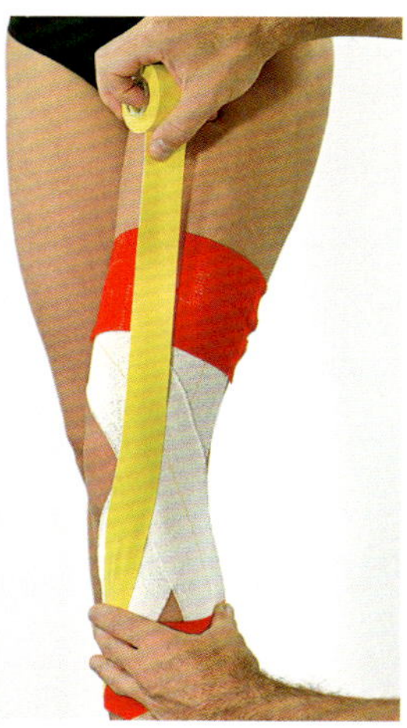

9

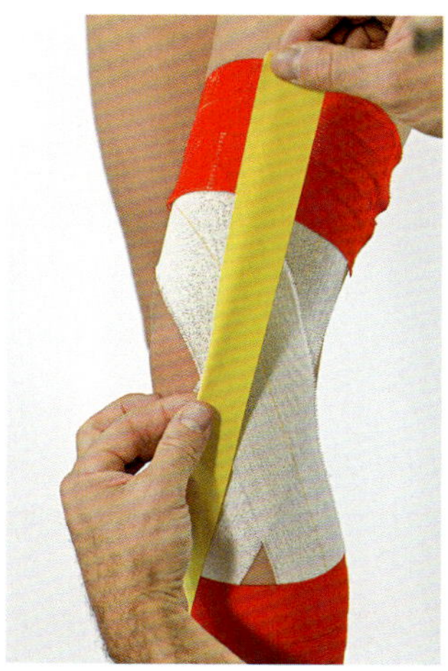

10

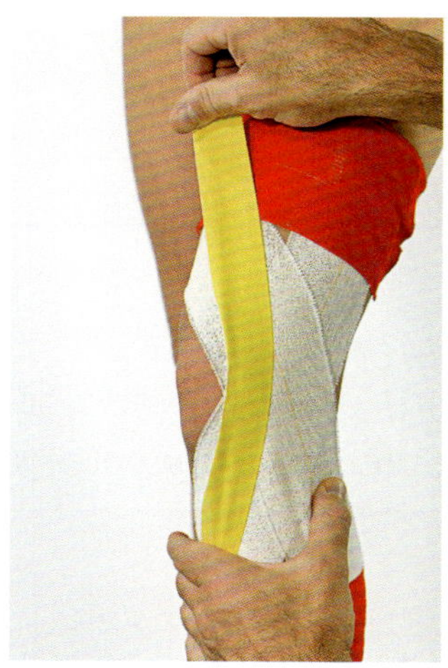

11

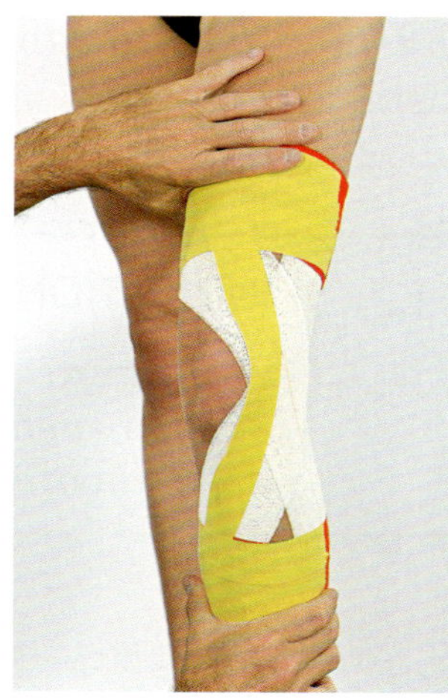

12

Recentering of the patella

MATERIAL

✓ Cotton fabric porous elastic adhesive bandage that can be stretched lengthwise, 7.5 cm in width
✓ Inelastic adhesive tape

APPLICATION

1 The subject, standing, keeps the lower limb to be treated in slight semi-flexion. Bandaging begins by preparing base bandaging with a porous elastic adhesive bandage; the proximal and distal anchoring points are secured, respectively, at the middle third of the thigh and the middle third of the lower leg.

2-3 Two strips of adhesive elastic bandage are applied such that they cross in the area bordering on the lateral portion of the patella, in order to provide a force in the lateral-medial direction aimed at correcting the position of the patella.

4-5-6-7 The distal and proximal anchoring points are then secured, applying several inelastic adhesive tape strips in a semicircle.

8-9 A strip of inelastic adhesive tape is applied with corrective and retentive action on the patella, starting from the medial portion of the distal anchoring point on the lower leg. From here, the bandage is directed upward to border on the lateral portion of the patella.

10-11 The bandage must be folded near the area of contact with the lateral portion of the patella, and is then secured over the proximal anchoring point.

12 Bandaging finishes by securing the anchoring points with several strips of bandage applied in a semicircle.

INDICATIONS

✓ *Effects of lateral subluxation*
✓ *Patellar instability*

KNEE JOINT

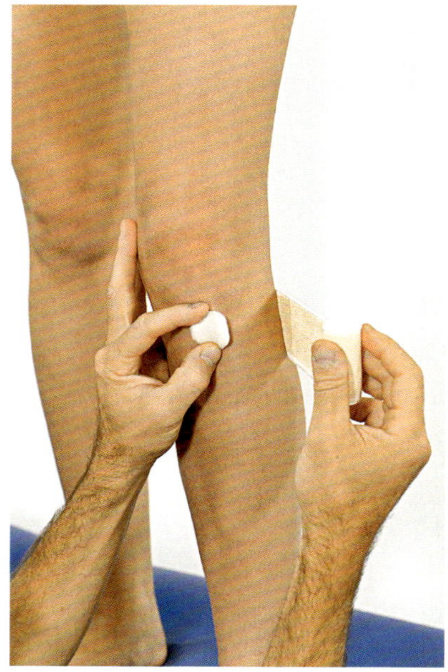

1

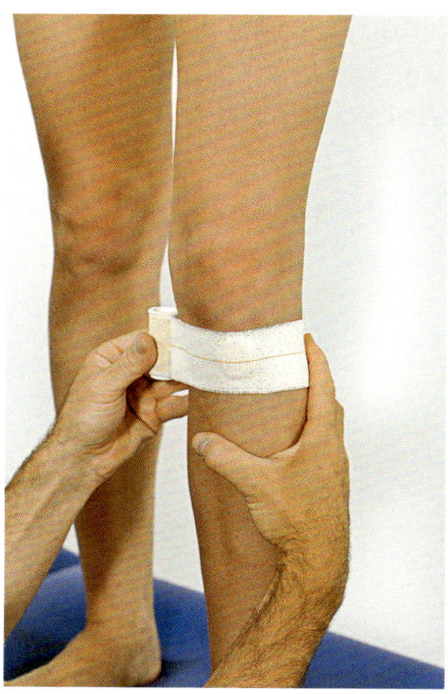

2

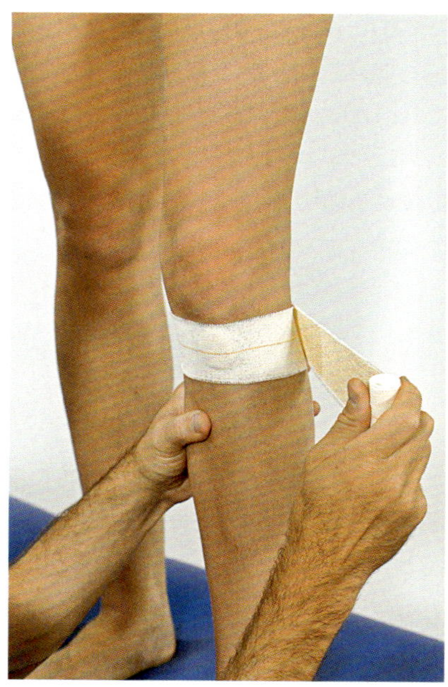

3

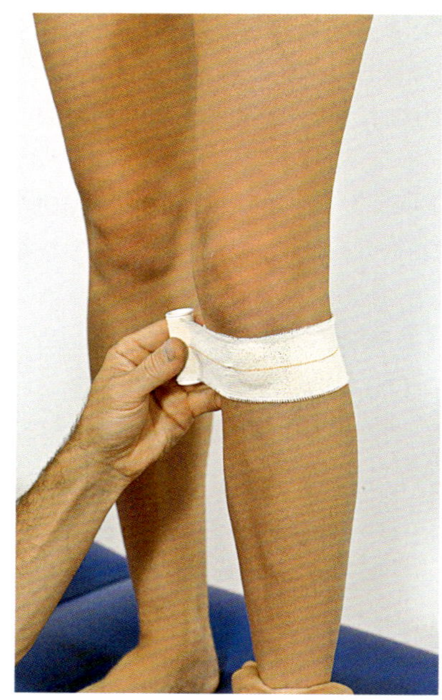

4

Unloading of the patellar tendon with a pad

MATERIAL

- ✓ Cotton fabric porous elastic adhesive bandage that can be stretched lengthwise, 5 cm in width
- ✓ Pre-tape or foam rubber compress for creating a compressive unloading pad

APPLICATION

1 A soft unloading pad is placed at the skin projection of the insertion of the patellar tendon on the tibial tuberosity.

2-3-4 The bandaging is done by applying a full wrap of bandage beginning from the skin projection of the head of the fibula and going on to cover, with the bandage in tension, the unloading pad in direct compression.

Alternatively, this bandaging may be made using a roll of elastic adhesive tape.

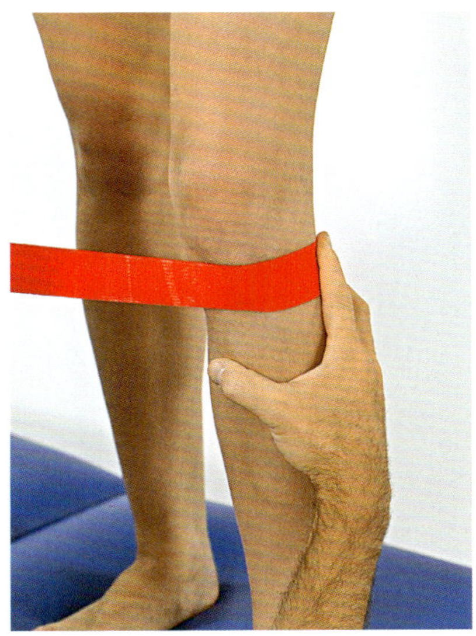

INDICATIONS

✓ *Inflammation of the insertion of the patellar tendon (or patellar ligament)*

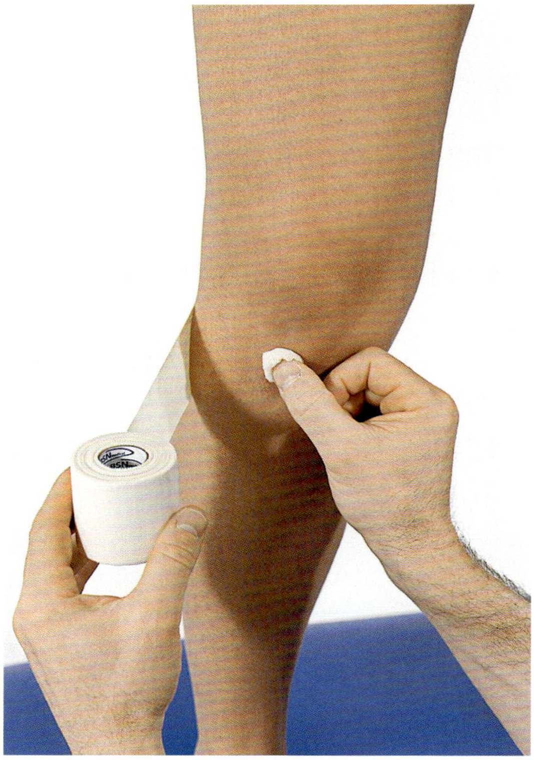
1

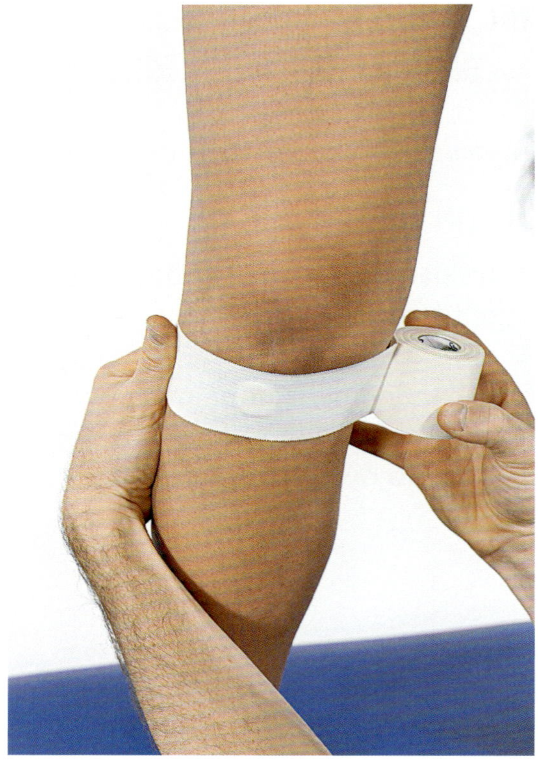
2

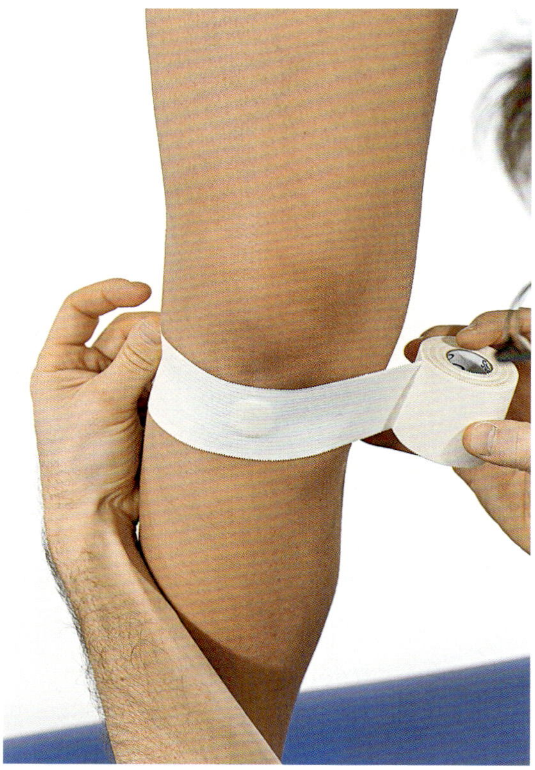
3

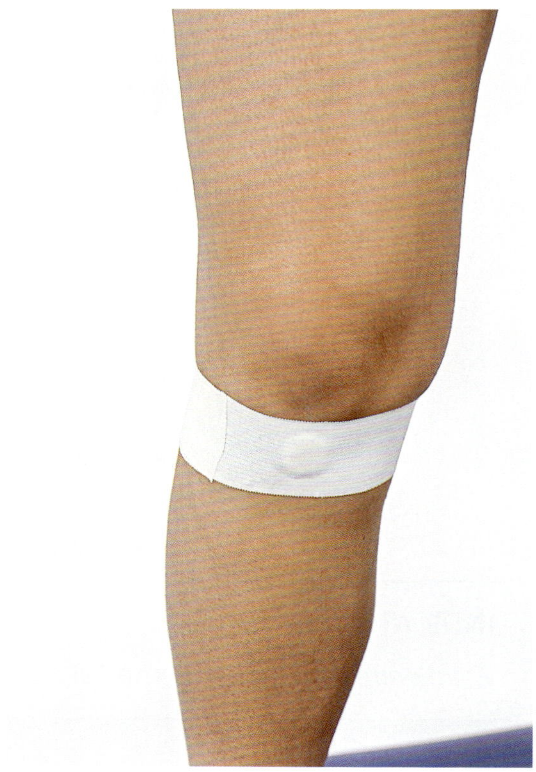
4

Unloading of the patellar tendon with inelastic adhesive tape

MATERIAL

- ✓ Inelastic adhesive tape, 5 cm in width
- ✓ Foam rubber or pre-tape compress for creating a compressive unloading pad

APPLICATION

1 A foam rubber or pre-tape unloading compress is placed over the skin projection of the insertion of the patellar tendon on the tibial tuberosity.

2-3 The bandaging is done by applying a full wrap of inelastic adhesive tape, beginning from the skin projection of the head of the fibula and going on to cover the unloading pad.

4 Bandaging is complete.

INDICATIONS

- ✓ *Inflammation of the insertion of the patellar tendon (or patellar ligament)*

KNEE JOINT

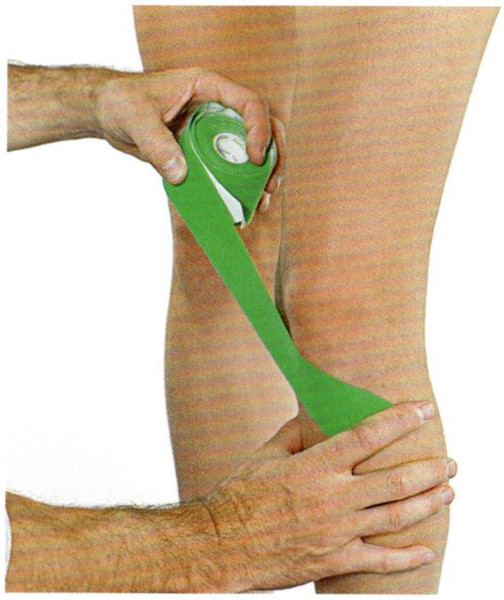

1

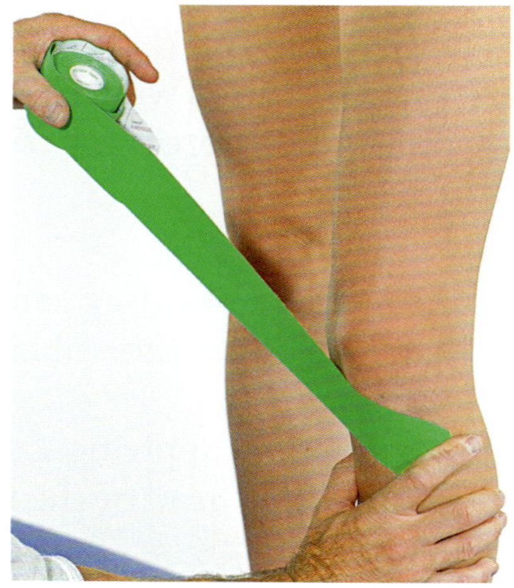

2

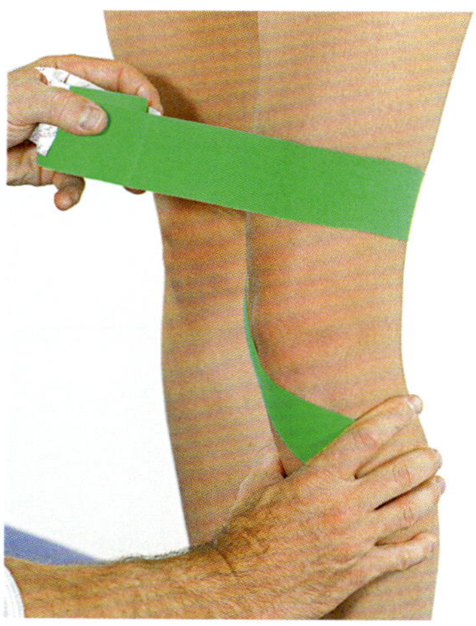

3

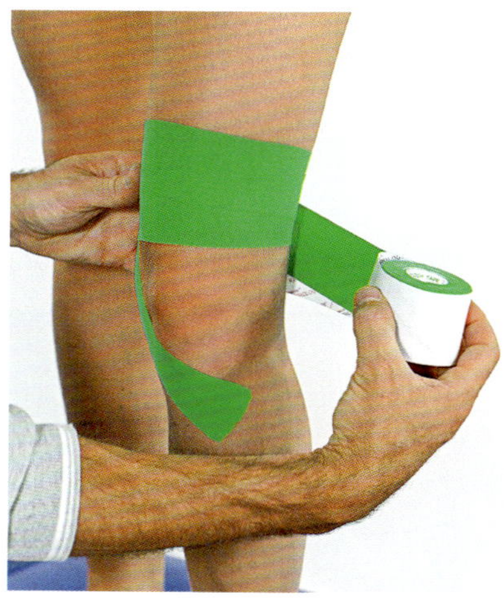

4

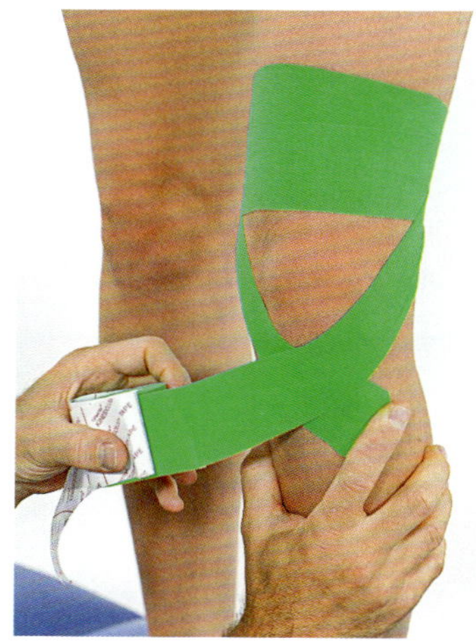

5

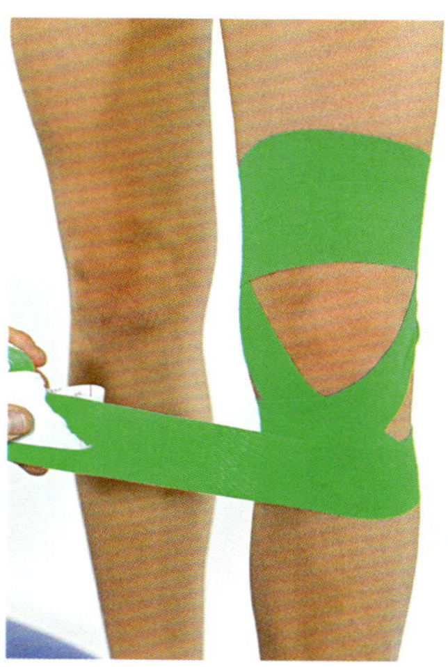

6

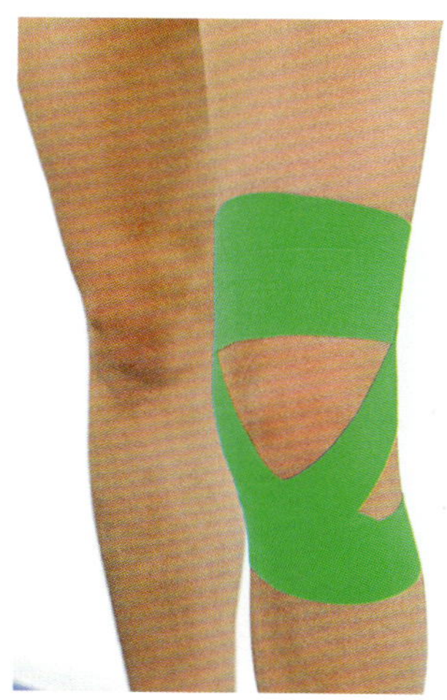

7

Unloading of the patellar tendon with elastic adhesive tape

MATERIAL

✓ Elastic adhesive tape, 5 cm in width

APPLICATION

1 The subject stands with one heel supported on a 2-4 cm lift (see page 139), the quadriceps muscle relaxed, the knee in semi-flexion, and the weight of the body resting on the opposite limb. A piece of elastic adhesive tape is applied from the proximal third of the tibia lateral to the point of tendinous insertion.

2 The bandage is placed one-third on the projection of the point of tendinous insertion and the other two-thirds on the body of the tendon itself below the tip of the patella, and is put under tension.

3-4 After stretching the bandage distally to proximally and anteriorly to posteriorly in order to have it medially border on the lower edge of the patella, three spiral wraps of bandage are made around the thigh from its middle third, going in the proximal to distal direction. These wrappings should overlap by 50%.

5 The bandage is anteriorly brought to border on the lower edge of the patella on its lateral portion, then is put under tension and made to pass over the anterior tibial tuberosity and cross the previous path.

6 Bandaging proceeds with a complete wrapping of the bandage around the proximal third of the lower leg.

7 Bandaging is complete.

With this type of bandaging, not only the patellar tendon but also the quadriceps muscle and the quadriceps tendon are relieved.

INDICATIONS

✓ *Inflammation of the insertion of the patellar tendon*
✓ *Inflammation of the patellar tendon*

KNEE JOINT

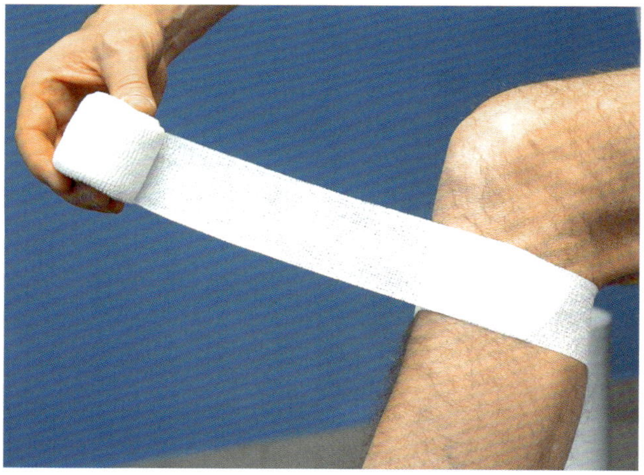

1

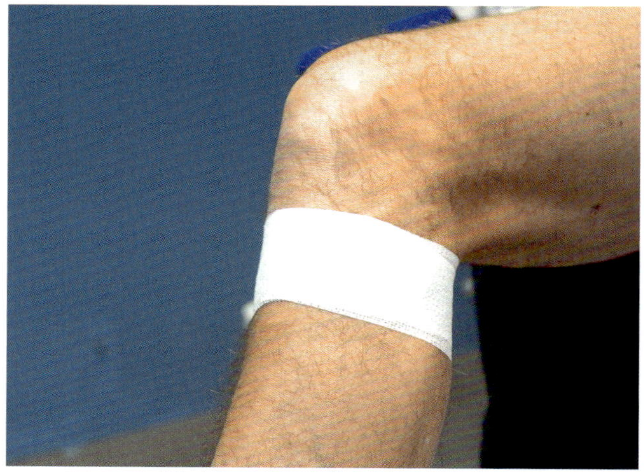

2

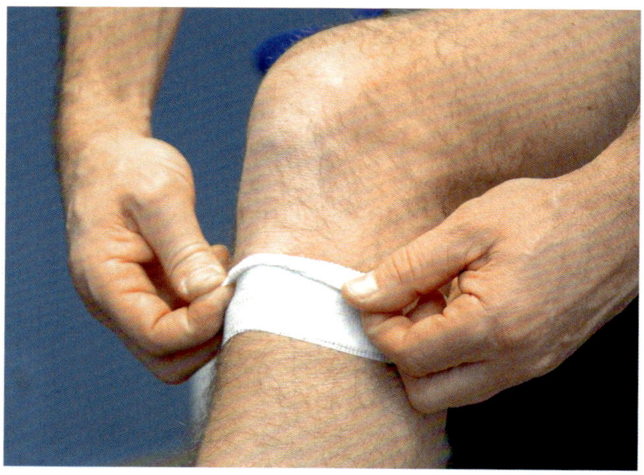

3

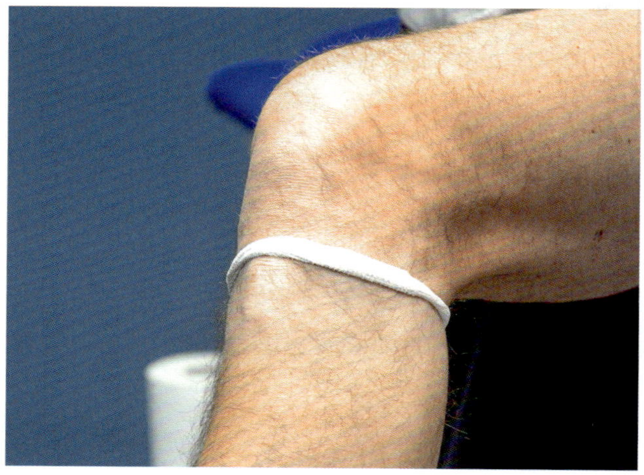

4

Support of the patellar tendon

MATERIAL

✓ 2.5 or 5 cm wide elastic cohesive bandage

APPLICATION

1-2 A full wrap of cohesive bandage is made around the axis of the lower leg, covering the point of insertion of the patellar tendon.

3-4 The bandage must be unrolled over itself and placed above the point of insertion of the patellar tendon, supported on the tibial crest.

INDICATIONS

✓ *Preventative sports treatment*
✓ *Insertional tendinous inflammation*

POSTERIOR MUSCLES OF THE LOWER LEG

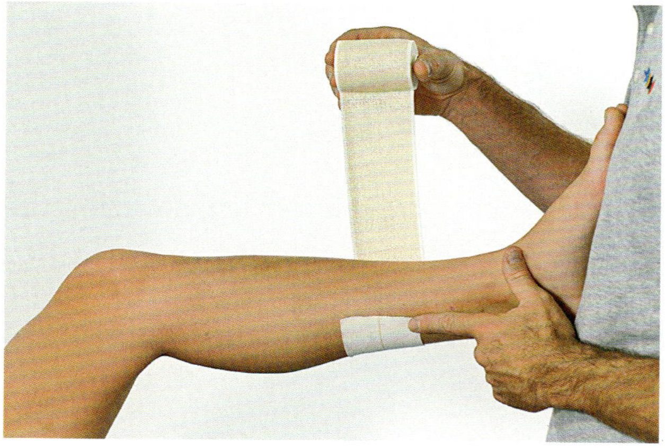

1

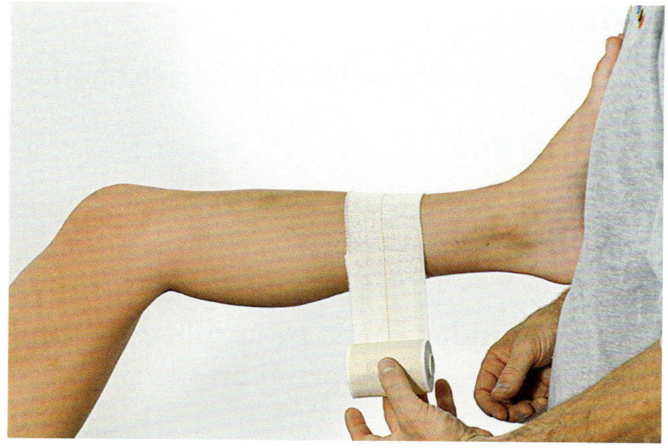

2

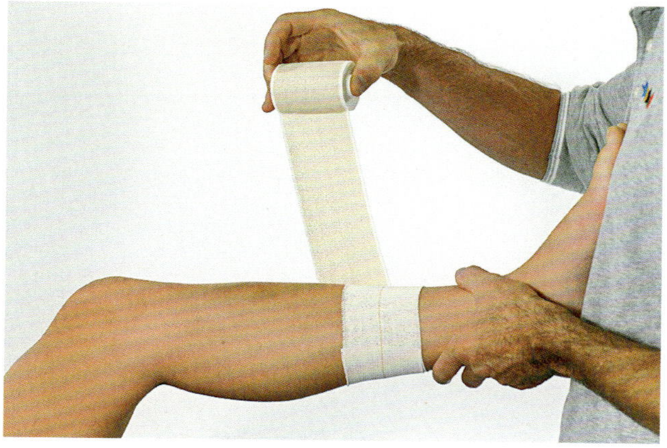

3

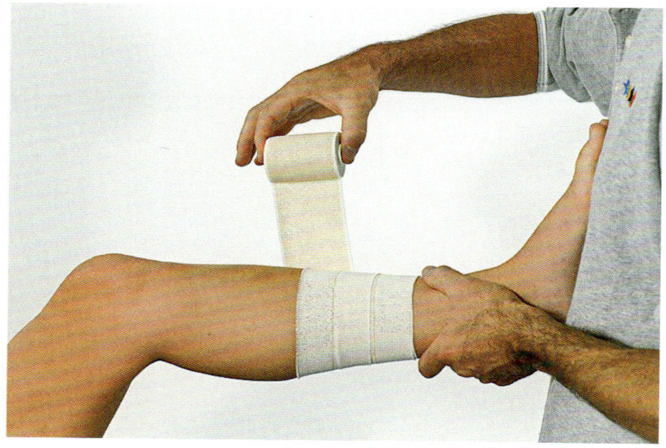

4

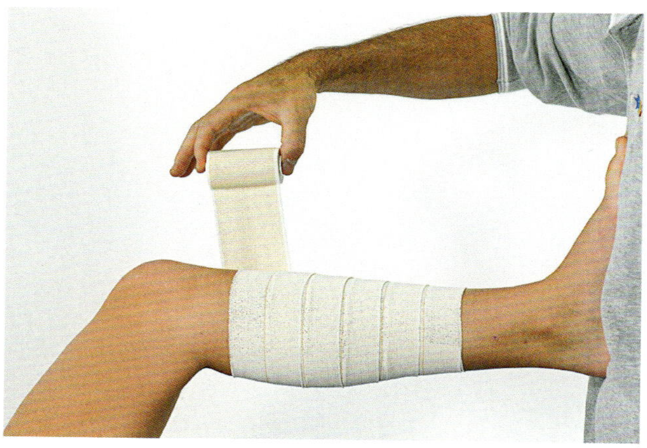

5

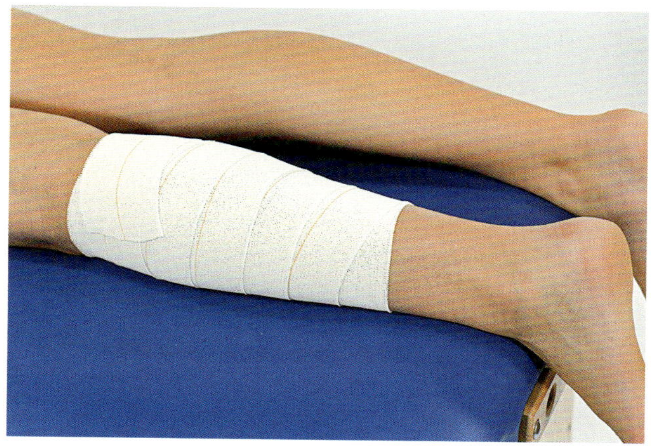

6

Muscular unloading via compressive bandaging

MATERIAL

- ✓ Cotton fabric porous elastic adhesive bandage that can be stretched lengthwise, 7.5 cm in width
- ✓ Inelastic adhesive tape

APPLICATION

1-2 The subject is in the supine decubitus position with the foot resting on the attendant's thorax. The application of the base elastic bandaging begins by covering the lower leg at the myotendinous junction of the gastrocnemius with a complete wrap of bandage.

3-4-5 Bandaging proceeds, covering the lower leg with spiral wraps overlapping by 50% moving in the distal-proximal direction until reaching the proximal third of the lower leg.

6 The subject enters the prone position for the application of the inelastic adhesive tape strips.

POSTERIOR MUSCLES OF THE LOWER LEG

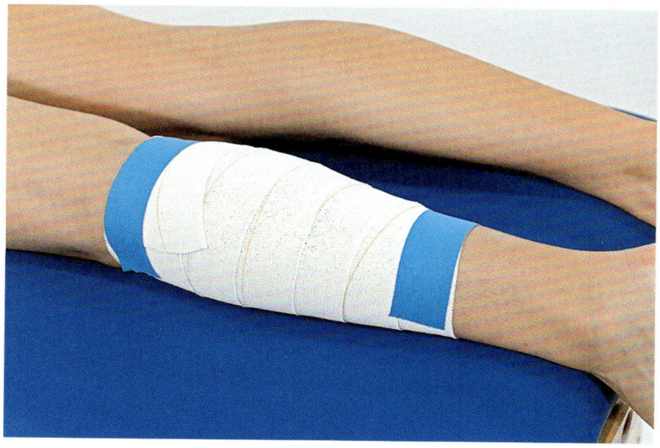

7

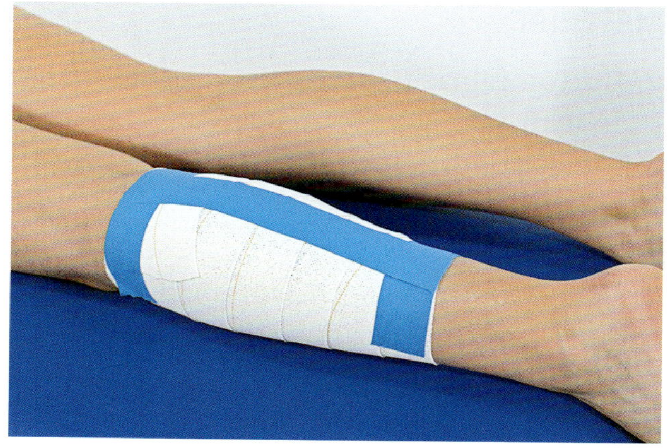

8

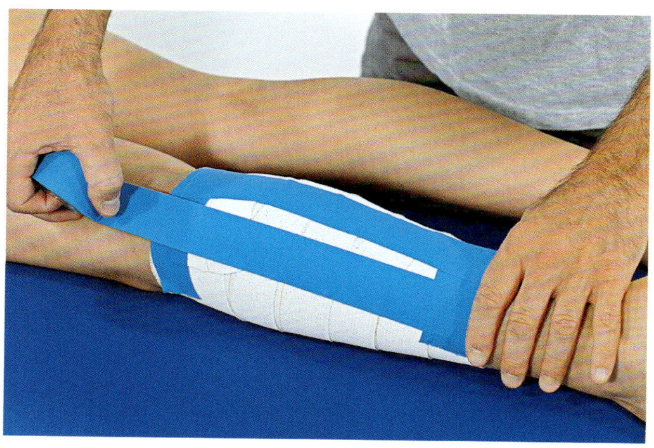

9

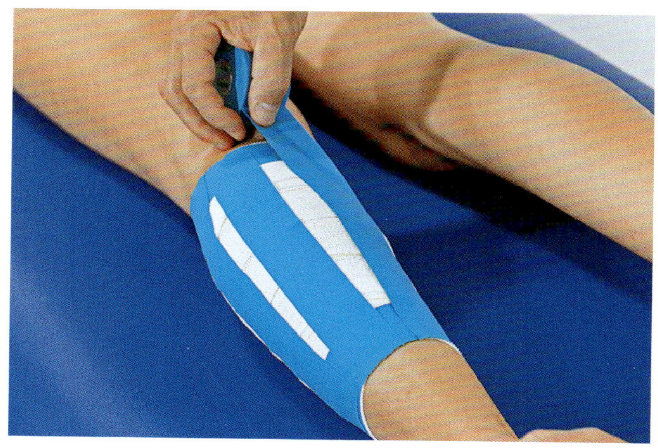

10

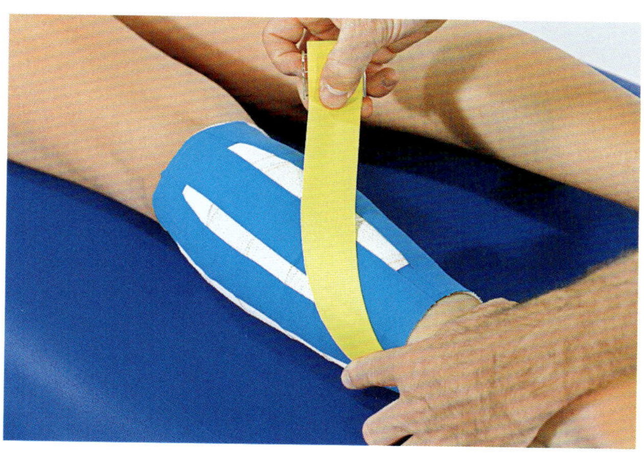

11

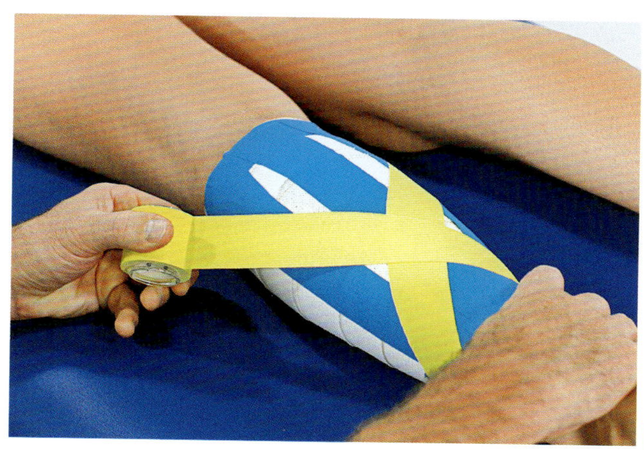

12

Muscular unloading via compressive bandaging

7 First, the proximal and distal anchoring points are secured: two strips of tape are applied in a semicircle perpendicular to the longitudinal axis of the lower leg.

8-9-10 Next, three strips of inelastic adhesive tape are longitudinally applied to the muscle fibers: a central strip passing over the area to be unloaded and two lateral ones as anchoring points for the subsequent fasteners.

11-12 Two strips cross over the central tape, such that the crossing point is located over the projection of the muscular area to be unloaded.

POSTERIOR MUSCLES OF THE LOWER LEG

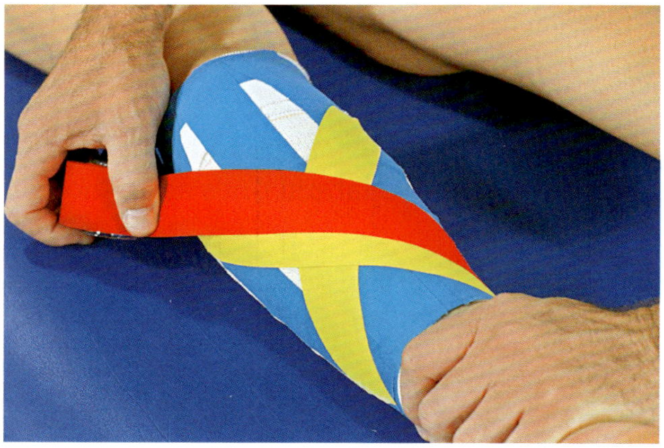
13

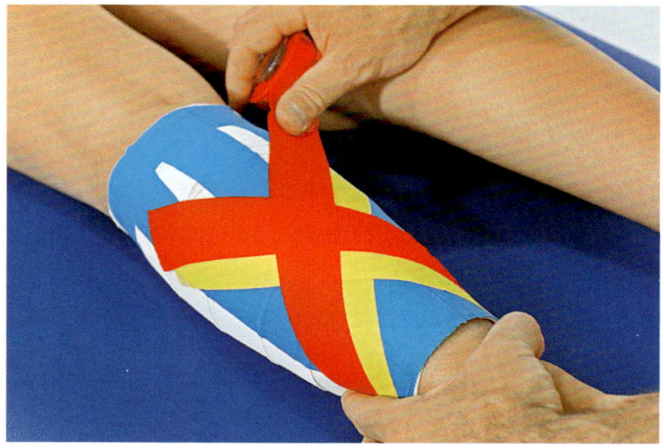
14

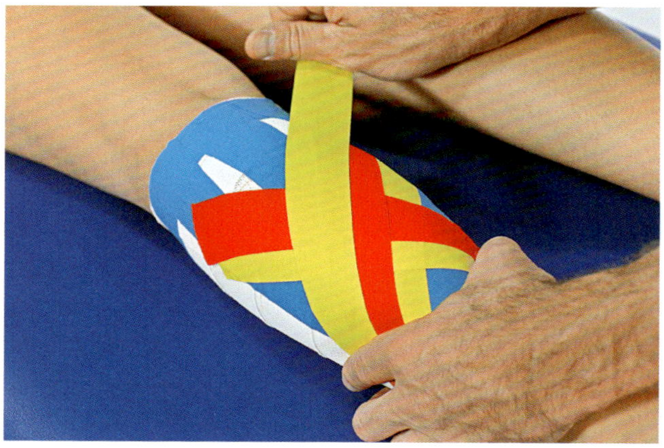
15

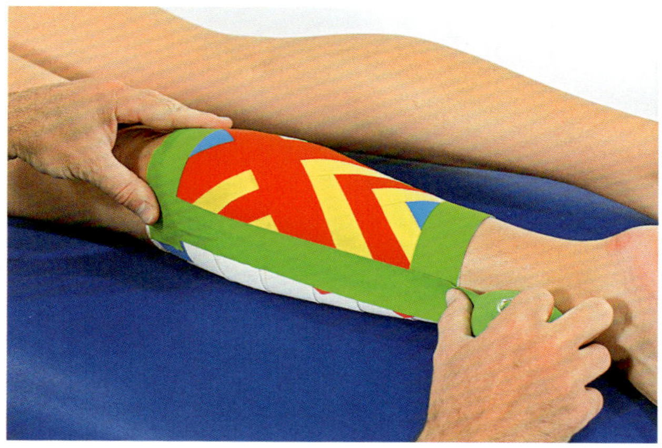
16

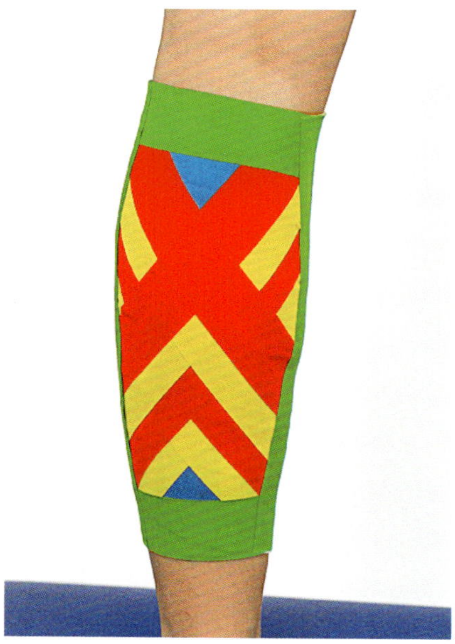
17

Muscular unloading via compressive bandaging

13-14-15 Bandaging proceeds by making subsequent crosses until the area of the injury is completely covered, overlapping the preceding strips by 30-50% and moving in the distal-proximal direction.

16 Bandaging is finished with vertical and horizontal strips that secure the anchoring points it started from.

17 Bandaging is complete.

INDICATIONS

Effects of muscular injuries such as:

- ✓ *Contractures*
- ✓ *Strains*
- ✓ *Elongations*

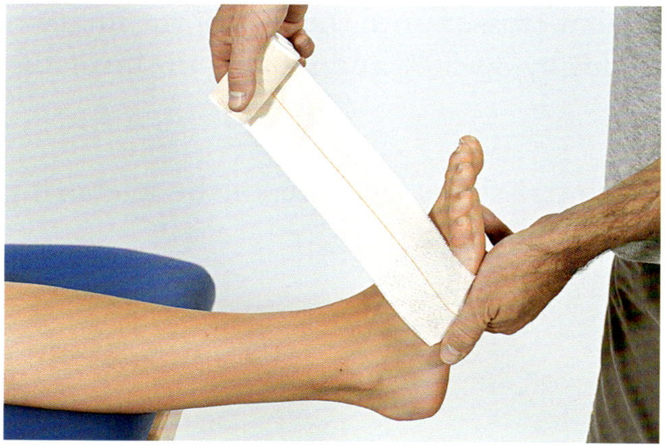

1

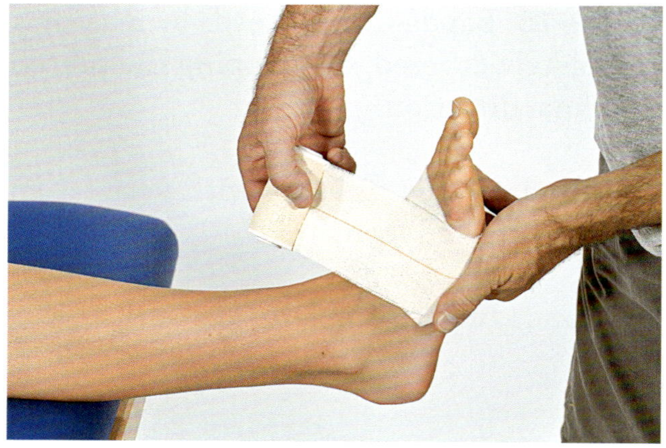

2

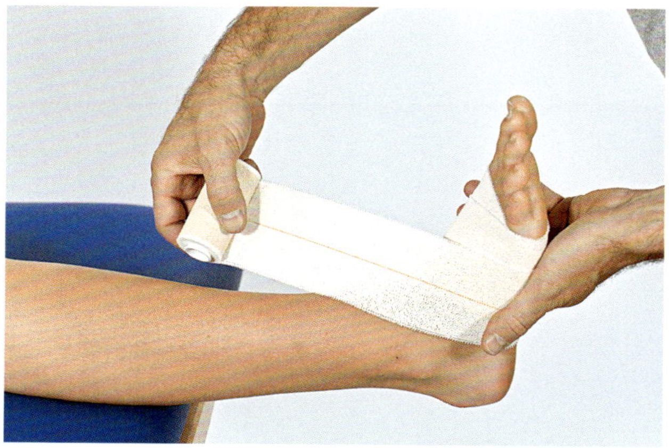

3

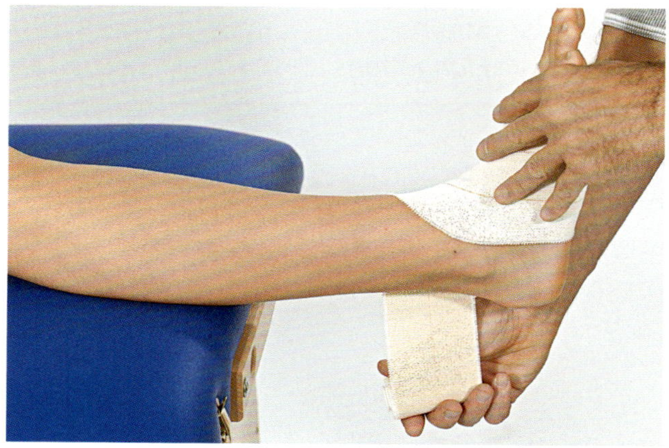

4

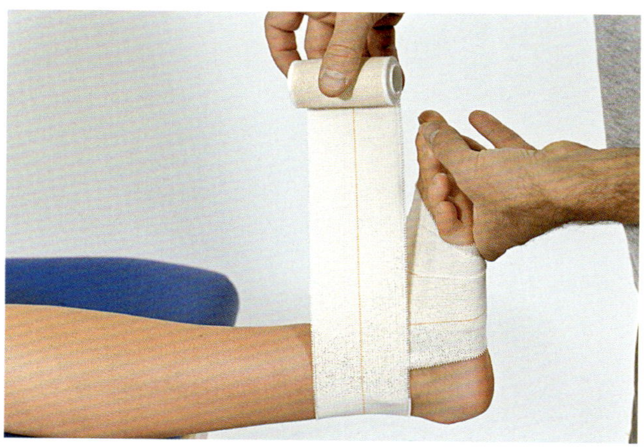

5

Base bandaging

MATERIAL

✓ Cotton fabric porous elastic adhesive bandage that can be stretched lengthwise, 7.5 cm in width

APPLICATION

1-2 The subject, in supine position, keeps the foot in dorsal flexion in the neutral position at 90 degrees and in slight eversion. A full wrap of bandage is made to cover the metatarsal heads beginning from the lateral edge of the forefoot on the dorsal skin projection of the fifth metatarsal.

3 Bandaging proceeds with the application of several spiral wraps in the distal-proximal direction to cover the midfoot.

4-5 The bandage is directed toward the medial malleolus, and after having wrapped around the Achilles tendon, toward the skin projection of the lateral malleolus.

If the bandaging has to be kept in place for several days, remember to apply two foam rubber or pre-tape compresses in order to protect the regions corresponding to the skin projection of the Achilles tendon and the anatomical structures of the anterior compartment of the ankle.

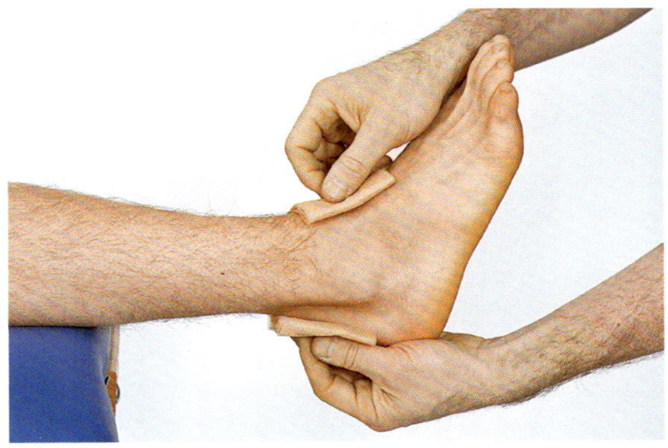

For base bandaging in cases of sprain trauma of the medial area, the same procedure is done; however, the bandage starts from the dorsal skin projection of the first metatarsal with the foot in a position of slight inversion.

On this base bandaging, articular support can be provided via the placement of inelastic adhesive strips that protect the ligaments of the wounded capsuloligamentous area from exertion.

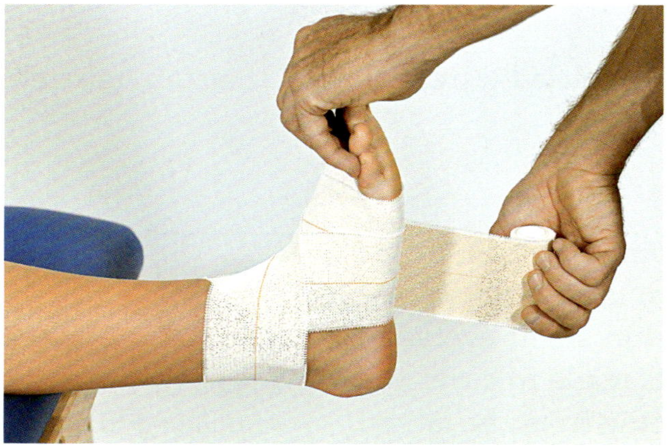

6

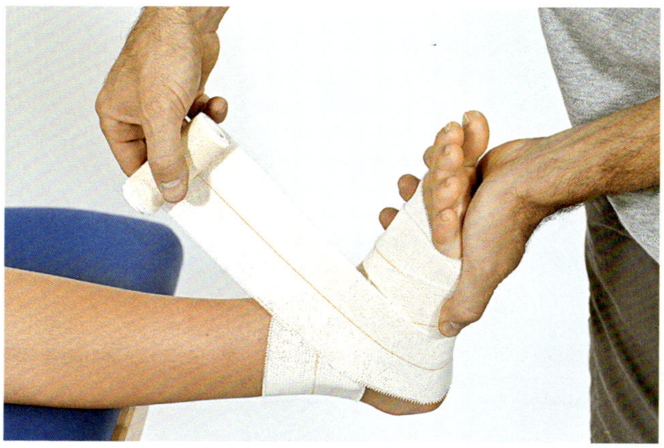

7

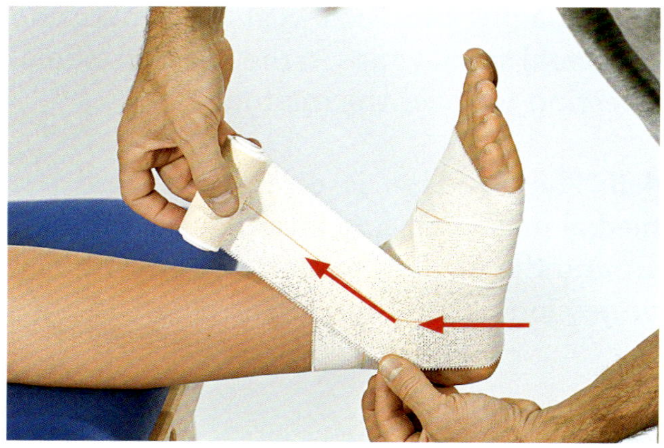

8

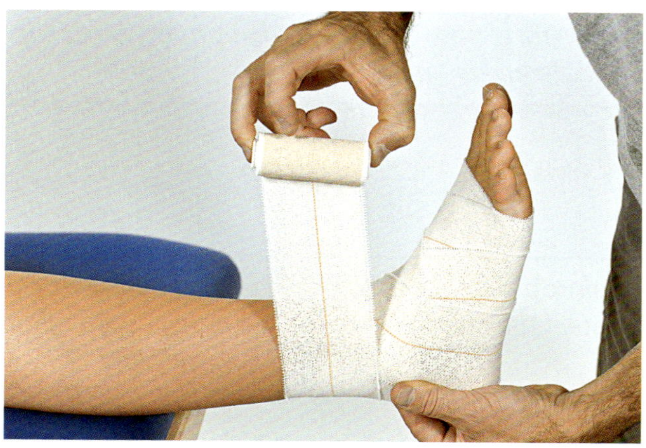

9

6 From the lateral malleolus, the bandage is brought to wrap dorsally around the tibiotarsal joint.

7-8 The bandage is then passed below the heel and then toward the lateral malleolus. It should be pinched between the thumb and forefinger in order to improve its corrective effect on the back of the foot.

9 The bandaging finishes by wrapping the distal third of the lower leg.

In cases of significant intra-articular effusion, it is necessary to wrap all of the anatomical structures of the tibiotarsal joint. For this reason, an additional wrapping of bandage must be made that completely covers the heel before finishing bandaging by wrapping the distal third of the lower leg.

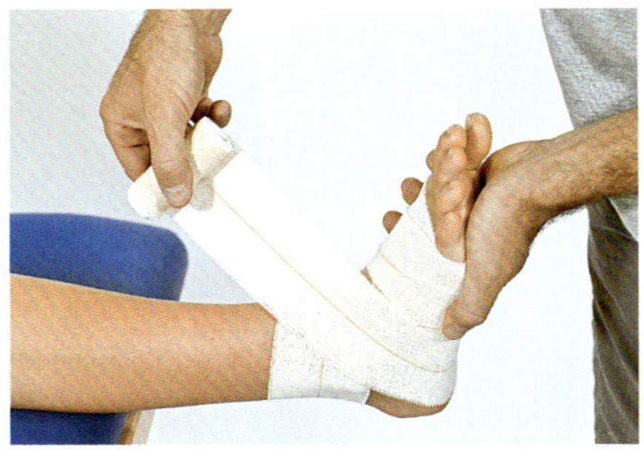

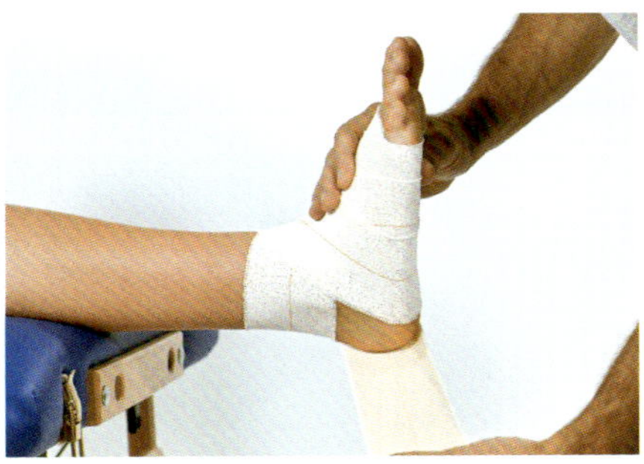

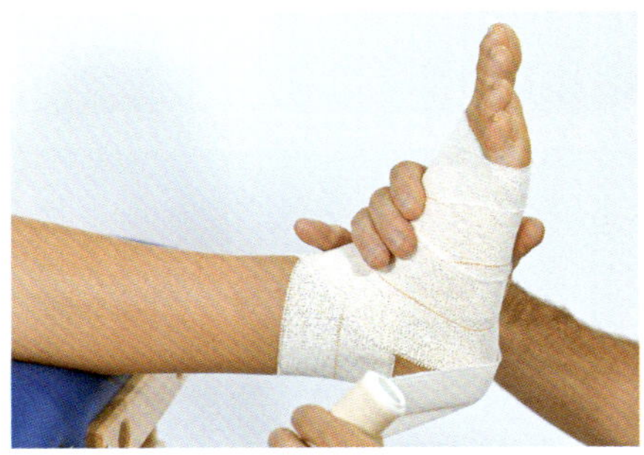

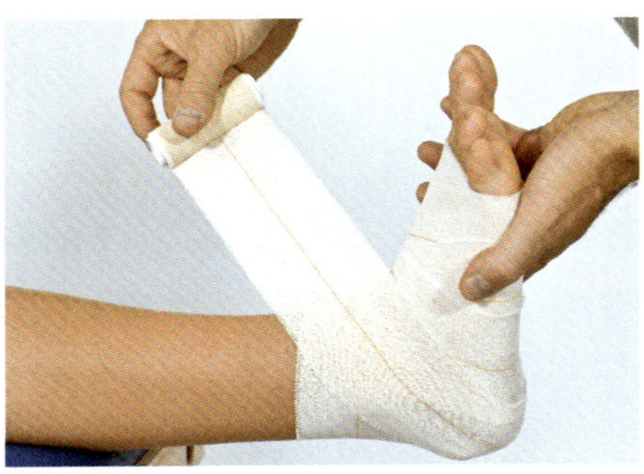

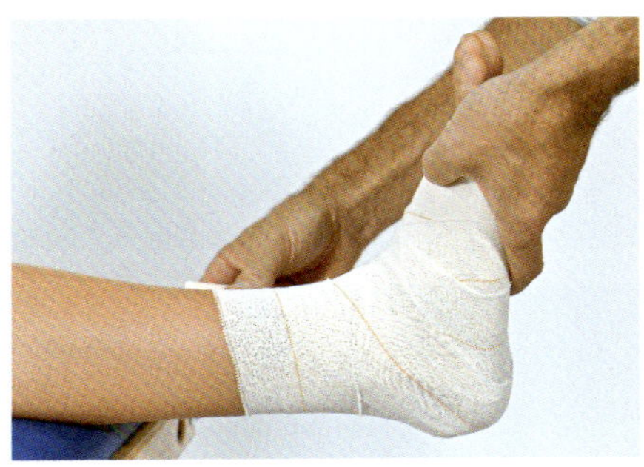

INDICATIONS

- ✓ *Sprain trauma of the lateral or medial compartments*
- ✓ *Therapeutic and sports bandaging*

TIBIOTARSAL JOINT

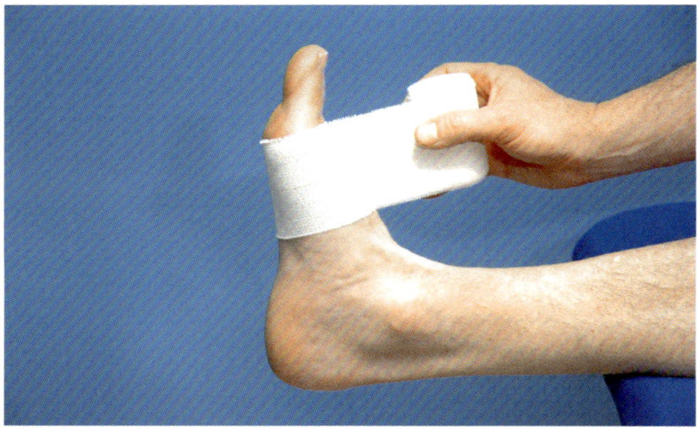

1

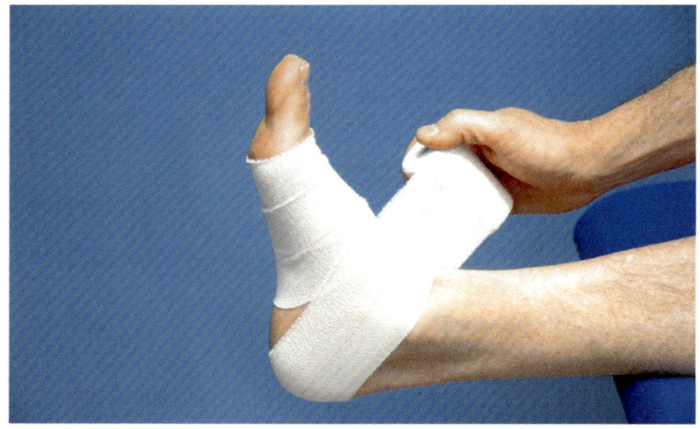

2

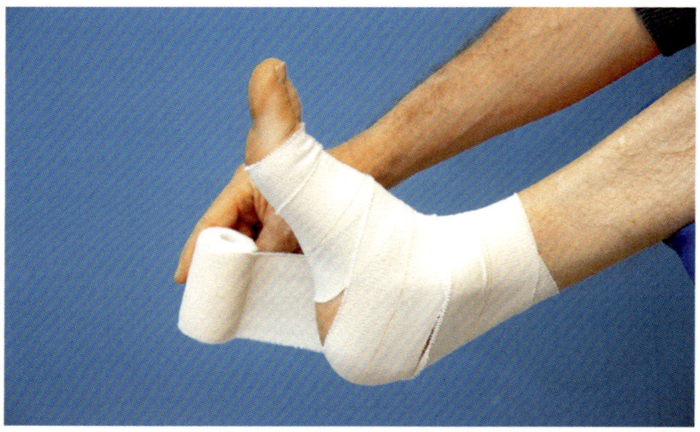

3

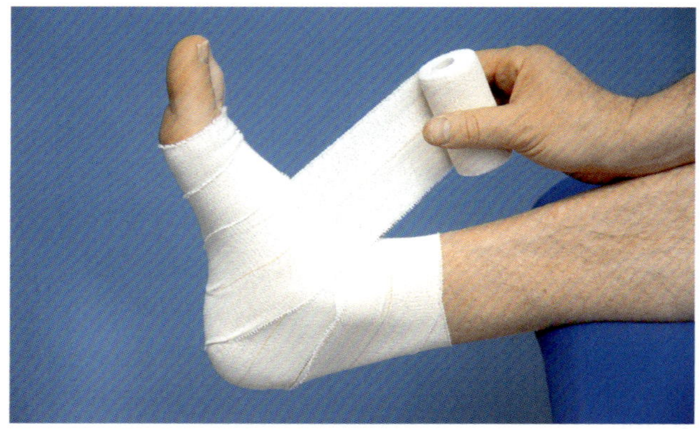

4

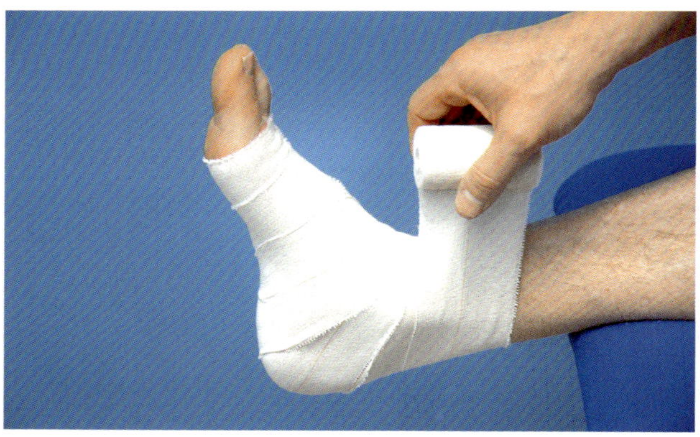

5

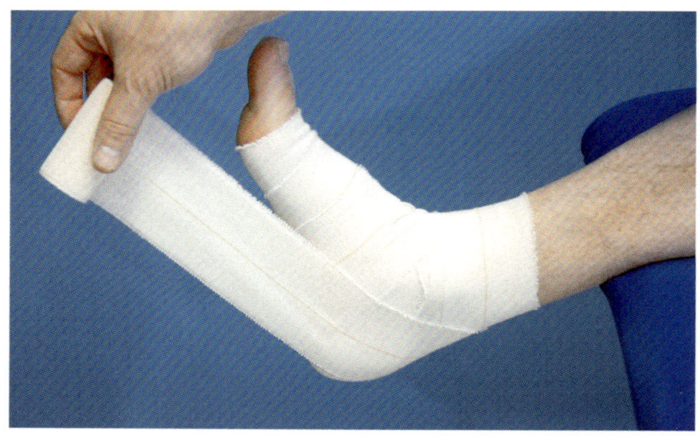

6

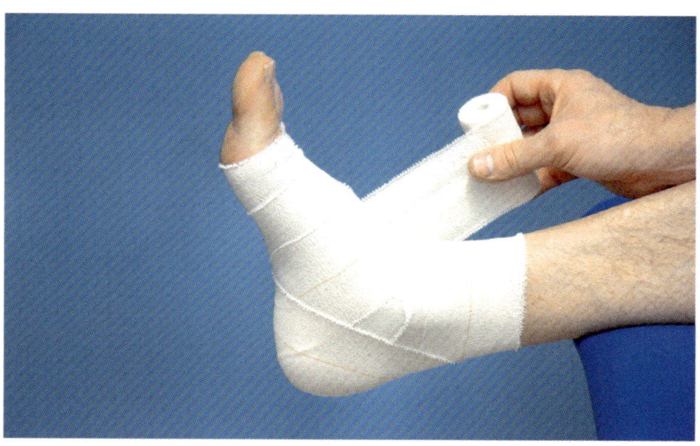

7

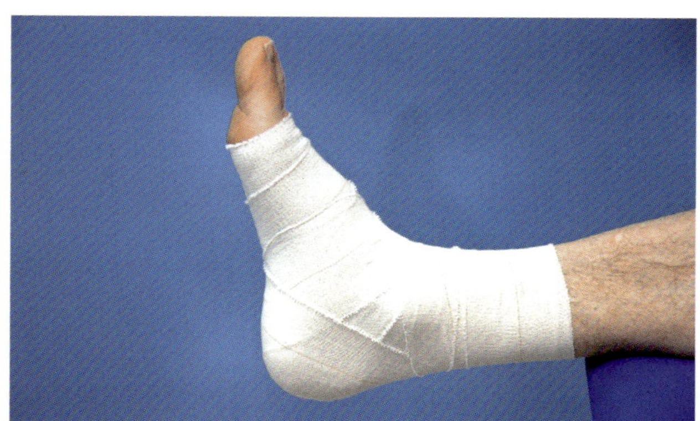

8

Retention base bandaging

MATERIAL

✓ Cotton fabric porous elastic adhesive bandage that can be stretched lengthwise, 7.5 cm in width

APPLICATION

1 The subject positions the foot off the end of the table. The mono-extensible adhesive elastic bandage is wrapped around the metatarsal heads.

2 Bandaging proceeds with several spiral wraps applied in the distal-proximal direction, wrapping the foot until the heel is covered.

3 Bandaging proceeds with a wrap of bandage around the axis of the lower leg, covering the Achilles tendon; then the bandage is brought diagonally over the lateral area of the heel.

4 The bandage is brought below the plantar arch and made to dorsally cover the tibiotarsal joint.

5 A wrap of bandage is made around the axis of the lower leg.

6 The bandage is brought diagonally to cover the medial part of the heel.

7 The bandage is brought again below the plantar arch and directed toward the dorsal surface of the tibiotarsal joint.

8 The bandaging finishes with several spiral wraps around the axis of the lower leg.

TIBIOTARSAL JOINT

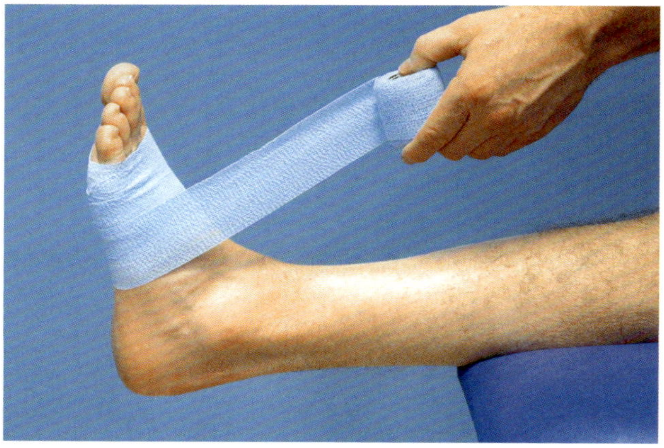

1

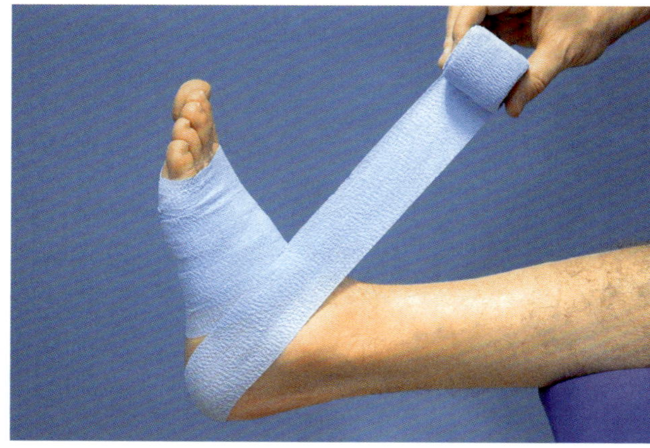

2

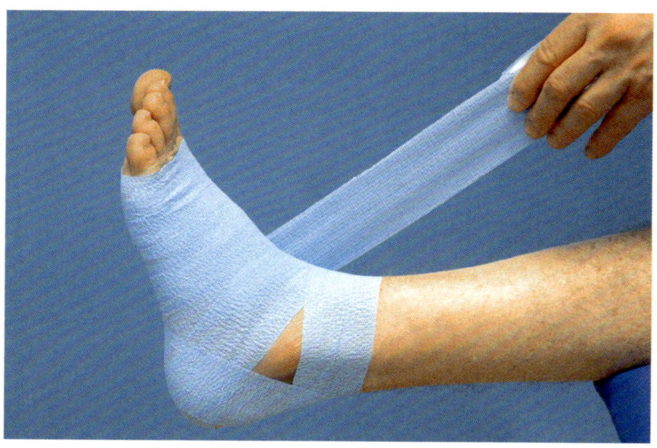

3

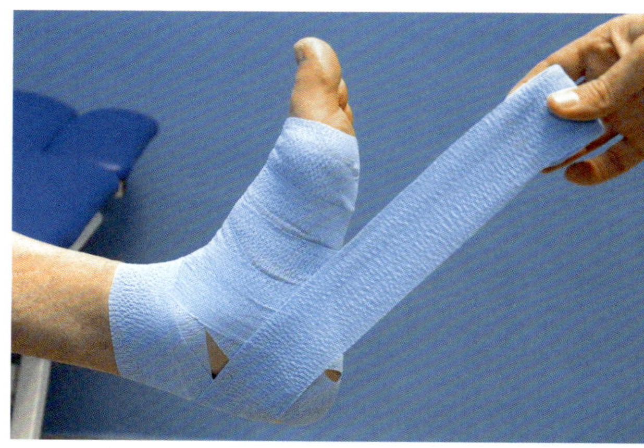

4

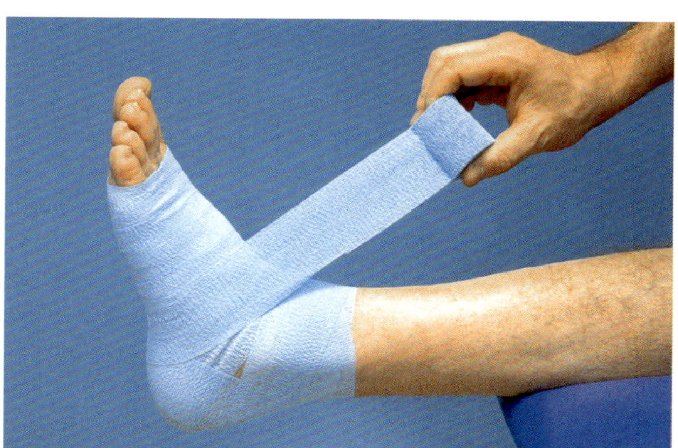

5

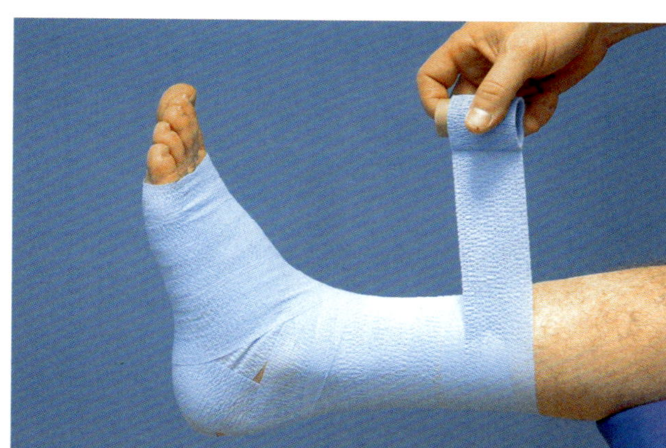

6

Base bandaging with cohesive elastic bandage

MATERIAL

✓ Elastic cohesive bandage, 7.5 cm in width

APPLICATION

1 The subject positions the foot off the end of the table. To begin, a full wrap of cohesive bandage covers the foot distally, then goes toward the tibiotarsal joint with several spiral wraps.

During the application of the bandage, the foot must always be kept in a neutral position at 90 degrees dorsal flexion.

2 The bandage now covers the heel.

3 With a full wrap completed around the distal third of the lower leg, the bandage is brought down diagonally along the skin projection of the lateral and then inferior portion of the heel.

4 Another wrap is made around the axis of the lower leg, later going down diagonally along the skin projection of the medial border of the heel.

5 The bandage is passed below the plantar arch and dorsally directed to cover the tibiotarsal joint.

6 The bandage covers the distal third of the lower leg with several spiral wraps, remaining below the myotendinous junction of the gastrocnemius.

TIBIOTARSAL JOINT

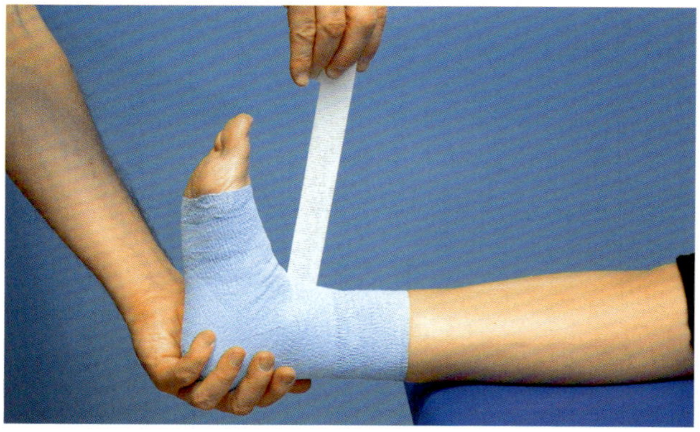

1

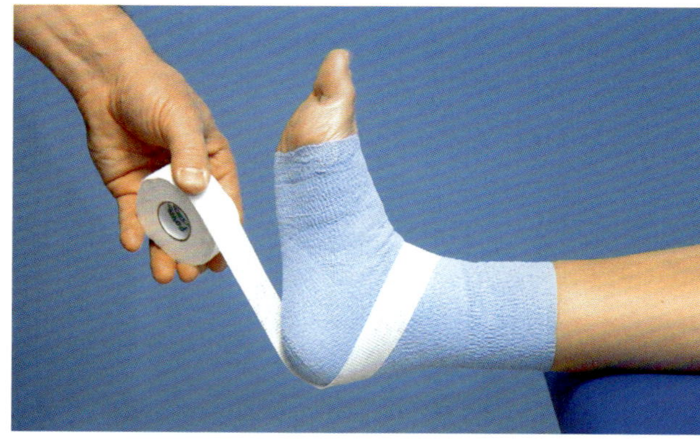

2

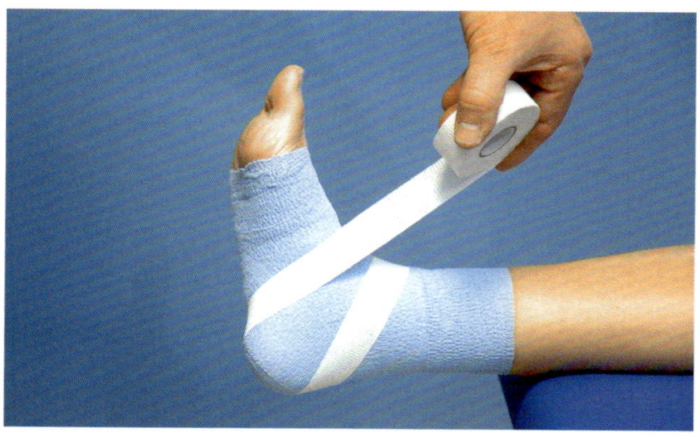

3

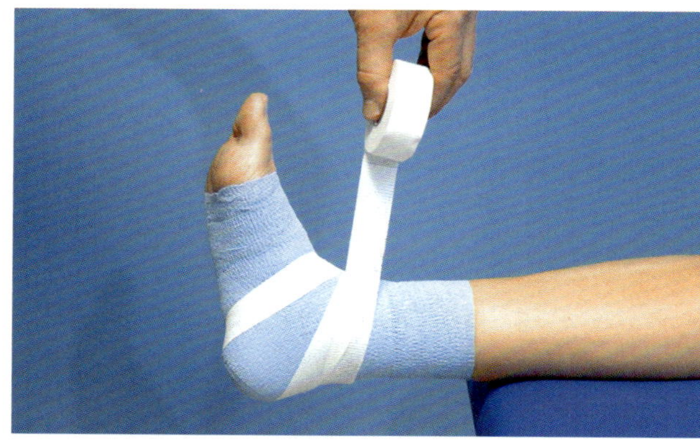

4

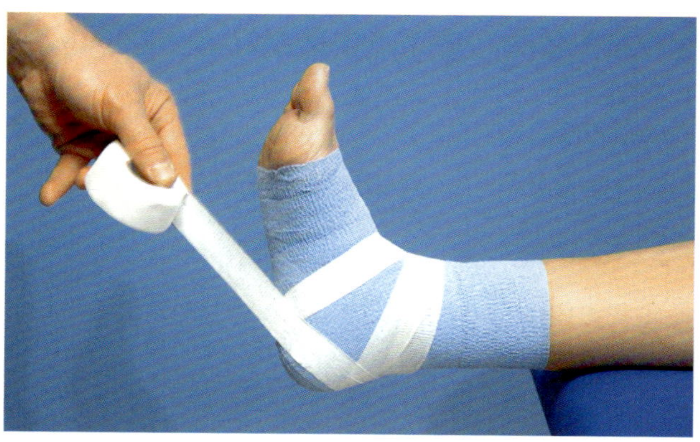

5

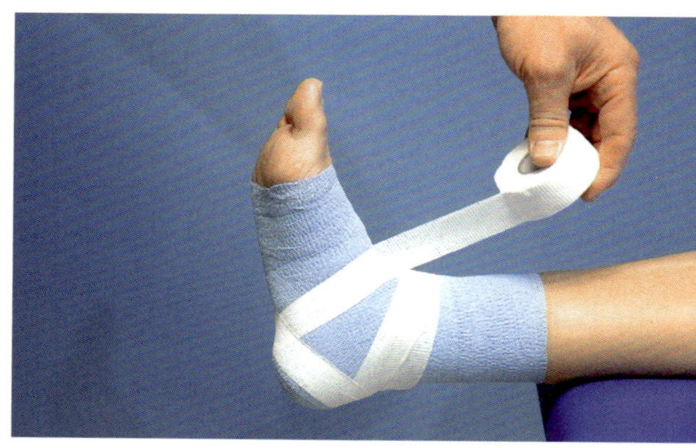

6

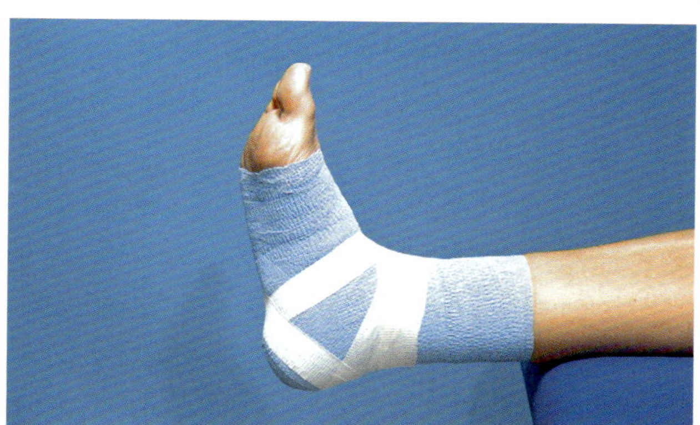

7

Fast bandaging with stabilization of the hindfoot

MATERIAL

✓ Cohesive elastic bandage for base bandaging, 7.5 cm wide
✓ Inelastic cohesive tape, 2 cm in width

APPLICATION

1 Several figure-eight bandagings are applied on base bandaging made with a cohesive elastic bandage (see pages 184-185), covering the tibiotarsal joint to stabilize the hindfoot. To begin, the inelastic adhesive bandage is placed on the skin projection of the fibular malleolus.

> *During the application of the bandaging, the subject positions the foot off the end of the table and keeps it in a neutral position at 90 degrees dorsal flexion.*

2 The tibiotarsal joint is then dorsally covered and the bandaging proceeds toward the heel.

3 The heel is wrapped, passing under the plantar arch, and then the bandage is proximally brought onto the dorsal surface of the tibiotarsal joint.

4 Once a wrap is made around the lower leg, the bandage is in a perpendicular position to the axis of the tibia at the skin projection of the tibial malleolus.

5 Another wrap of bandage is made around the axis of the lower leg, passing over the Achilles tendon and then brought diagonally over the medial area of the heel.

6 The heel is wrapped, passing under the plantar arch, then the bandage is proximally brought onto the dorsal surface of the tibiotarsal joint.

7 After a wrap is made around the axis of the lower leg, the bandage is cut and secured onto the bandaging.

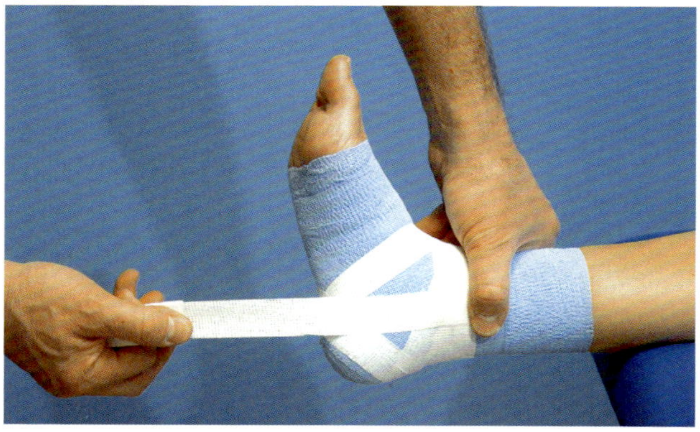
8

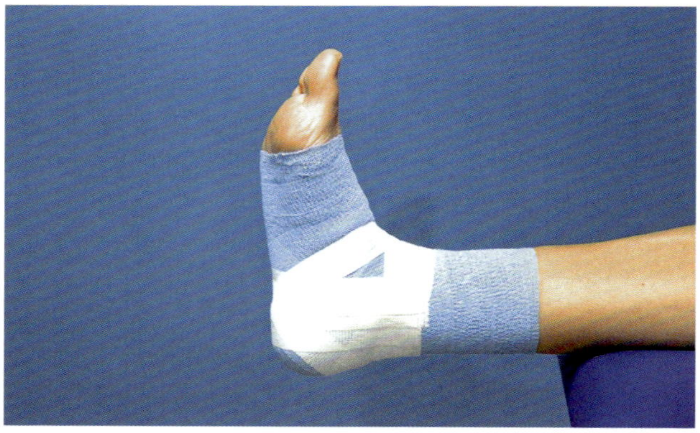
9

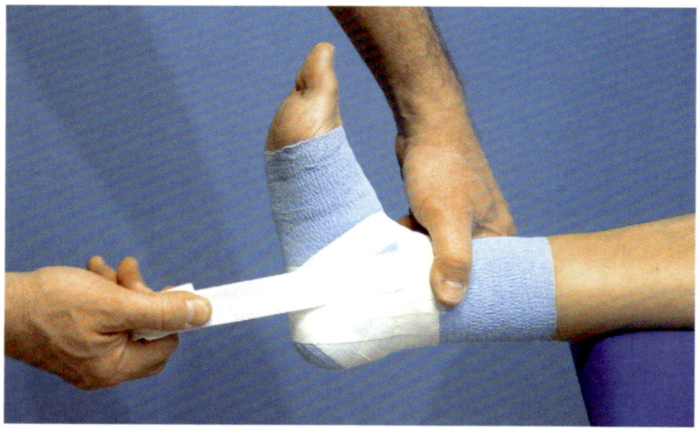
10

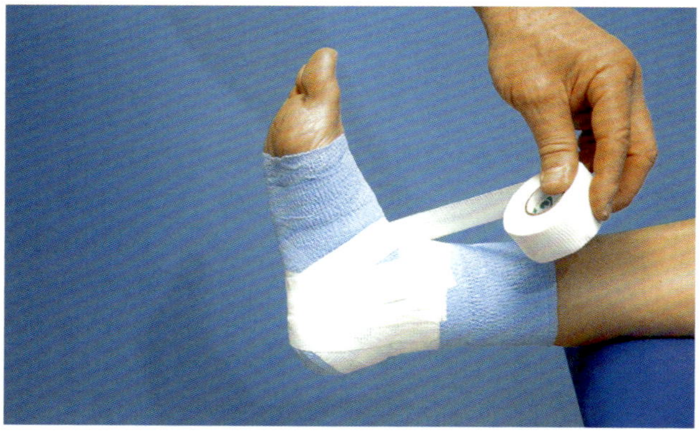
11

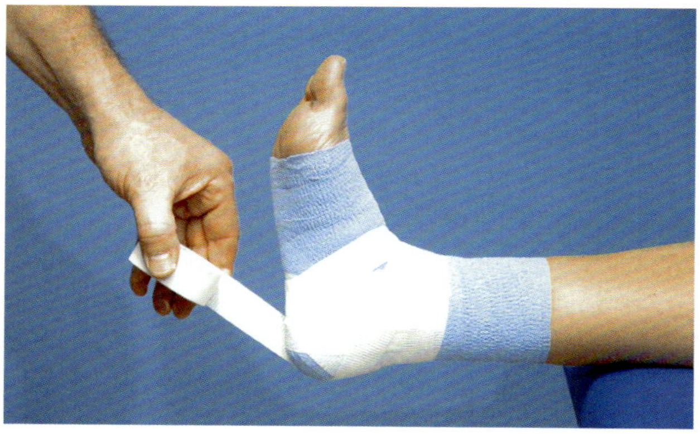
12

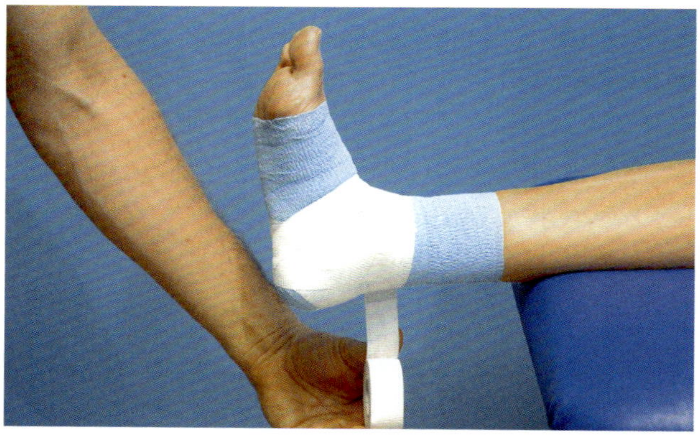
13

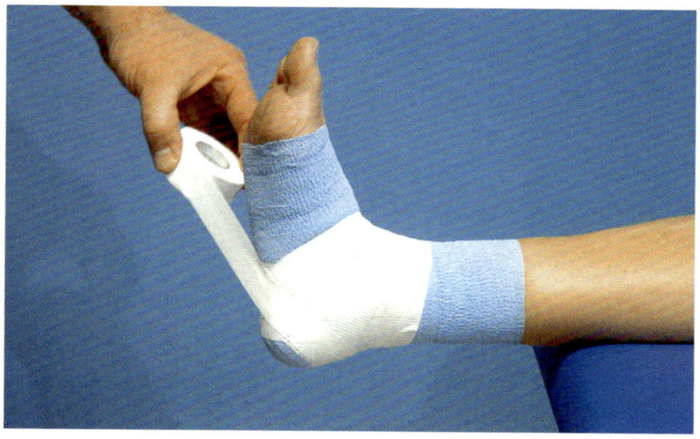
14

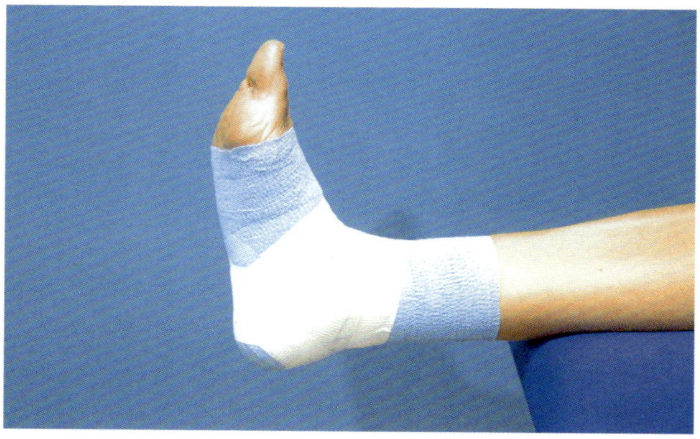
15

Fast bandaging with stabilization of the hindfoot

8-9 Three fasteners are prepared to be applied in horseshoe fashion so as to cover the heel from below. First, one fastener is applied starting from the tibial malleolus and going to the fibular malleolus, then the other two fasteners are placed parallel to the first, one anterior and one posterior to it.

10 Next, a figure-eight bandage is made to additionally reinforce the stabilization of the hindfoot, applying several wraps of inelastic bandage starting from the tibial malleolus.

11 The heel is wrapped, passing under the plantar arch, then the bandage is proximally brought onto the dorsal surface of the tibiotarsal joint.

12 After completing a wrap around the axis of the lower leg, the bandage is diagonally directed over the lateral area of the heel.

13 Bandaging proceeds by passing the bandage under the plantar arch to then bring it onto the dorsum of the tibiotarsal joint and make a full wrap around the axis of the lower leg.

14 The bandage is diagonally brought over the medial area.

15 Once it has passed over the plantar arch, the bandage proximally runs over the dorsal surface of the tibiotarsal joint, where it is cut and secured. Bandaging is complete.

INDICATIONS

✓ *Preventative sports treatment*

TIBIOTARSAL JOINT

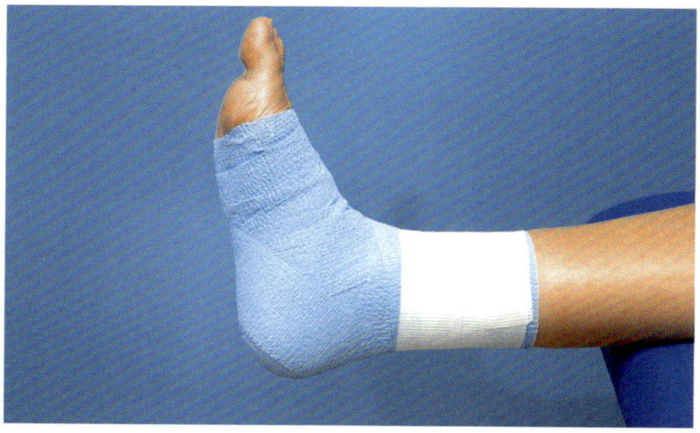

1

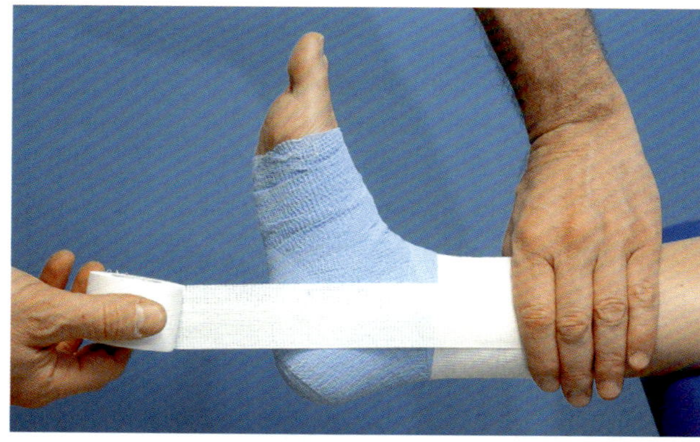

2

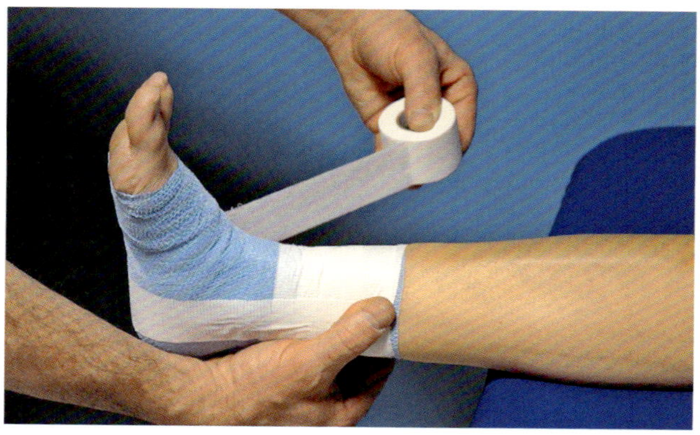

3

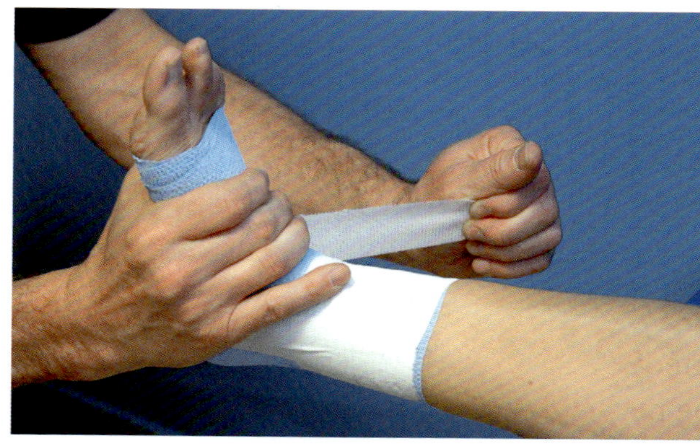

4

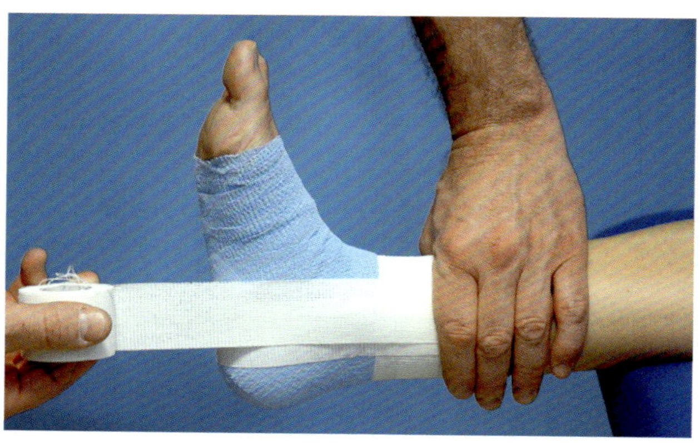

5

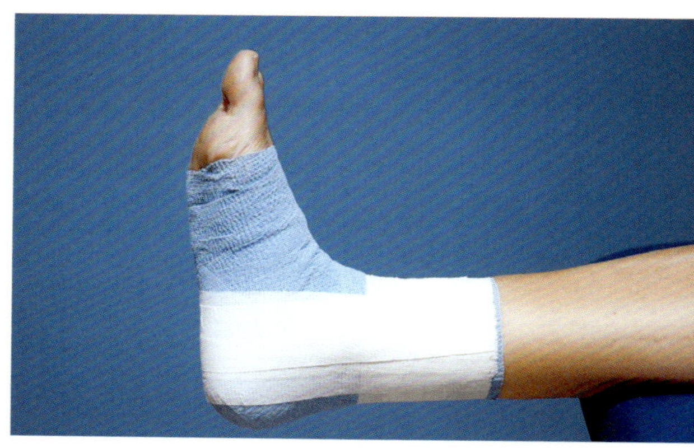

6

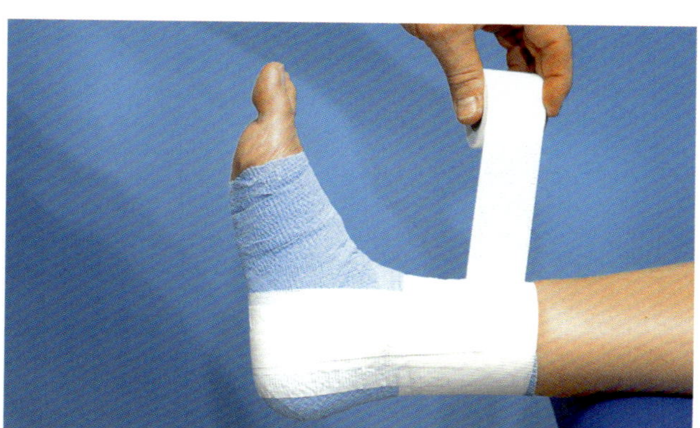

7

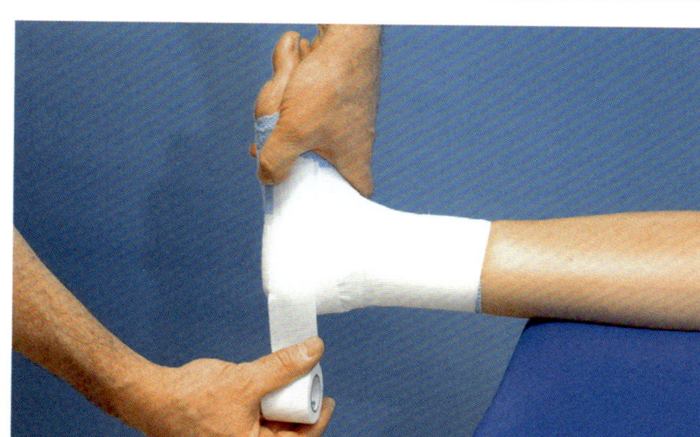

8

Stabilization of the hindfoot and support at the lateral space

MATERIAL

✓ Cohesive elastic bandage for base bandaging, 7.5 cm wide
✓ Inelastic cohesive tape, 2 cm in width

APPLICATION

1 The subject, in the supine position, places the foot off the end of the table. The foot is prepared by applying base bandaging with a cohesive elastic bandage (see pages 184-185), on which an anchoring point is made with several wraps of inelastic bandage at the distal third of the lower leg.

> *During the application of the bandaging, the subject positions the foot off the end of the table and keeps it in a neutral position at 90 degrees dorsal flexion.*

2-3-4 A strip of inelastic bandage is applied on the anchoring point in horseshoe fashion, medially to laterally, in such a way as to cover the lower part of the heel. The fastener should be made to pass directly over the bone "landmark" points of the fibular and tibial malleolus.

5-6 Another three strips of bandage are applied parallel to the first, placed anterior and posterior to it.

7 The support fasteners are secured with several wraps of inelastic bandage running in the proximal-distal direction.

8 The hindfoot is wrapped with several strips of bandage applied in horseshoe fashion.

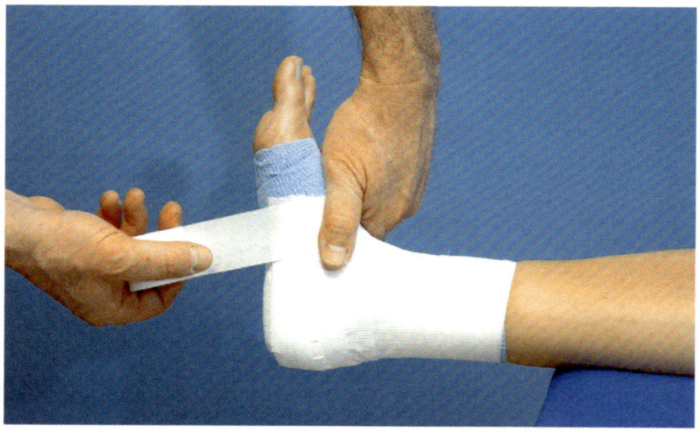
9

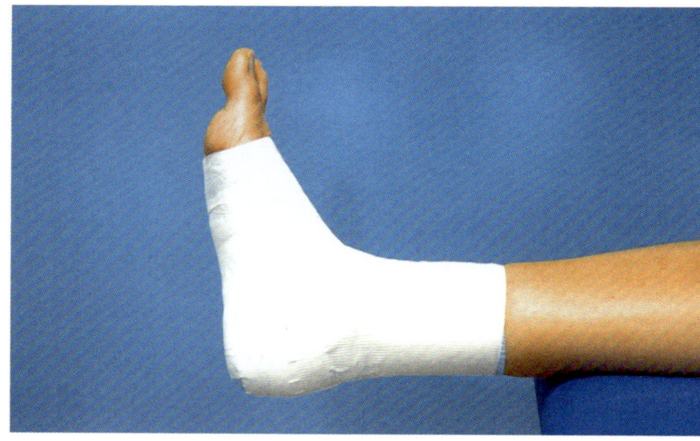
10

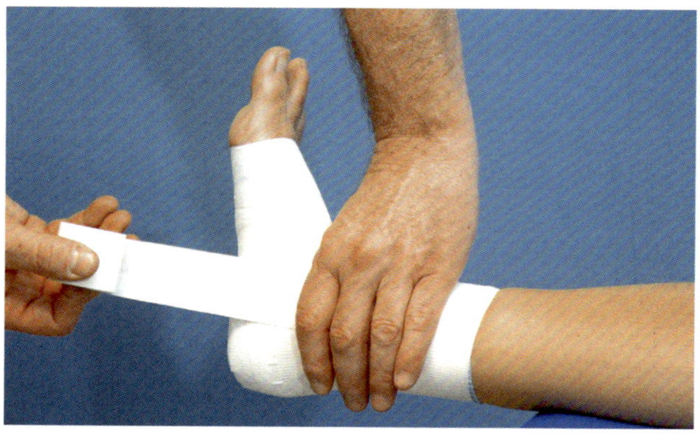
11

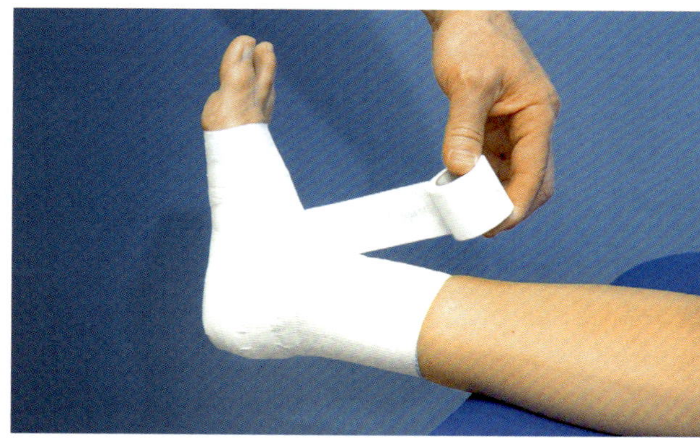
12

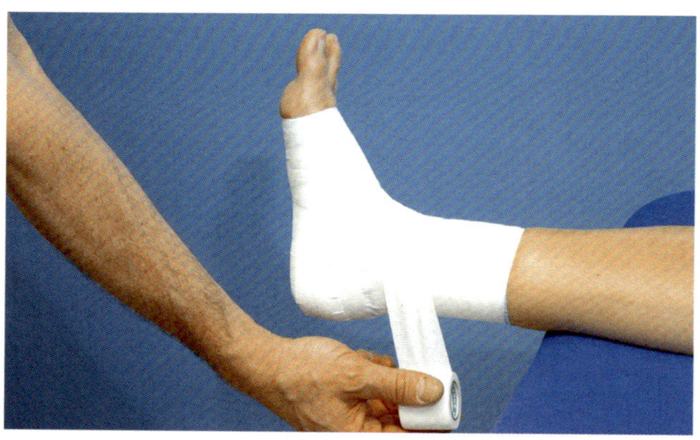
13

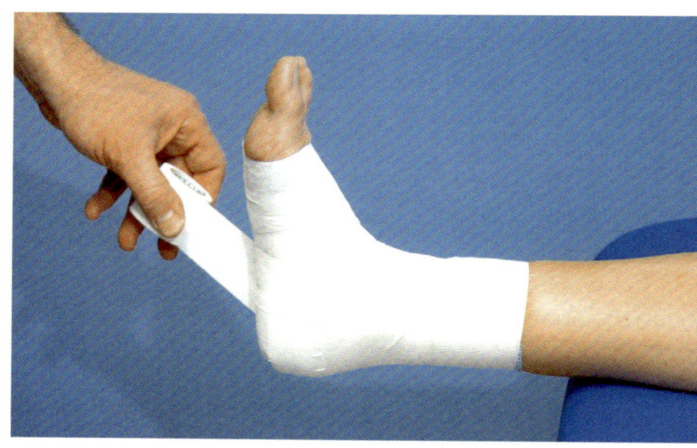
14

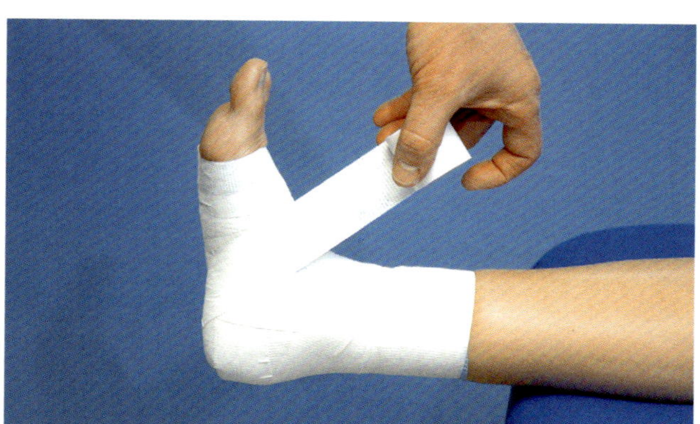
15

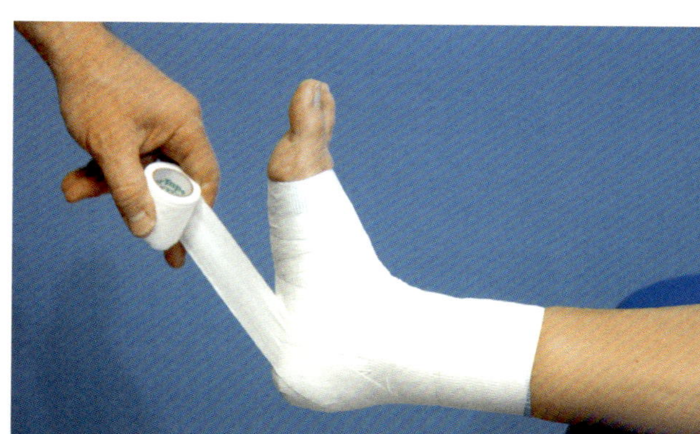
16

Stabilization of the hindfoot and support at the lateral space

9-10 The midfoot and forefoot are also wrapped by the bandaging, using several complete bandage wraps.

11 The bandaging for the stabilization of the hindfoot proceeds with the application of two figure-eight wraps of inelastic bandage. The bandage starts from the medial malleolus.

12 The bandage is brought to wrap the plantar arch.

13 Next, the bandage runs over the dorsum of the foot, covering the tibiotarsal joint.

14 Having made a complete wrap of bandage around the axis of the lower leg, the bandage is diagonally brought down in the direction of the lateral area of the heel.

15 The bandage is again brought below the plantar arch and then directed toward the dorsum of the foot, covering the tibiotarsal joint.

16 A wrap of bandage is made around the axis of the lower leg, and the bandage is diagonally brought toward the heel to cover the medial area.

TIBIOTARSAL JOINT

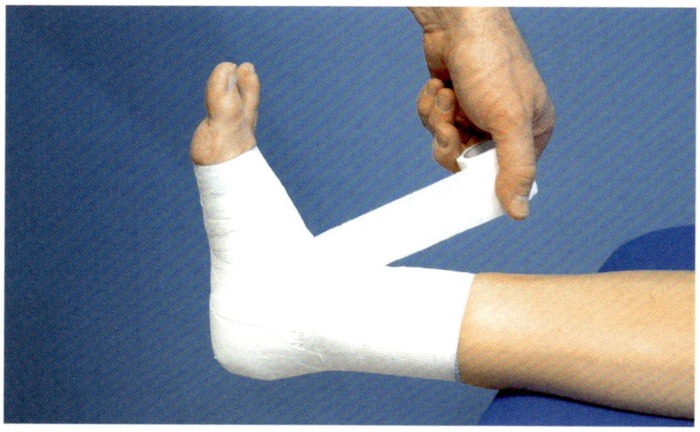

17

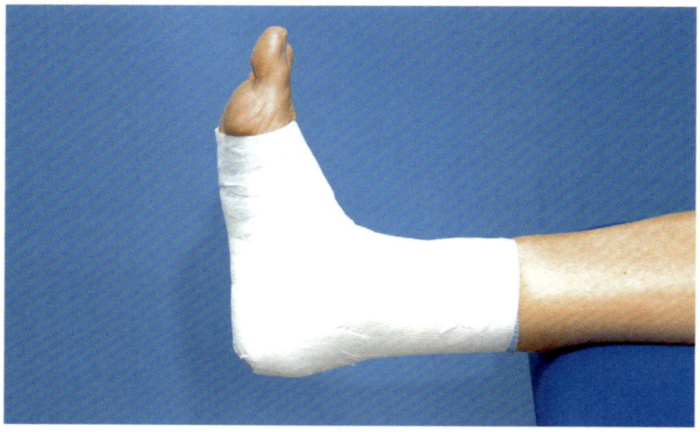

18

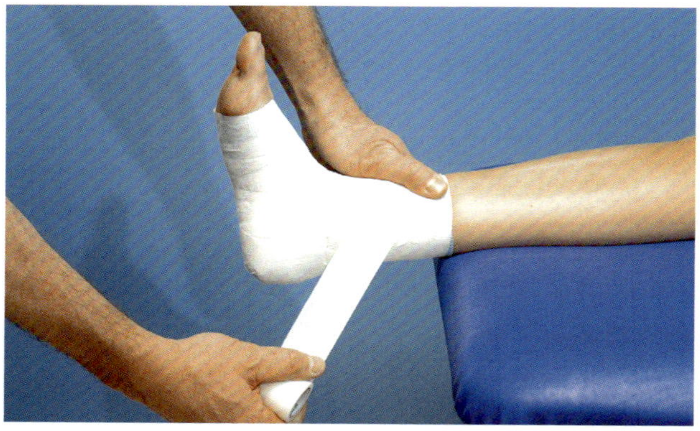

19

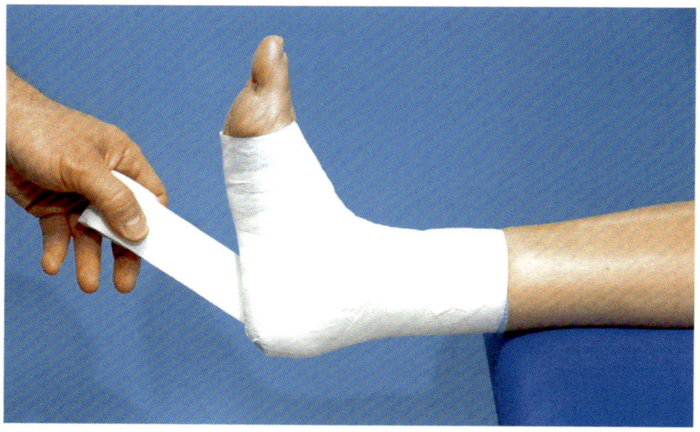

20

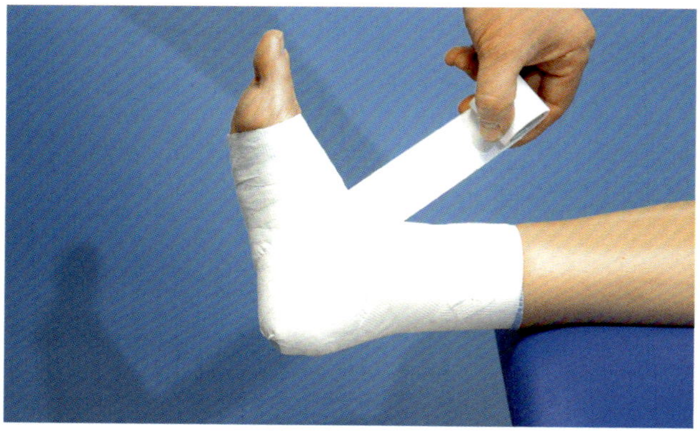

21

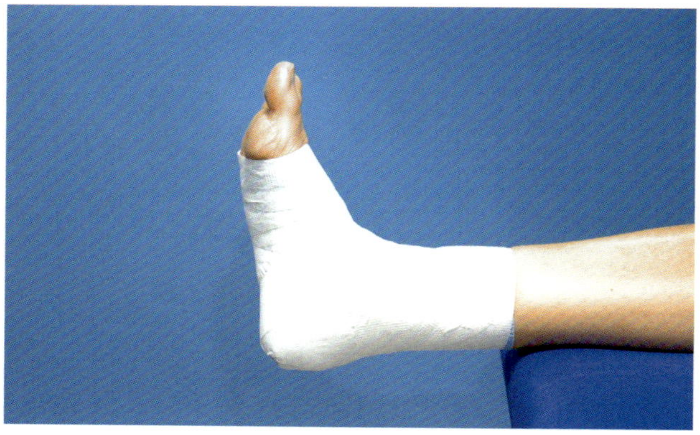

22

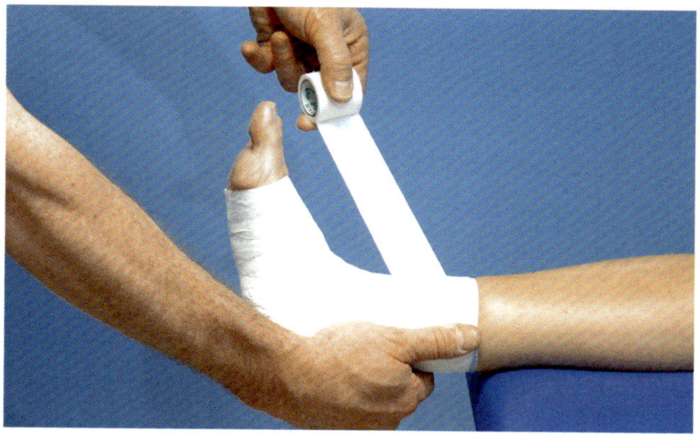

23

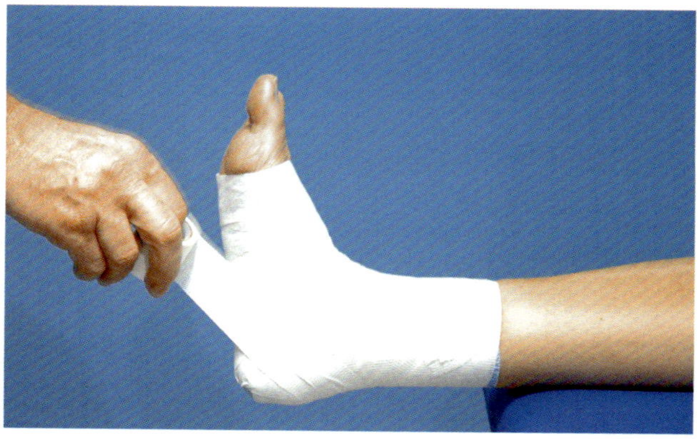

24

Stabilization of the hindfoot and support at the lateral space

17-18 Next, the heel is covered and the bandage is brought toward the lower leg, where it is cut and secured to the bandaging.

19-20 The hindfoot is additionally stabilized with the application of two strips of bandage that pass laterally to the heel. The first strip is applied with a pulling force laterally to medially, then it is passed behind the Achilles tendon to wrap the lateral part of the heel.

21 From here, the bandage passes below the plantar arch and is directed toward the tibiotarsal joint.

22 The bandage is now cut and adhered to the bandaging.

23 The second strip of bandage is applied with a medial-to-lateral pulling force.

24 After it has passed behind the Achilles tendon, the bandage covers the medial part of the heel.

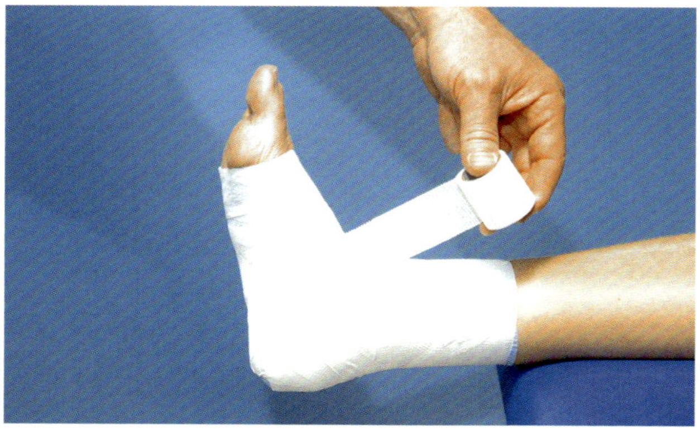

25

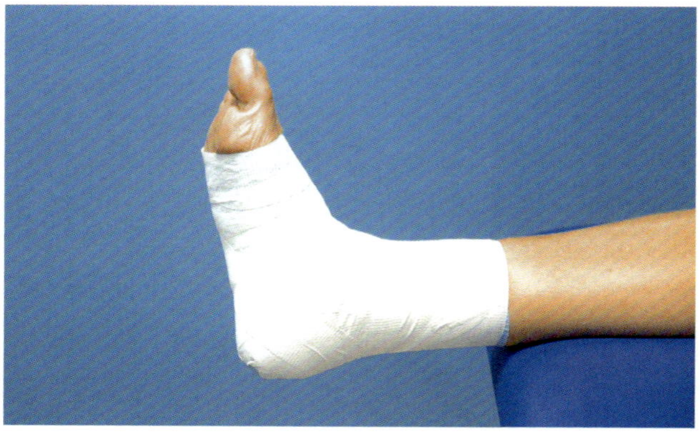

26

Stabilization of the hindfoot and support at the lateral space

25 The bandage crosses the plantar arch and runs toward the dorsum of the tibiotarsal joint, where it is finally cut and adhered to the bandaging.

26 Bandaging is complete.

INDICATIONS

✓ *Preventative sports treatment*

TIBIOTARSAL JOINT

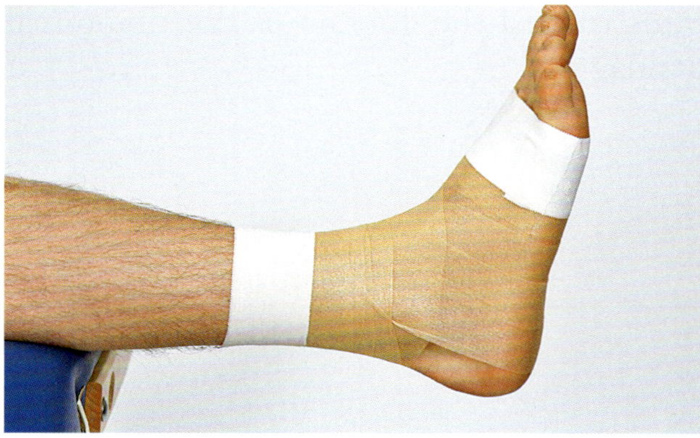

1

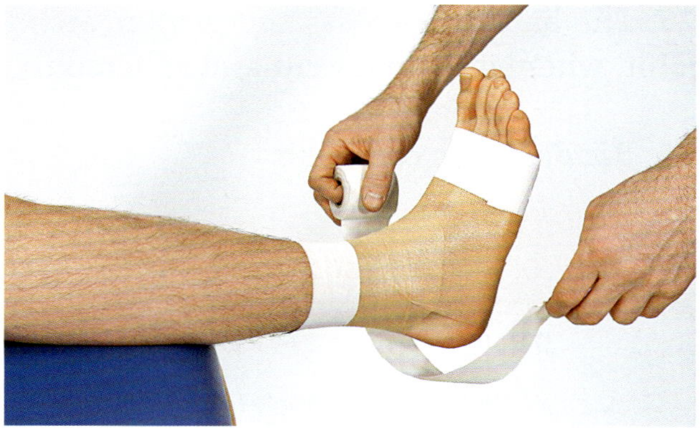

2

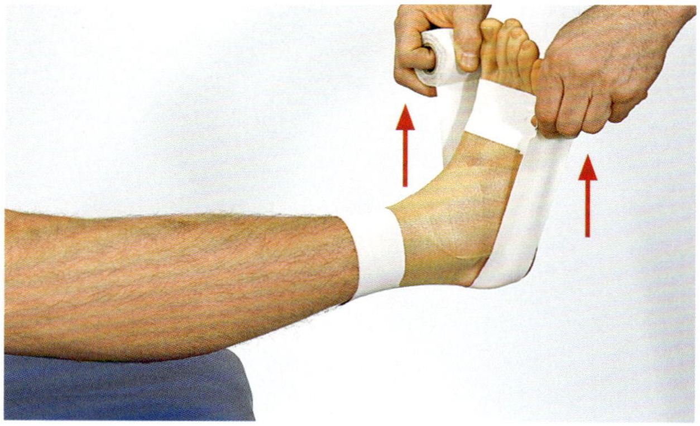

3

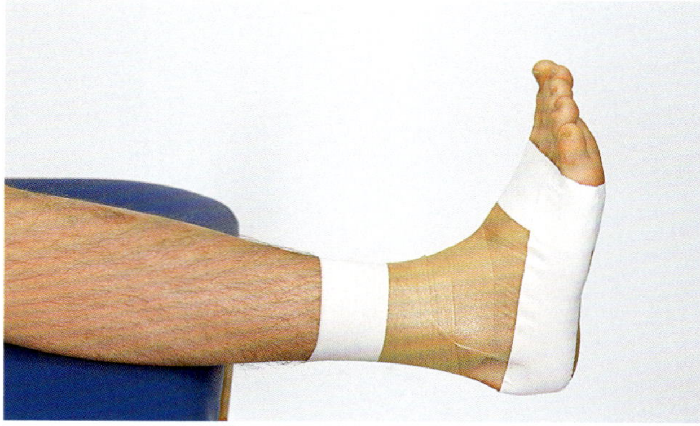

4

Support via inelastic bandage

MATERIAL

- ✓ Inelastic adhesive tape, 5 cm in width
- ✓ Pre-tape bandage

APPLICATION

1 The subject, in the supine position, places the foot off the end of the table and keeps it in 90 degrees dorsal flexion. The foot is prepared by applying base bandaging (see pages 178-181) made with pre-tape bandage. The proximal and distal anchoring points are prepared on the bandaging using two strips of inelastic adhesive tape.

2-3-4 A strip of inelastic adhesive tape is placed so as to cover the hindfoot. After adhering it to the heel, it is placed under tension by pulling it toward the toes, and is then applied to the distal anchoring point.

> *Before starting this bandaging, the tendinous projections must be protected by preparing pre-tape or foam rubber pads (see page 179).*

> *The bandaging may also be applied directly onto the skin, without using the pre-tape bandage.*

TIBIOTARSAL JOINT

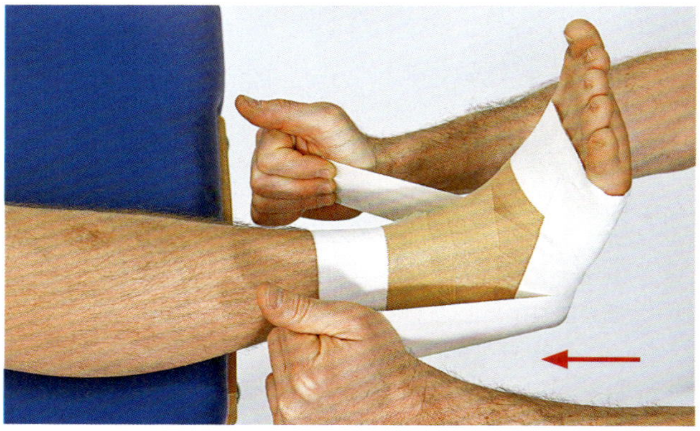

5

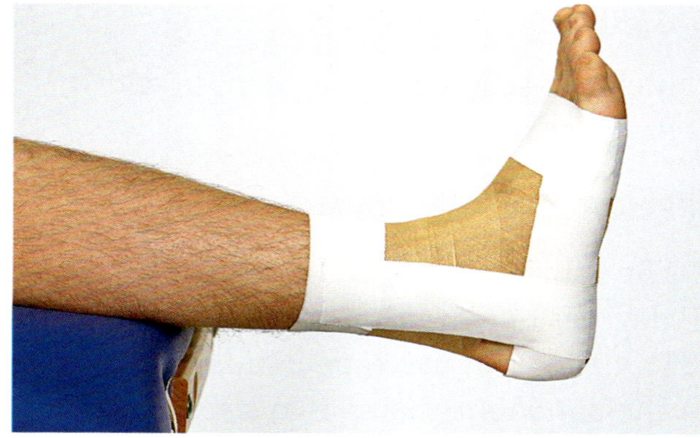

6

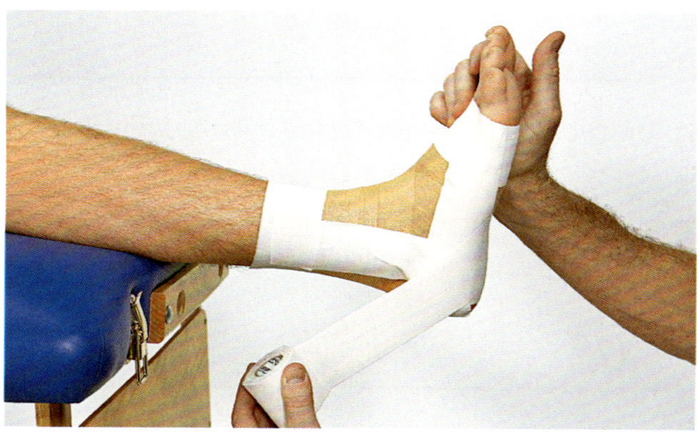

7

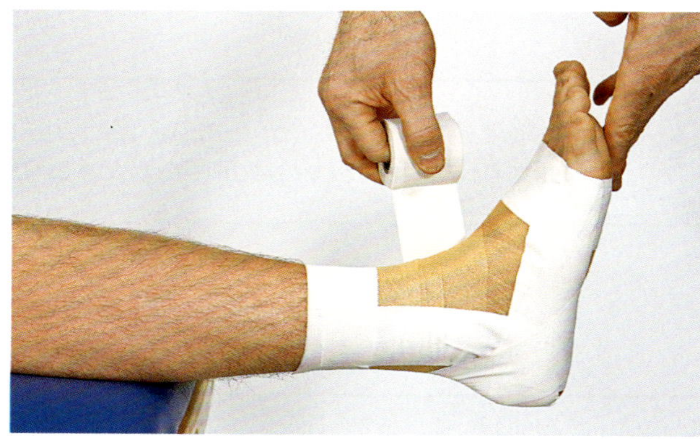

8

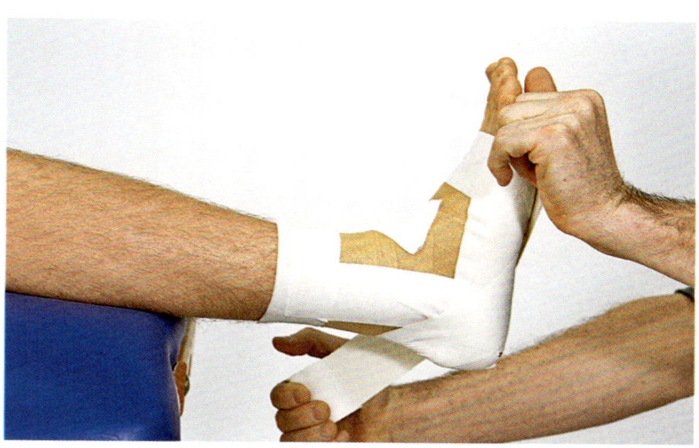

9

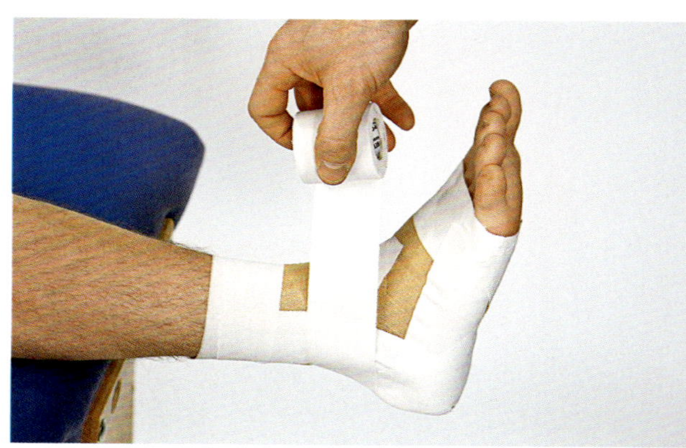

10

Support via inelastic bandage

5-6 Another strip of inelastic adhesive tape is placed so as to cover the inferior area of the heel. After putting it under tension, it is adhered to the proximal anchoring point.

7-8 A piece of tape is then applied starting from the distal anchoring point at the metatarsal head of the first toe to direct it over the lateral region of the heel, then under the lateral malleolus, behind and over the Achilles tendon, and finally over the dorsal area of the tibiotarsal joint.

9-10 Another piece of tape starts from the distal anchoring point at the metatarsal head of the fifth toe and is then directed over the medial part of the heel, then under the medial malleolus, behind and over the Achilles tendon, and finally over the dorsal area of the tibiotarsal joint.

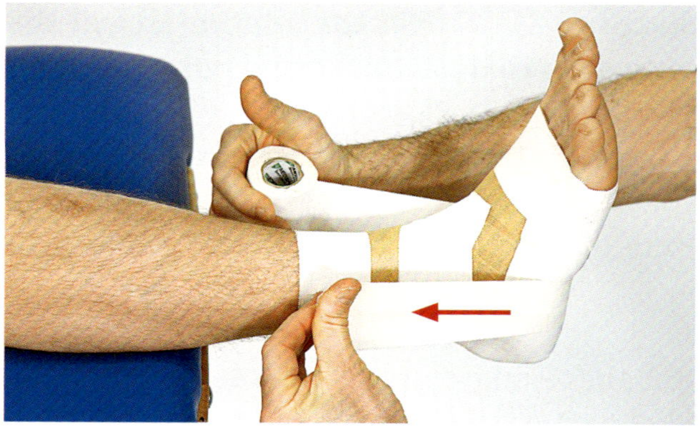

11

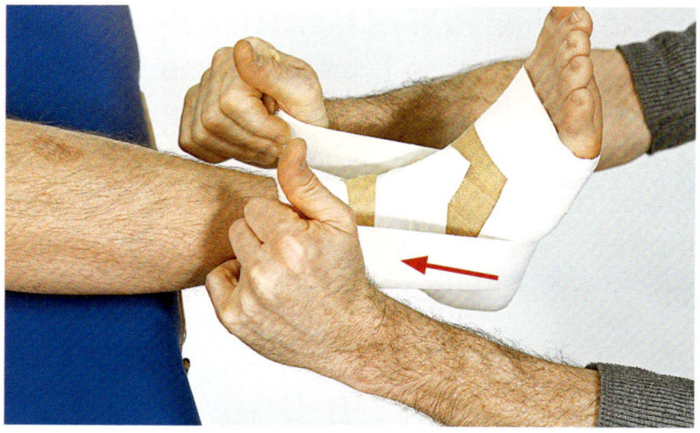

12

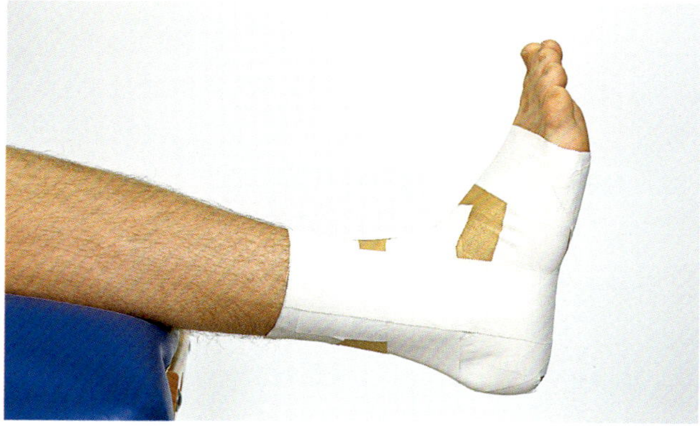

13

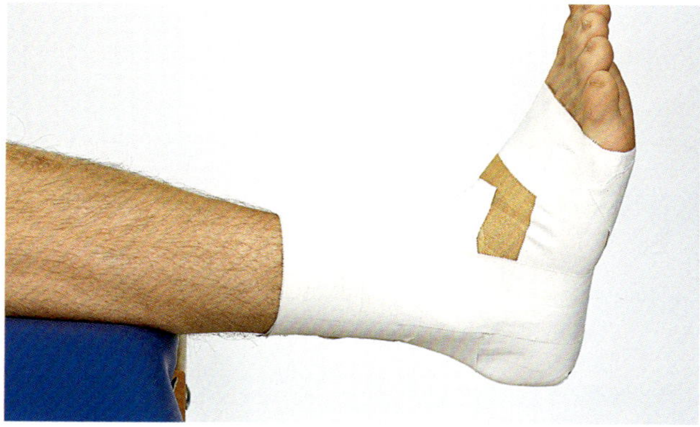

14

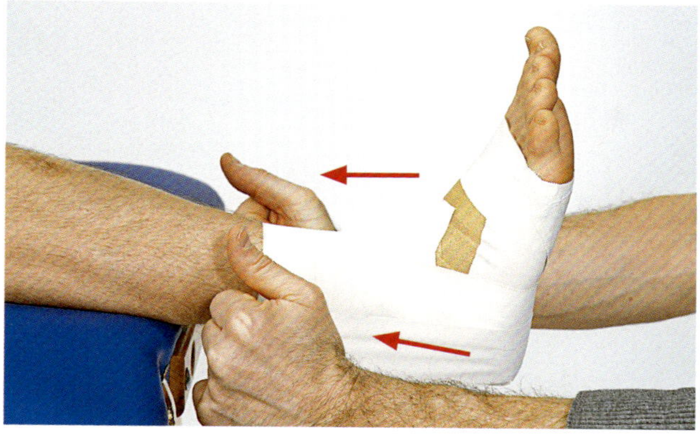

15

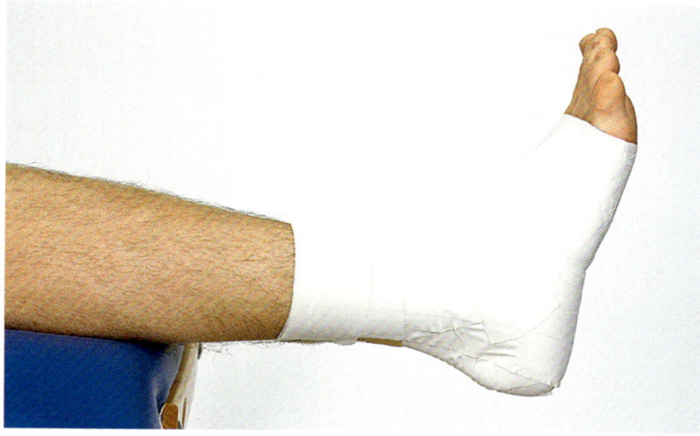

16

Support via inelastic bandage

11-12-13 A strip of tape is adhered over the one previously applied to cover the inferior area of the heel, overlapping it by 50%; this strip, after covering the inferior region of the heel, passes anteriorly to the medial and lateral malleoli and ends over the proximal anchoring point.

14 The bandaging is held in place with pieces of tape applied in a semicircle on the proximal anchoring point.

15 A third strip of tape is adhered to those previously applied to cover the inferior region of the heel; this piece of tape overlaps the first by 50%, passing posteriorly to the medial and lateral malleoli and always ending on the proximal anchoring point.

16 The bandaging is finished and secured by applying several strips of tape in a semicircle until all free spaces are covered.

INDICATIONS

✓ *Preventative sports treatment*

TIBIOTARSAL JOINT

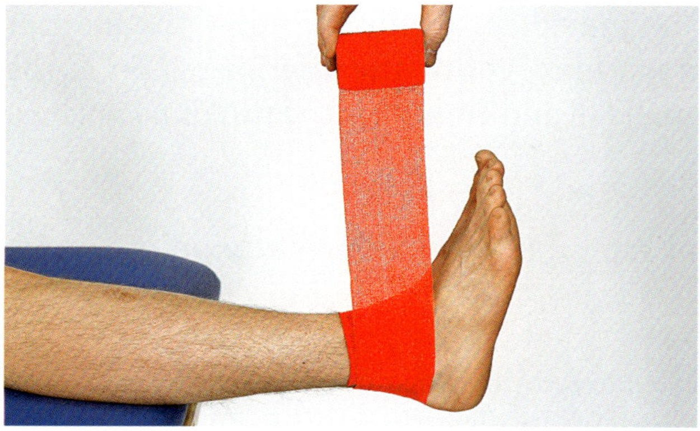
1

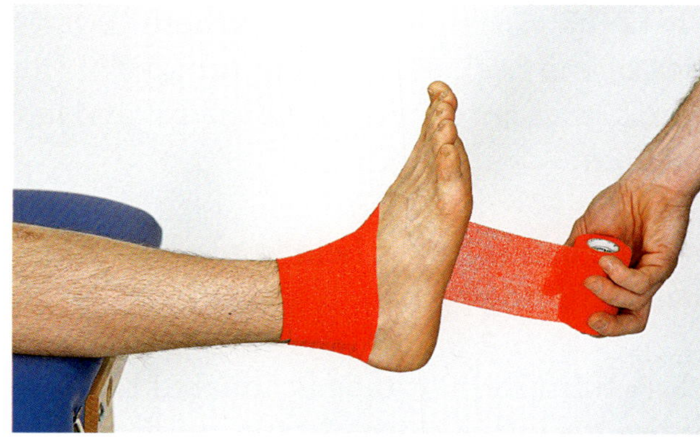
2

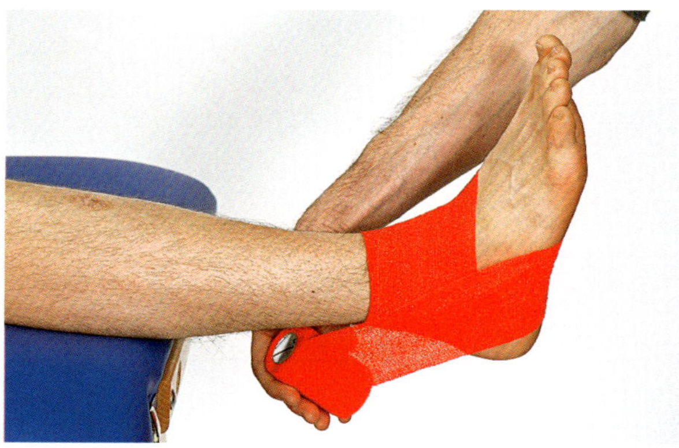
3

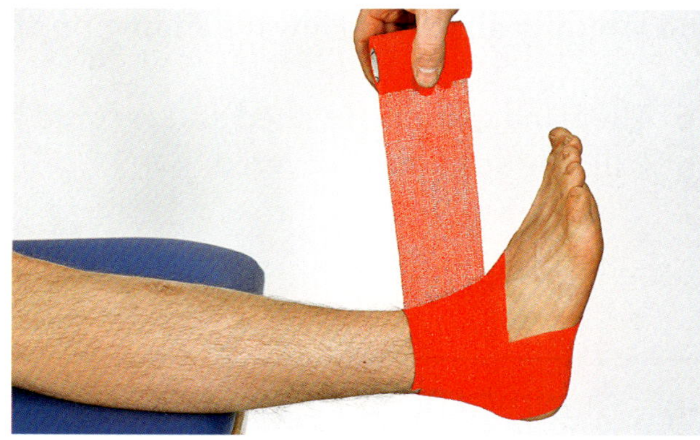
4

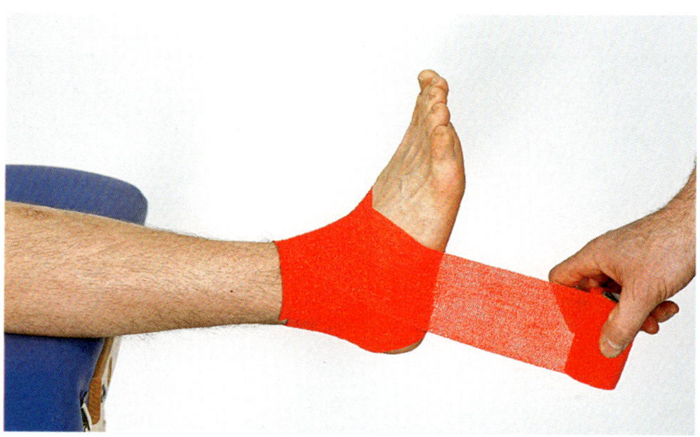
5

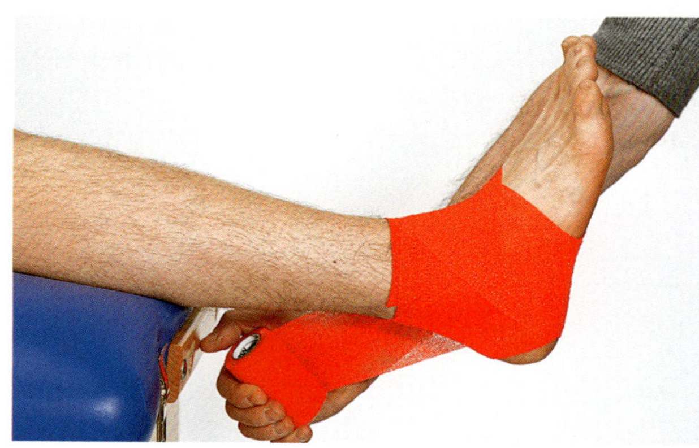
6

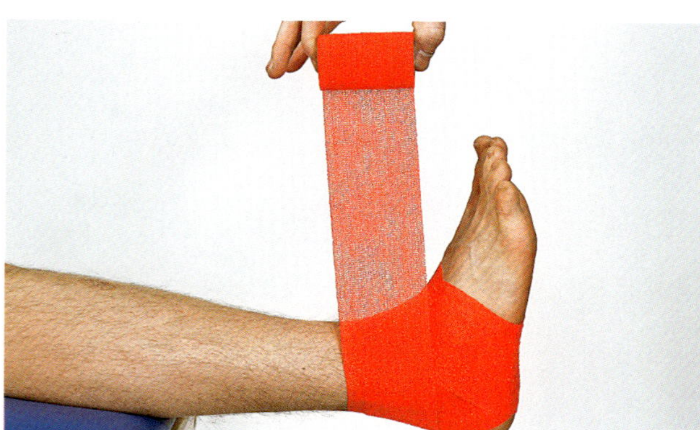
7

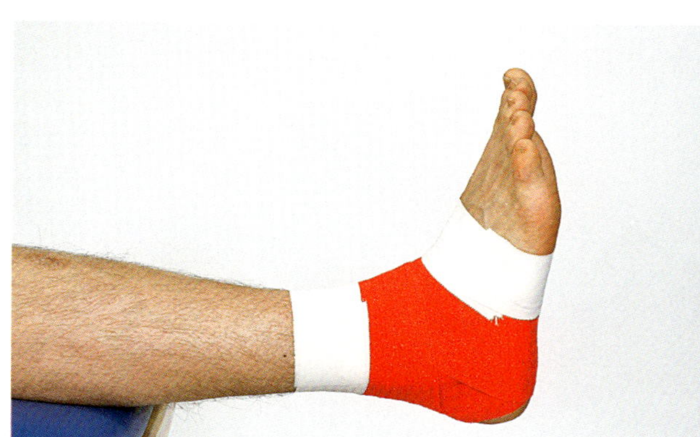
8

Stabilization of the hindfoot

MATERIAL

✓ 5 or 7.5 cm wide cohesive bandage
✓ Inelastic adhesive tape for affixing the bandage

APPLICATION

1 The subject, in the supine position, places the lower leg off the end of the table, keeping it in 90 degrees dorsal flexion. To begin, a wrap of bandage is made to cover the distal tibiofibular joint.

2-3 The bandage is brought under the plantar arch in a direction parallel to the axis of the lower leg, where it goes on to cover two thirds of the heel at its inferior and lateral portions.

4-5 After covering the Achilles tendon, the bandage runs perpendicular to the axis of the lower leg and then passes over the dorsal portion of the tibiotarsal joint.

6 The bandage is brought under the plantar arch, where it goes on to cover two thirds of the heel at its inferior and medial portions.

7-8 After covering the Achilles tendon, the bandage runs perpendicular to the axis of the lower leg: from this position, it is possible to both repeat the bandage wrappings already done in order to additionally reinforce the bandaging, and to apply a complete wrap of bandage around the distal tibiofibular joint in order to then secure the bandaging with the distal and proximal anchoring points created with strips of inelastic adhesive tape.

INDICATIONS

✓ *Preventative sports treatment*

TIBIOTARSAL JOINT

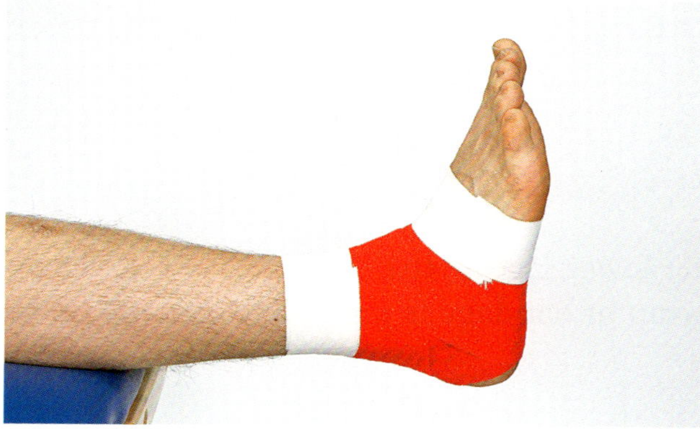

1

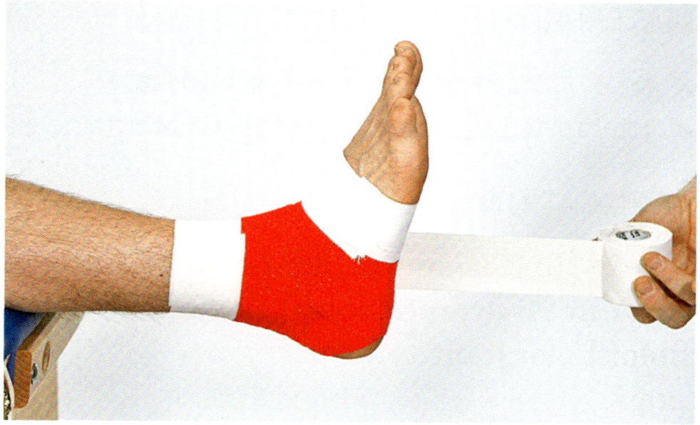

2

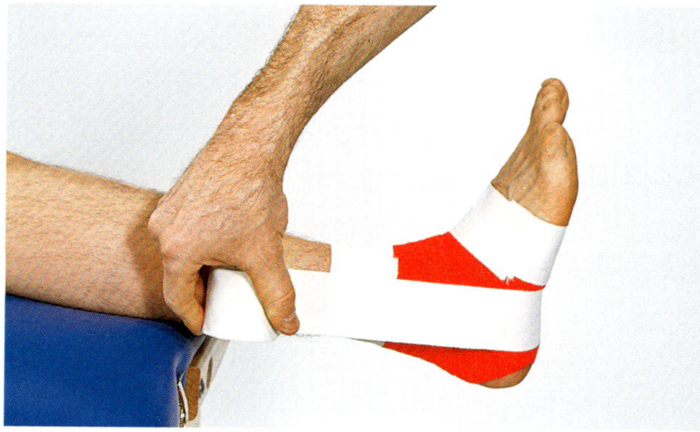

3

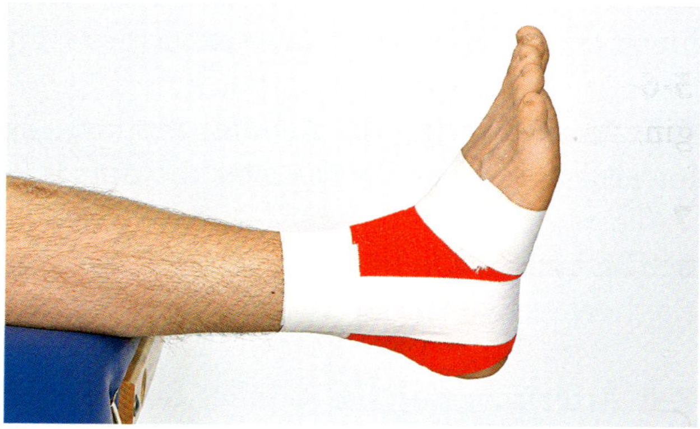

4

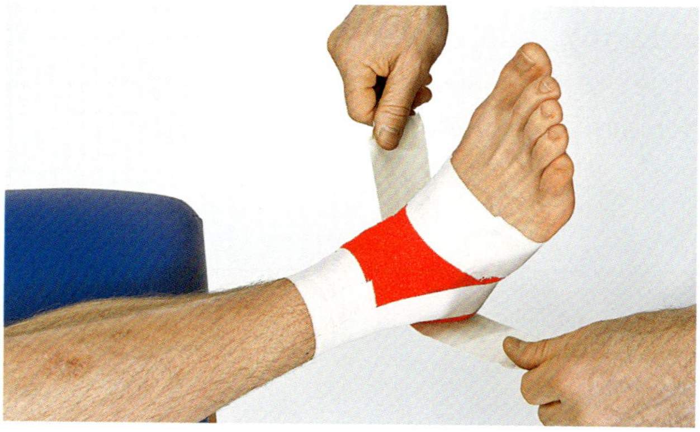

5

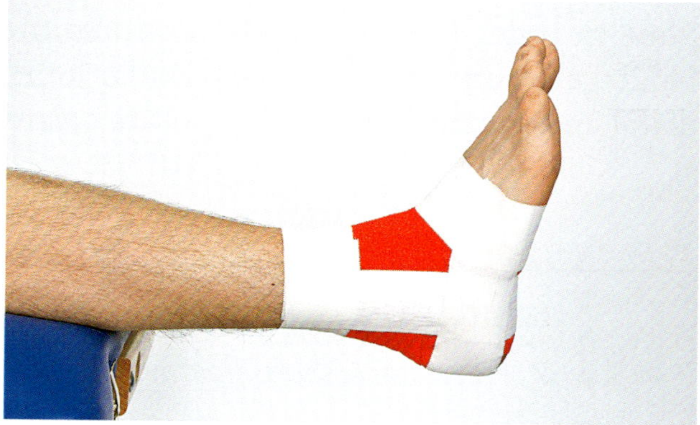

6

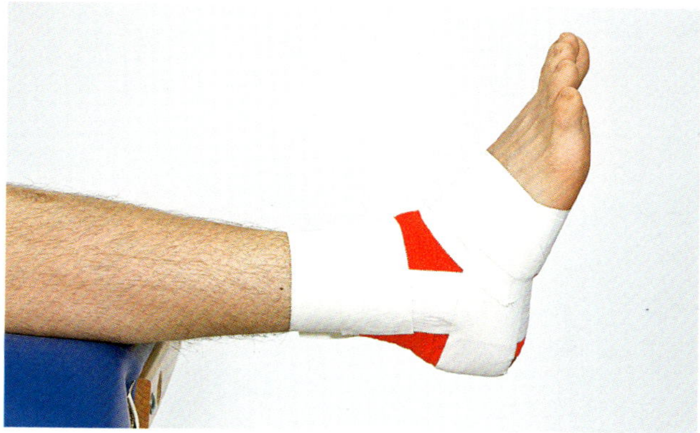

7

Stabilization of the hindfoot reinforced with tape

MATERIAL

✓ 5 or 7.5 cm wide cohesive bandage
✓ Inelastic adhesive tape, 5 cm in width

APPLICATION

1-2-3-4 After finishing a Louisiana-type bandaging of the ankle and preparing proximal and distal anchoring points (see pages 204-205), bandaging proceeds by applying a wrap of inelastic adhesive tape. The tape begins from the medial region of the proximal anchoring point and ends in its lateral region, reaching the medial malleolus, the heel, and the lateral malleolus. The tape must be placed under tension while it is being applied.

5-6 Another wrap of inelastic adhesive tape under tension posteriorly covers the heel, beginning and ending on the distal anchoring point.

7 The bandage is fixed in place with several strips of inelastic adhesive tape applied in a semicircle.

INDICATIONS

✓ *Preventative sports treatment*

TIBIOTARSAL JOINT

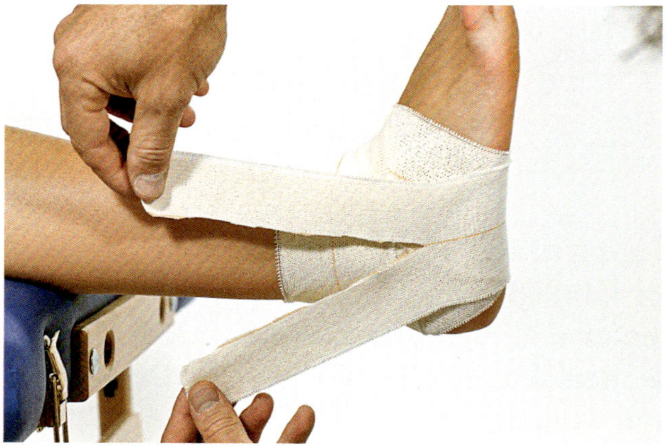

1

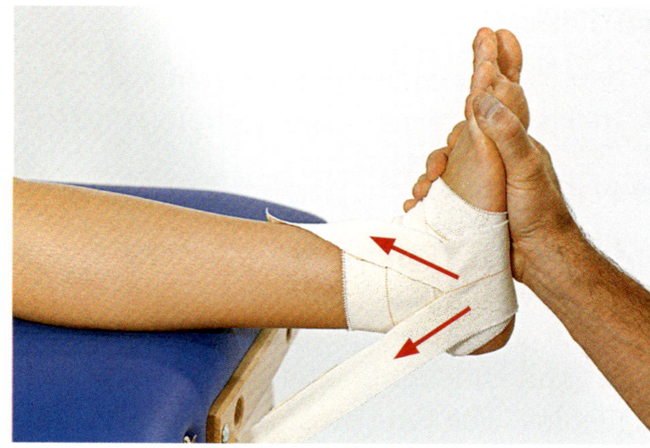

2

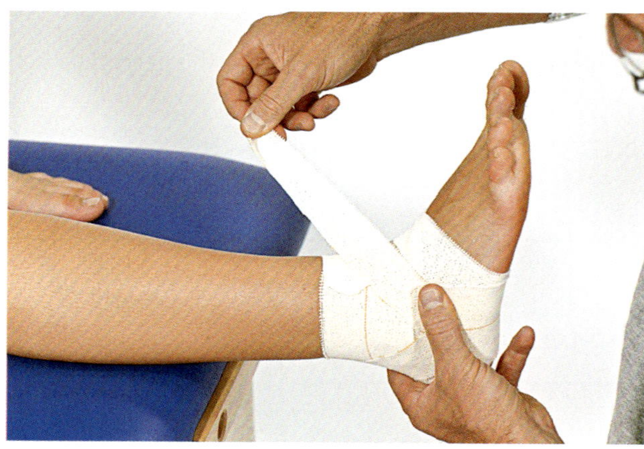

3

Retention of the lateral space

MATERIAL

✓ Cotton fabric porous elastic adhesive bandage that can be stretched lengthwise, 7.5 cm in width

APPLICATION

1 After finishing a figure-eight bandaging on the ankle, the end of the bandage is cut into a Y to form two strips to be used to finish bandaging. The part of the bandage where the two cut strips join is adhered below the fibular malleolus.

2 The two parts of the bandage that are still free are tensed by 70%. The first part is passed behind the Achilles tendon.

3 The second part is secured to the dorsal surface of the ankle.

INDICATIONS

✓ *Injuries of the ligaments of the lateral space in recovery*
✓ *Ankle instability*

TIBIOTARSAL JOINT

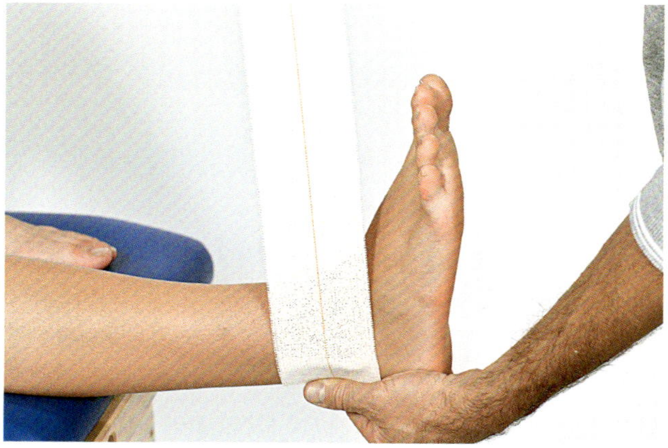

1

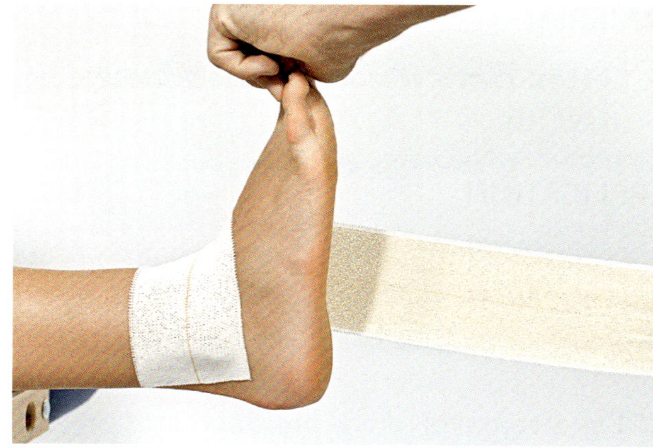

2

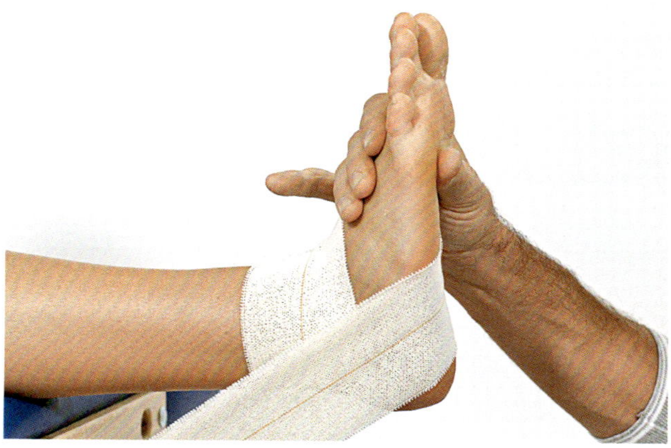

3

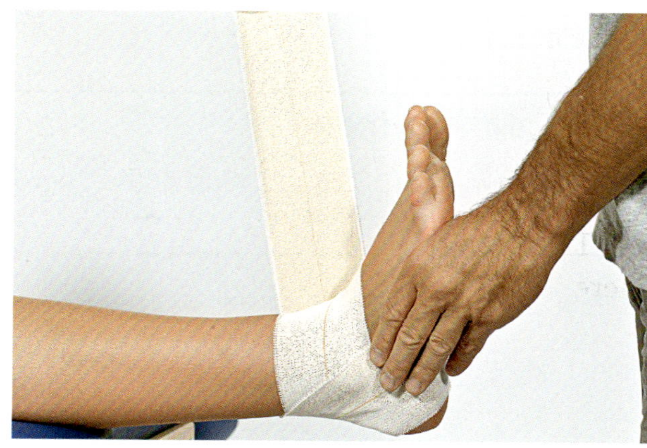

4

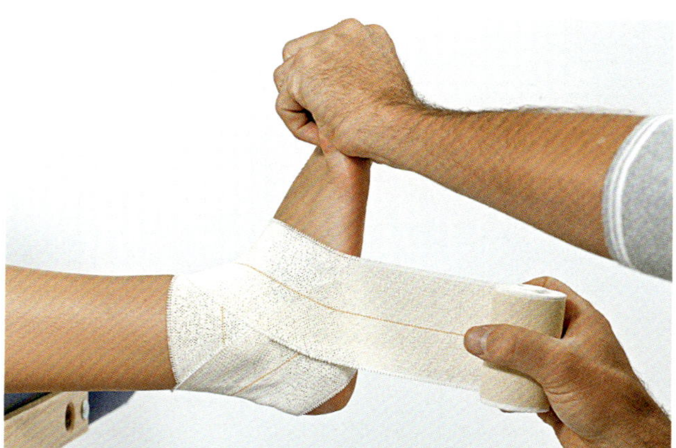

5

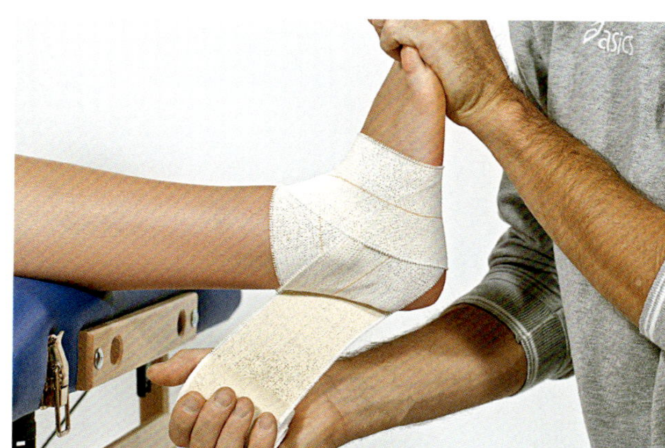

6

Stabilization of the lateral space

MATERIAL

- ✓ Cotton fabric porous elastic adhesive bandage that can be stretched lengthwise, 5 or 7.5 cm in width
- ✓ Inelastic adhesive tape for affixing the bandage

APPLICATION

1 The subject, in the supine position, places the foot off the end of the table, keeping it in 90 degrees dorsal flexion. Securing the bandage with the thumb posterior to the lateral malleolus, it is put under tension by pulling it in the direction perpendicular to the longitudinal axis of the fibula.

2 The bandage, after dorsally covering the tibiotarsal joint, is pulled in the direction perpendicular to the longitudinal axis of the foot.

3 The bandage then covers the heel, being brought in the direction of the lateral malleolus.

4 After adhering the bandage well to the Achilles tendon, it is run along the skin projection of the medial malleolus and tensed perpendicular to the longitudinal axis of the tibia.

5-6 The bandage dorsally crosses the tibiotarsal joint and runs toward the sole of the foot, where it crosses the previous path of bandage below the heel.

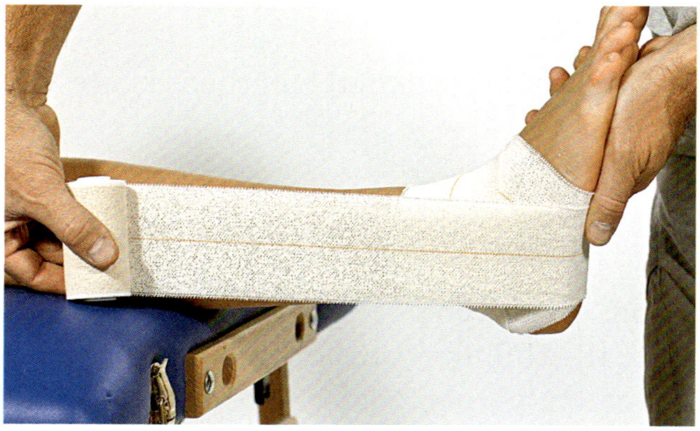
7

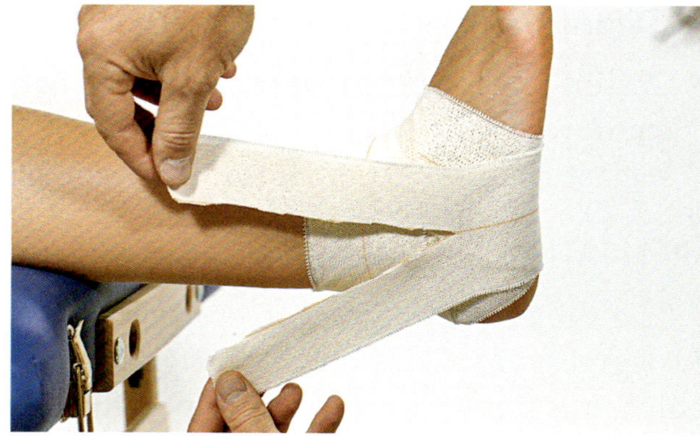
8

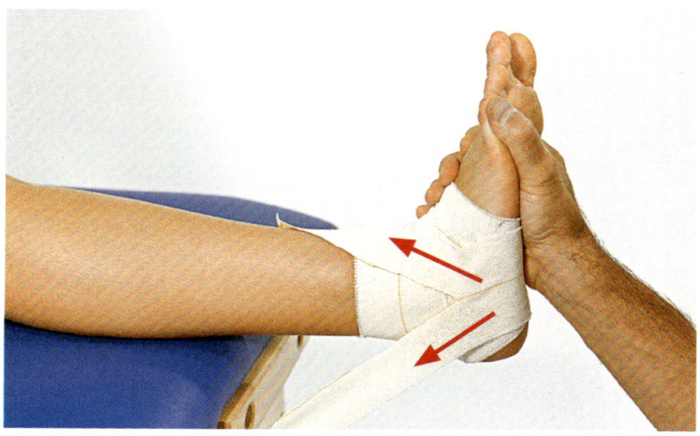
9

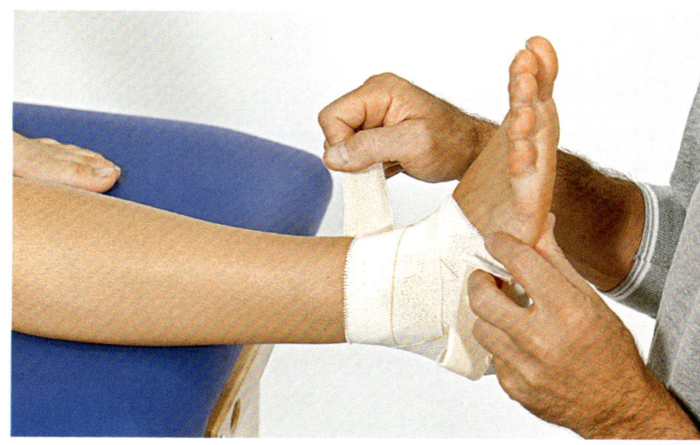
10

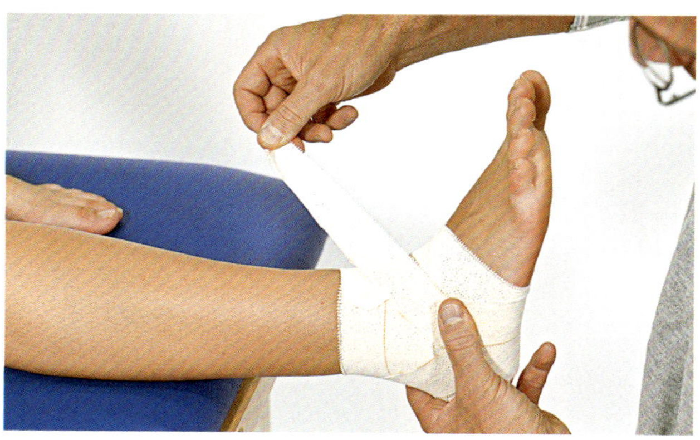
11

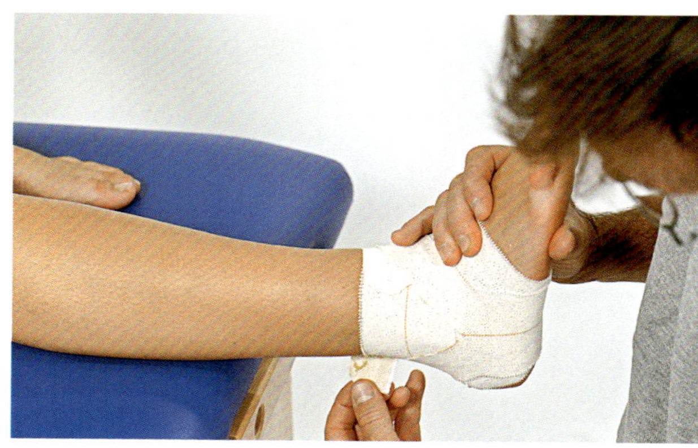
12

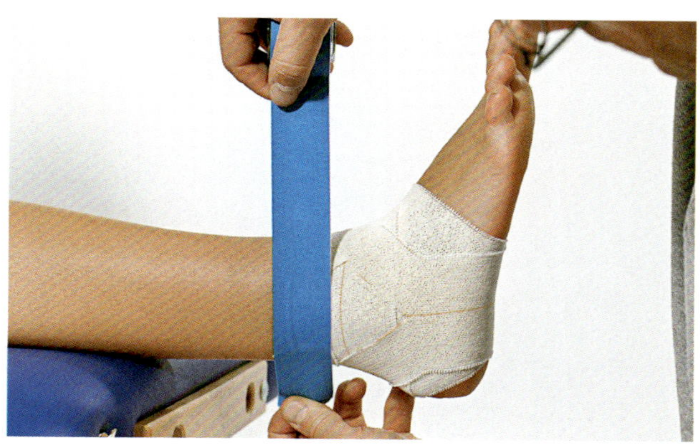
13

Stabilization of the lateral space

7 After dorsally covering the tibiotarsal joint and then the heel again, the bandage runs perpendicular to the axis of the fibula, passing over the projection of the lateral malleolus.

8 The bandage is then cut in half lengthwise until reaching the submalleolar projection of the fibula.

9-10-11-12 The two free pieces of bandage are put under tension around the distal third of the lower leg; one is made to pass behind the Achilles tendon and the other on the dorsal surface of the ankle.

13 The bandaging is secured with a wrap of inelastic adhesive tape.

INDICATIONS

✓ *Sprains of the tibiotarsal joint in the lateral space*

✓ *Preventative sports treatment*

TIBIOTARSAL JOINT

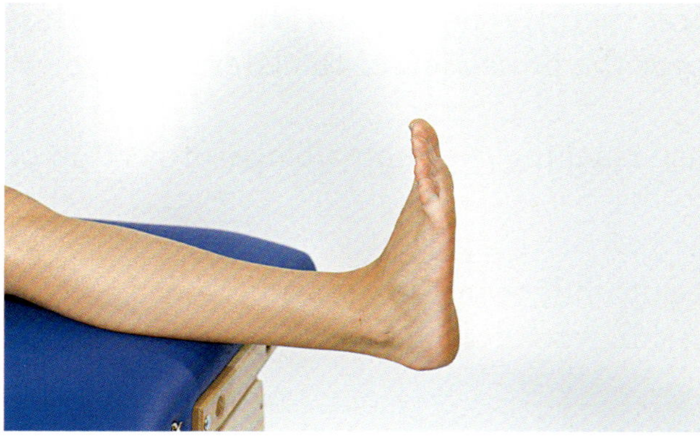
1

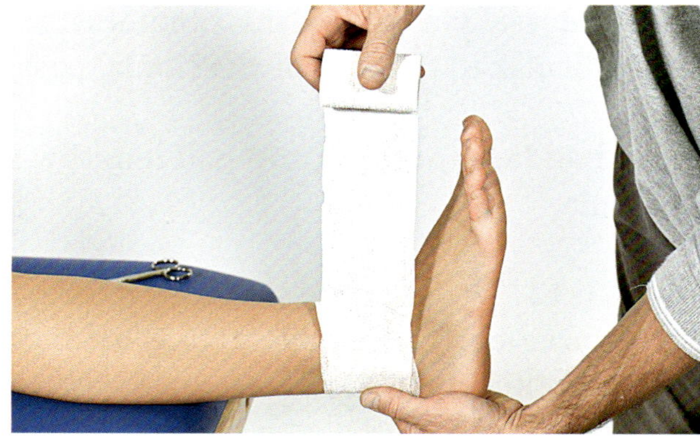
2

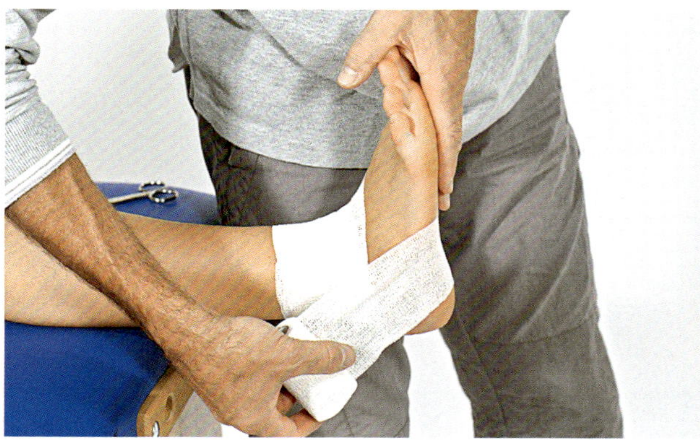
3

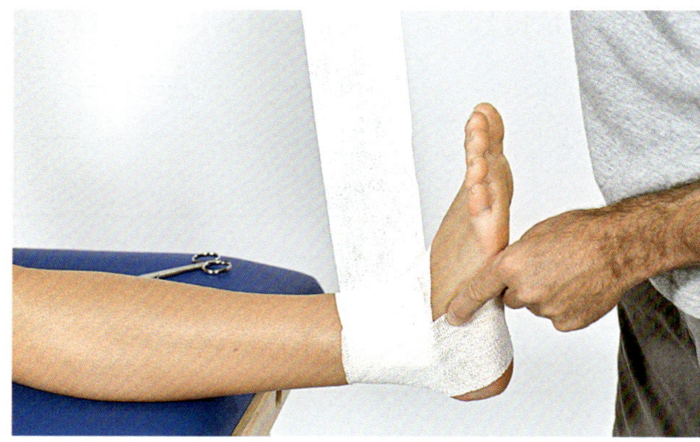
4

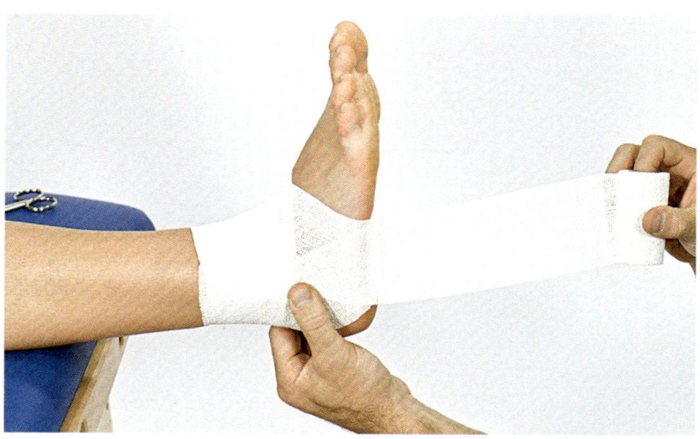
5

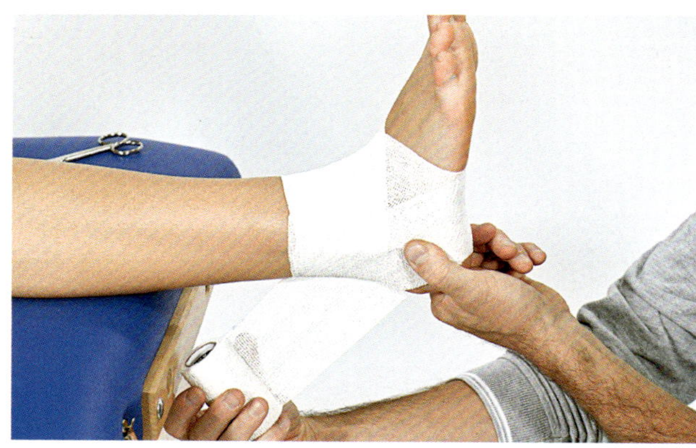
6

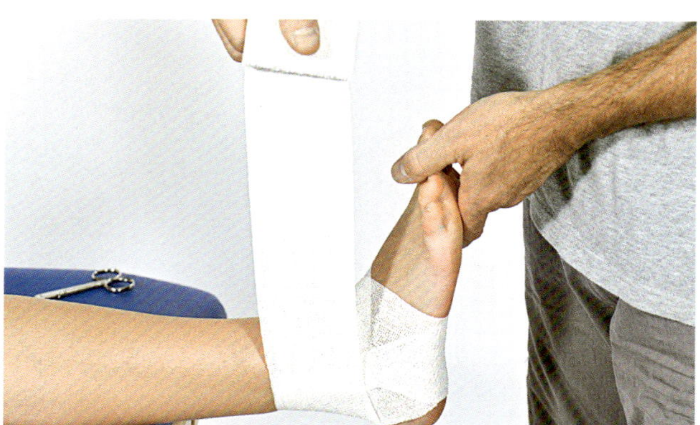
7

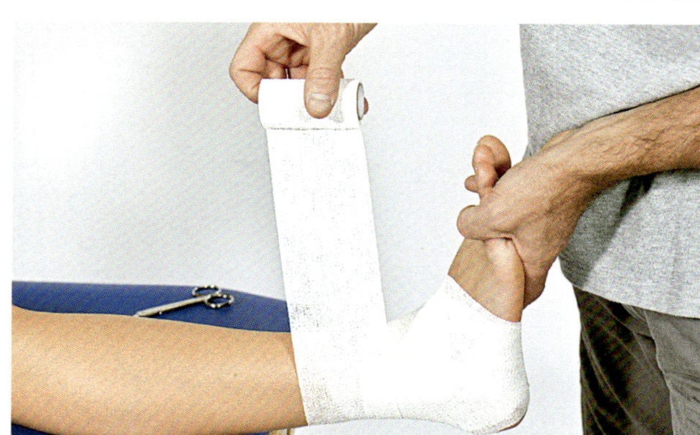
8

Stabilization of the lateral space with reinforcement

MATERIAL

- ✓ 7.5 cm wide cohesive bandage
- ✓ Inelastic adhesive tape

APPLICATION

1 The subject lies supine and keeps the foot in dorsal flexion at 90 degrees.

2 To begin, a complete wrap of the bandage is made at the distal third of the lower leg, starting from the lateral malleolus. With the wrap finished, the bandage is pulled perpendicular to the longitudinal axis of the lower leg.

3 The bandage is first medially brought to cover the dorsum of the foot, and is then directed under the plantar arch and made to run toward the lateral region of the heel.

4 The bandage passes behind the Achilles tendon and is again pulled perpendicular to the axis of the tibia.

5 After having covered the dorsal region of the tibiotarsal joint, the bandage is directed over the heel, having it pass over the lateral malleolus.

6 The bandage passes under the plantar arch, covering the hindfoot, and is then directed toward the Achilles tendon.

7-8 Next, several complete wraps of bandage are made at the distal third of the lower leg, and the bandage is then brought perpendicular to the axis of the fibula and cut.

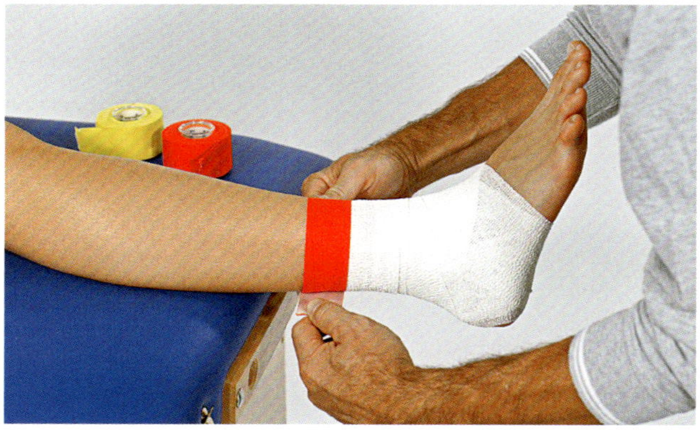

9

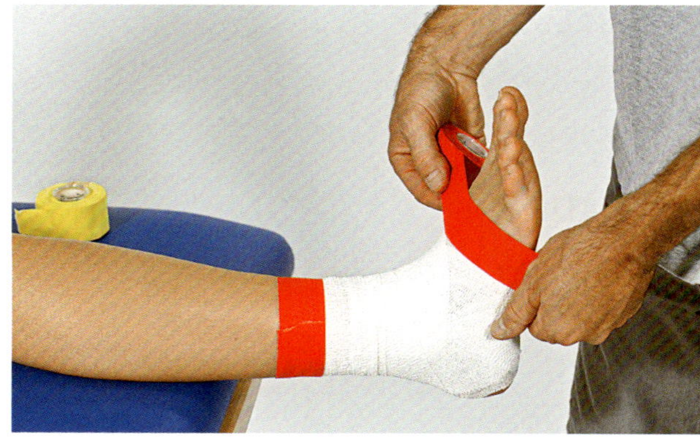

10

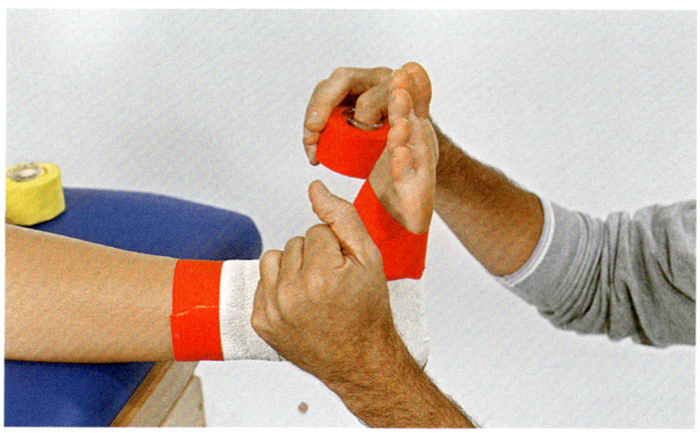

11

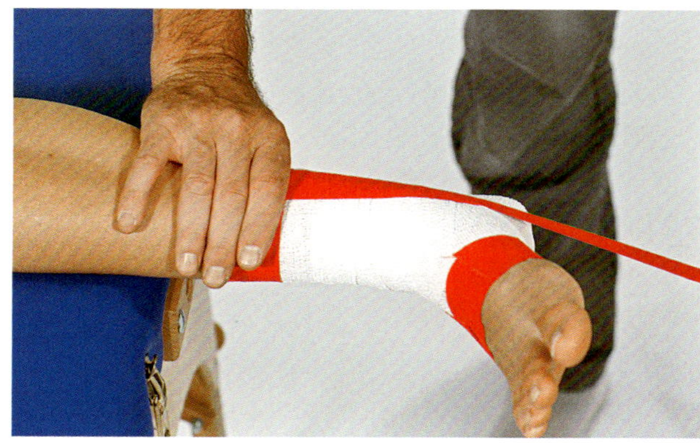

12

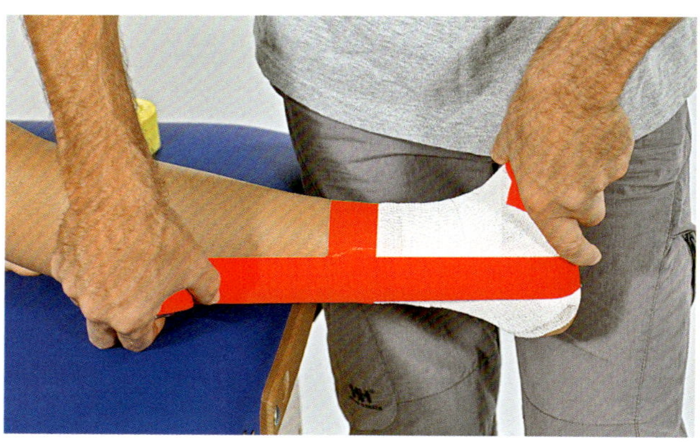

13

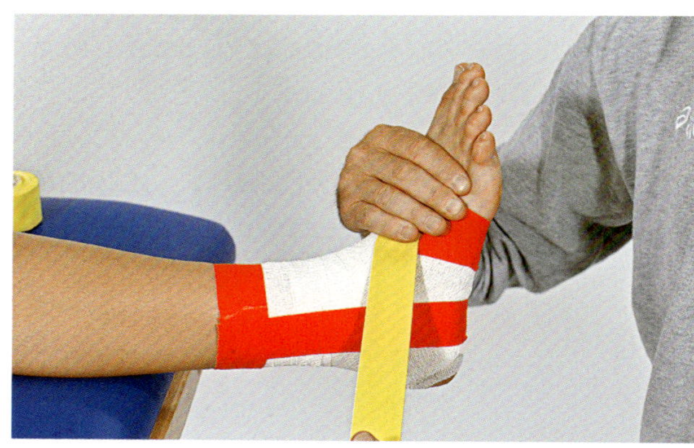

14

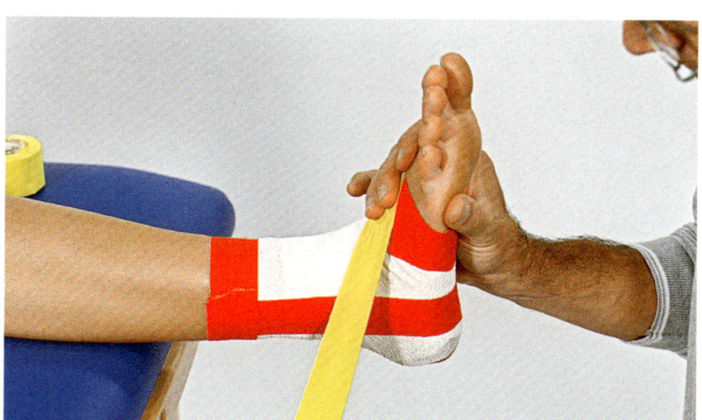

15

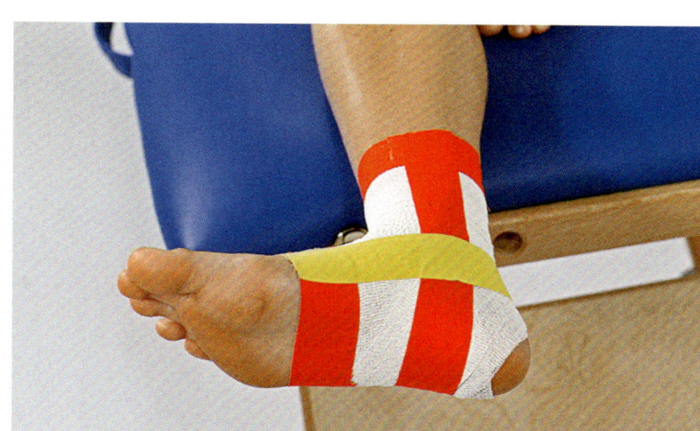

16

Stabilization of the lateral space with reinforcement

9-10-11 In order to prepare the proximal and distal anchoring points, strips of inelastic adhesive tape are used; rather than using a single strip of tape to do a full wrap around the lower leg or forefoot, it is recommended that two strips be used for each anchoring point, applying them in a semicircle.

12 Now the first inelastic adhesive strip is applied for the unloading of the calcaneofibular ligament: the tape leaves from the medial region of the proximal anchoring point and longitudinally goes directly to the axis of the tibia, to cover the tibial malleolus, which is a medial "landmark" of the path of tape for unloading. In this path, the tape is well adhered without being placed under tension.

13 After covering the heel, the tape passes over the skin projection of the fibular malleolus, which is the lateral "landmark" for the path of unloading tape. The hindfoot is put in talus valgus position, then a piece of tape is brought into tension along the longitudinal axis of the fibula and applied to the lateral portion of the proximal anchoring point.

14 Bandaging proceeds with the application of the first inelastic adhesive tape necessary for the unloading of the anterior talofibular ligament: the tape starts over the distal anchoring point at the ray of the first toe and is directed toward the fibular malleolus.

> *When applying the strips of inelastic adhesive tape, the compression of the styloid process of the fifth toe must be absolutely avoided.*

15-16 After putting the foot in eversion, the tape goes on to cover the hindfoot and turns to adhere over the distal anchoring point at the projection of the first digit.

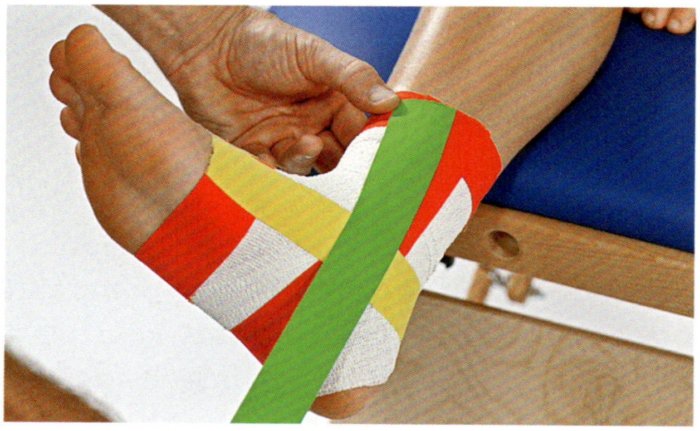

17

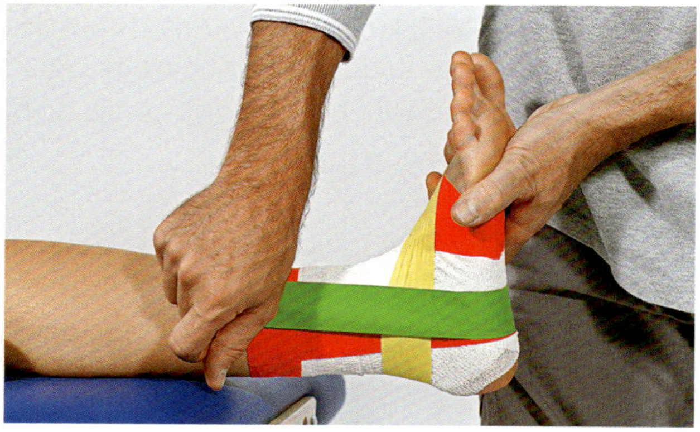

18

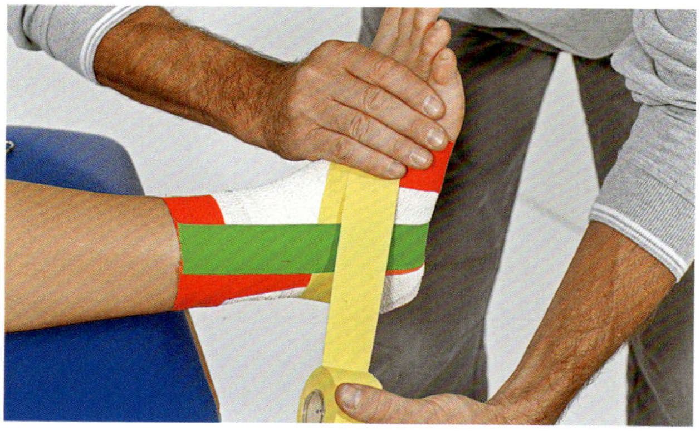

19

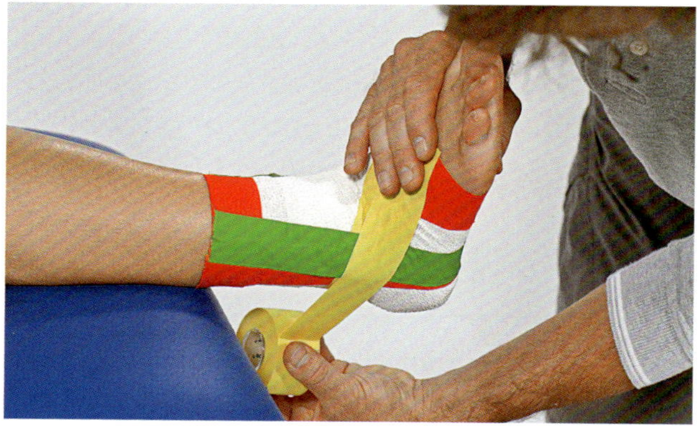

20

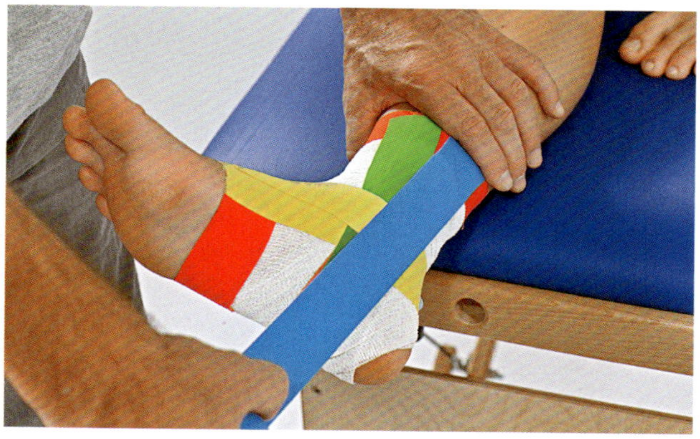

21

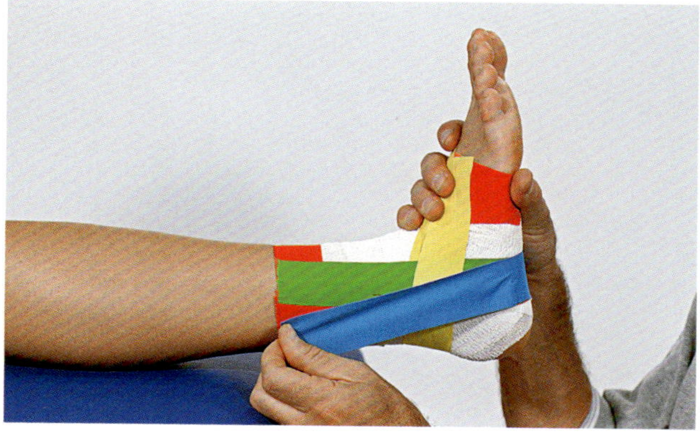

22

Stabilization of the lateral space with reinforcement

17-18 Next, the second piece of tape for the unloading of the calcaneofibular ligament is applied: the tape begins over the proximal anchoring point, in a more anterior position than that of the first strip, and overlaps the first by 50%; like the first strip, this one also passes over the tibial malleolus, covers the heel, passes over the fibular malleolus, and then goes on to adhere over the proximal anchoring point at a more anterior point than the first piece of tape (which is covered by 50%).

19-20 The second piece of tape for the unloading of the anterior talofibular ligament begins over the distal anchoring point at the projection of the rays of the second and third digits; after having put the foot in eversion, the bandage is directed toward the fibular malleolus, covers the hindfoot, and is secured over the distal anchoring point.

> *Always remember to position the hindfoot in valgism before applying the tape to the lateral region of the lower leg.*

21-22 The third piece of tape for the unloading of the calcaneofibular ligament repeats the path of the two preceding strips: the tape begins over the proximal anchoring point, passes over the tibial malleolus, covers the heel, passes over the fibular malleolus, and is affixed over the proximal anchoring point. Note, however, that both points of fixation over the proximal anchoring point are located posterior to those of the first piece of tape, which is then overlapped by this tape by 50%.

TIBIOTARSAL JOINT

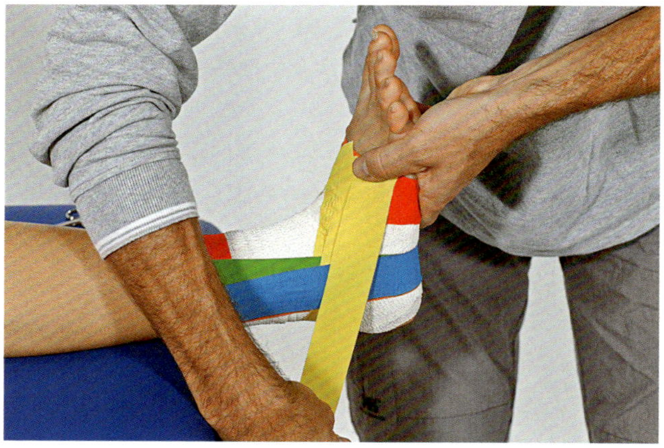
23

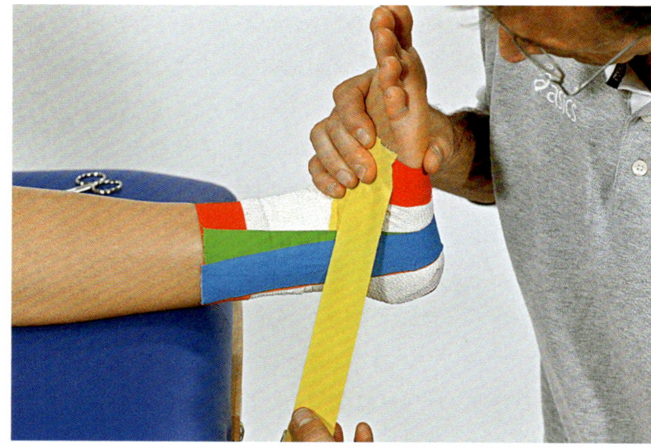
24

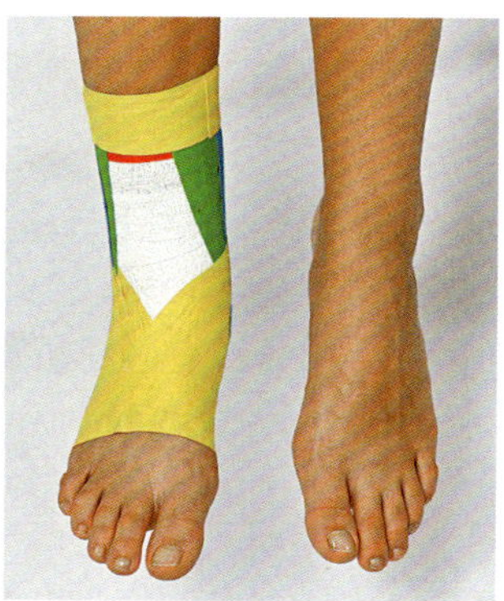
25

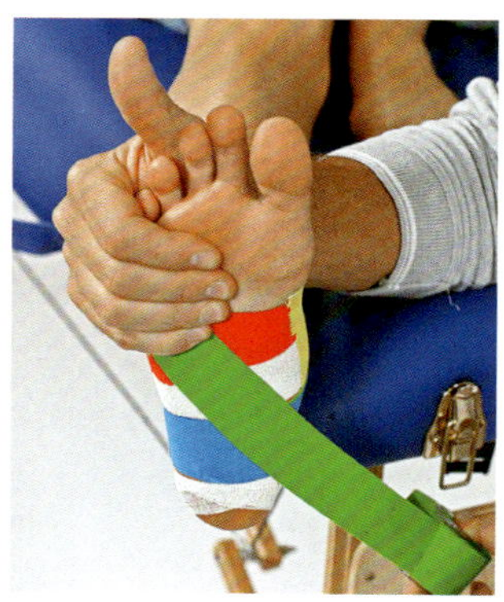
26

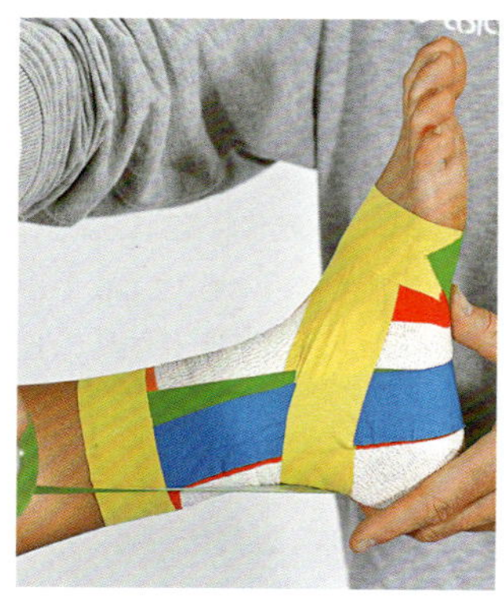
27

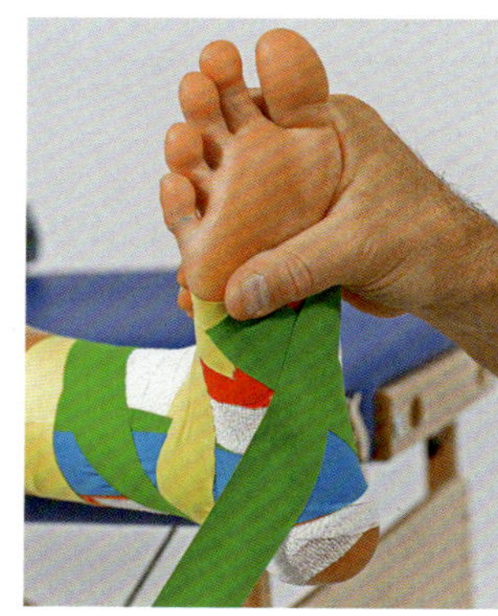
28

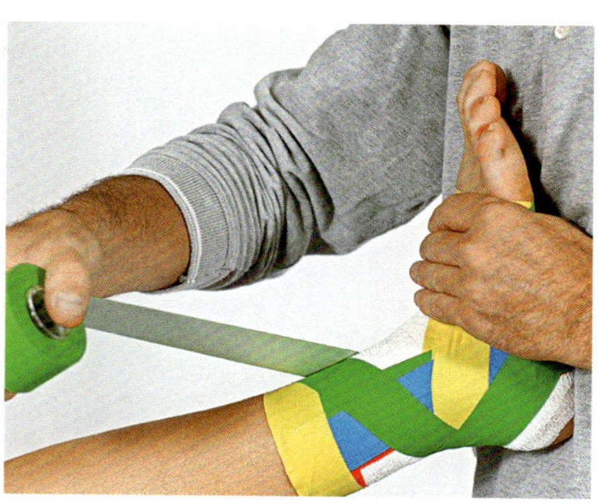
29

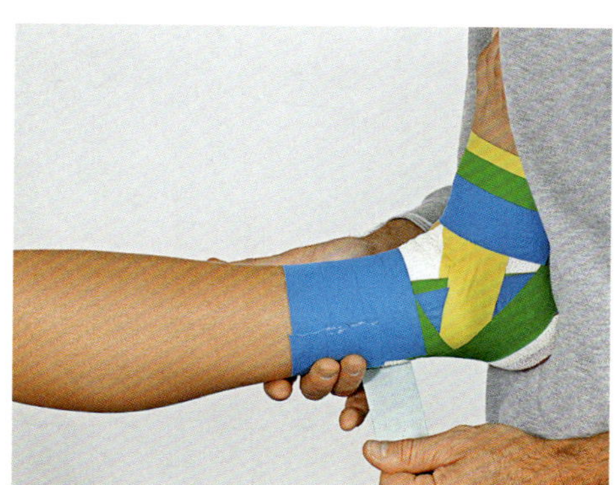
30

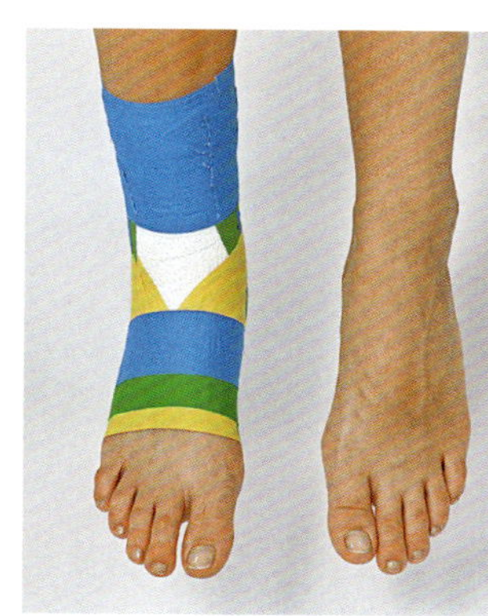
31

Stabilization of the lateral space with reinforcement

23 The third piece of tape for the unloading of the anterior talofibular ligament begins over the distal anchoring point at the projection of the rays of the fourth and fifth digits.

24 After putting the foot in eversion, the tape is directed toward the fibular malleolus, covers the hindfoot, and is then secured over the distal anchoring point.

25 The pieces of tape are now secured by wrapping the distal third of the lower leg and covering the forefoot at the metatarsal heads with strips applied in a semicircle.

26-27-28-29 Two strips of inelastic adhesive tape are used to stabilize the hindfoot. The first is applied over the distal anchoring point beginning from the plantar projection of the fifth digit; this piece of tape is then directed toward the medial projection of the heel in order to have it then run toward the proximal anchoring point after having covered the hindfoot. The second piece of tape begins over the distal anchoring point at the plantar projection of the first digit, is directed toward the lateral projection of the heel, covers the hindfoot, and then runs toward the proximal anchoring point.

30-31 The bandaging is secured and finished with the application of inelastic adhesive strips in a semicircle, which go on to cover the unloading tape.

INDICATIONS

- ✓ *Injuries of the lateral capsuloligamentous space*
- ✓ *Preventative sports treatment*
- ✓ *Capsuloligamentous instability*

TIBIOTARSAL JOINT

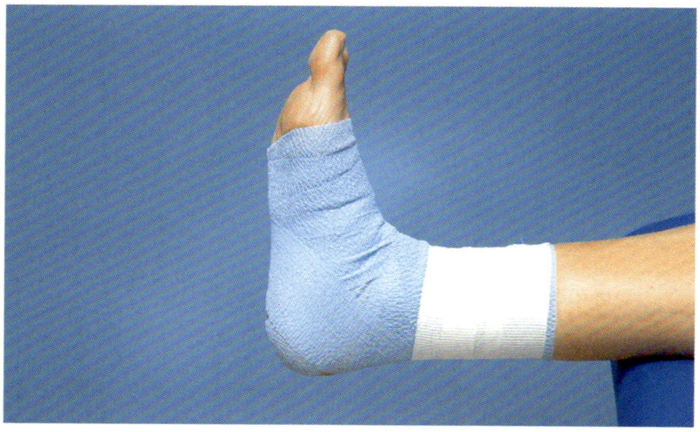
1

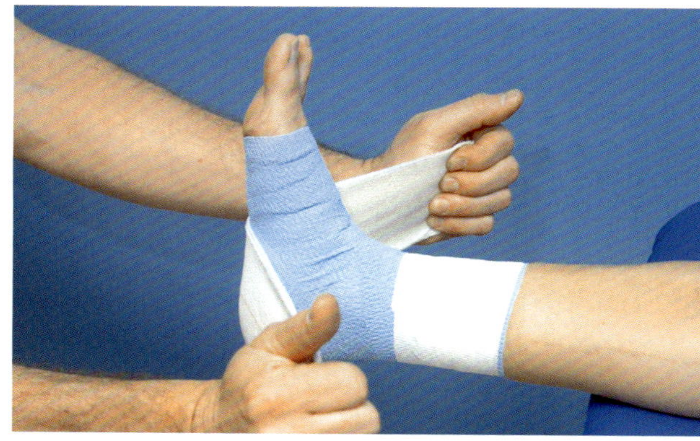
2

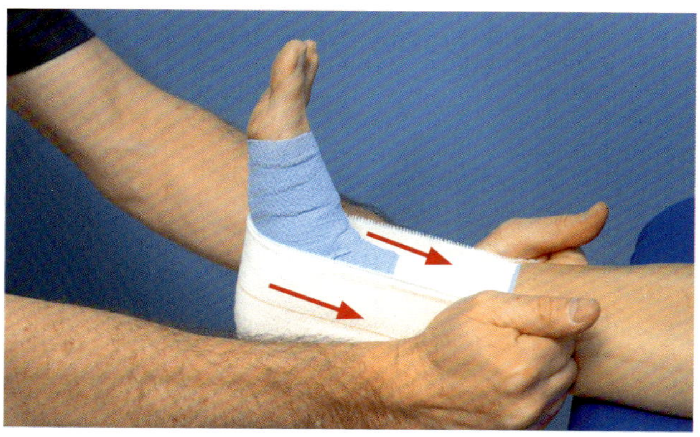
3

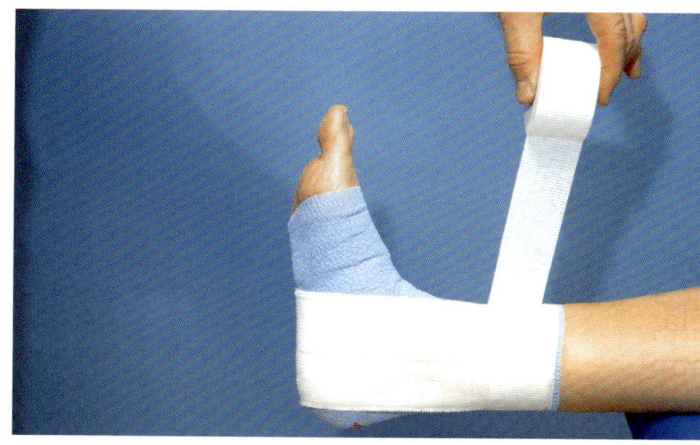
4

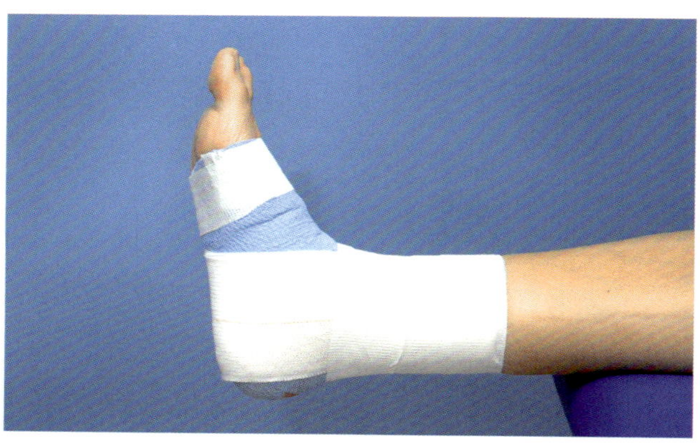
5

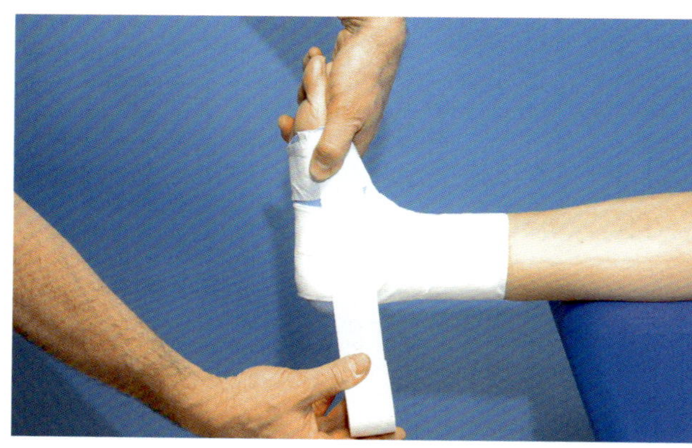
6

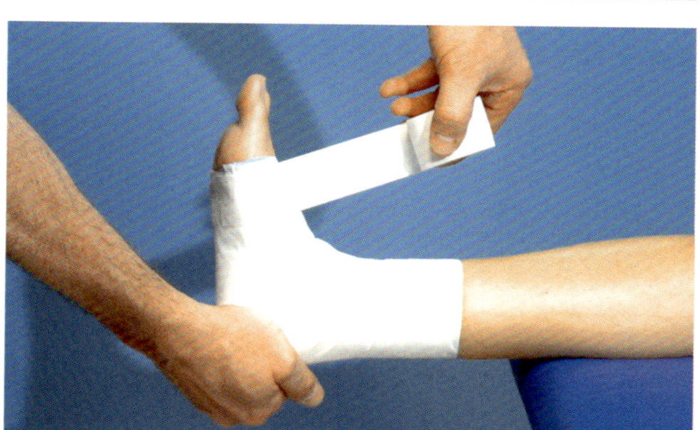
7

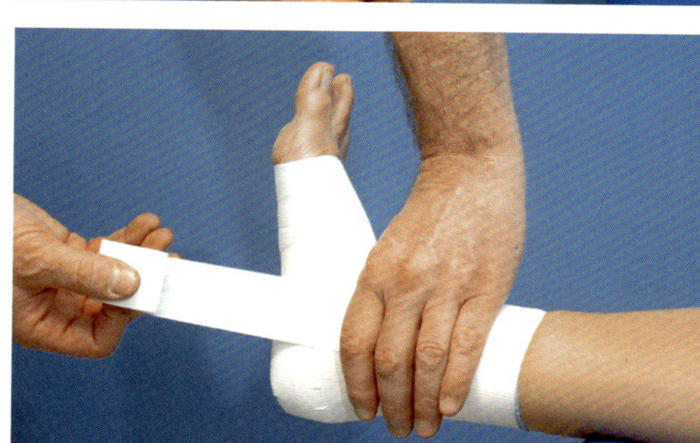
8

Limitation of inversion and eversion

MATERIAL

✓ 7.5 cm wide elastic cohesive bandage for base bandaging
✓ Cotton fabric porous elastic adhesive bandage that can be stretched lengthwise, 7.5 cm in width
✓ 2 cm wide adhesive inelastic bandage

APPLICATION

1 The subject, in the supine position, places the foot off the end of the table. The foot is prepared by applying base bandaging with a cohesive elastic bandage (see pages 184-185), on which an anchoring point is made with several wraps of inelastic bandage at the distal third of the lower leg.

The reinforced fastener must be made by overlapping two strips of mono-extensible elastic adhesive bandage of the proper length.

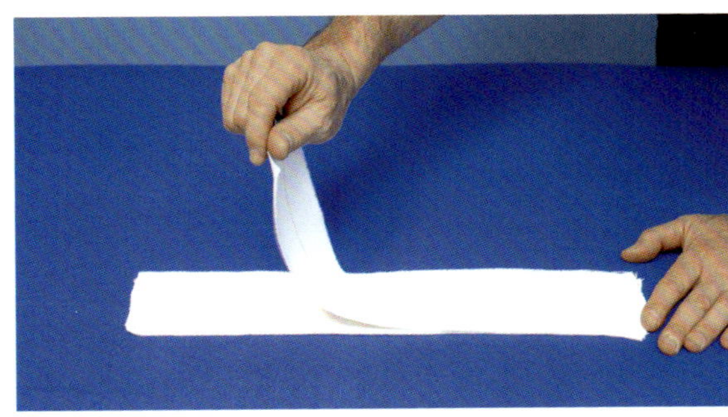

2 A strip of reinforced mono-extensible elastic adhesive bandage is prepared and applied in a horseshoe fashion to cover the heel.

3 The reinforced fastener must be tensed to nearly 100% of its elongation capacity to then be adhered over the proximal anchoring point.

4 The elastic fastener is secured with several wraps of adhesive inelastic bandage covering the axis of the lower leg.

5 Bandaging proceeds by preparing the distal anchoring point with a wrap of bandage around the forefoot at the metatarsals.

6 A fastener is applied in horseshoe fashion covering the heel, beginning and ending on the distal anchoring point.

7 The bandaging is secured with several wraps of inelastic adhesive bandage covering the midfoot and forefoot.

8 Bandaging for the stabilization of the hindfoot proceeds with the application of two figure-eight wraps of adhesive inelastic bandage. The bandage starts from the medial malleolus.

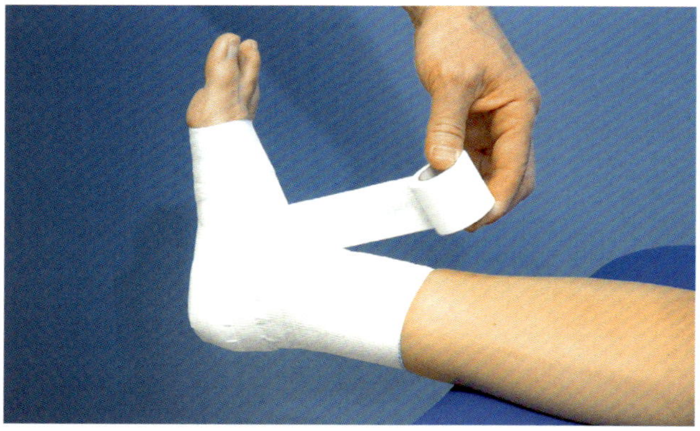

9

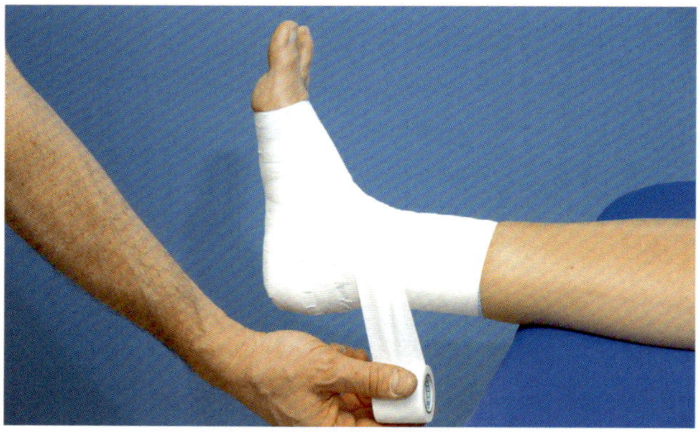

10

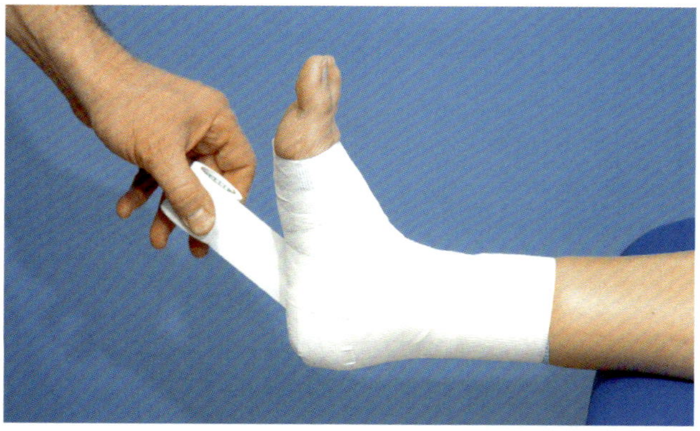

11

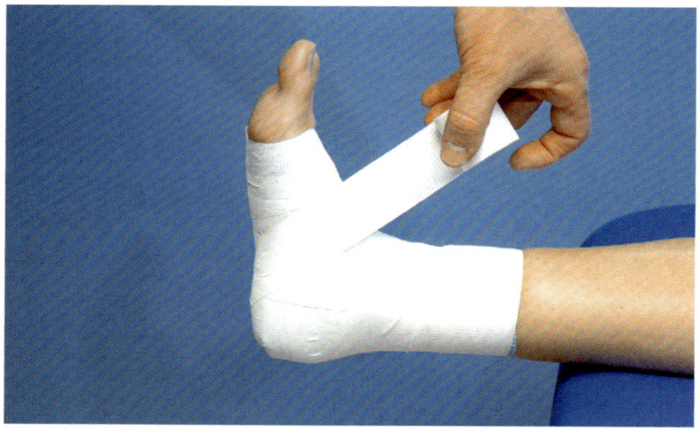

12

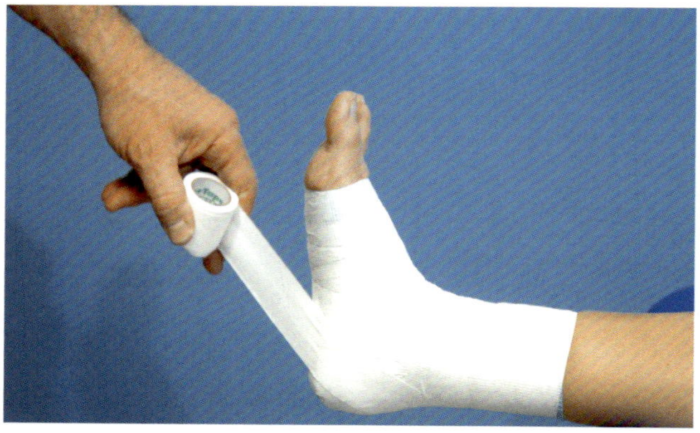

13

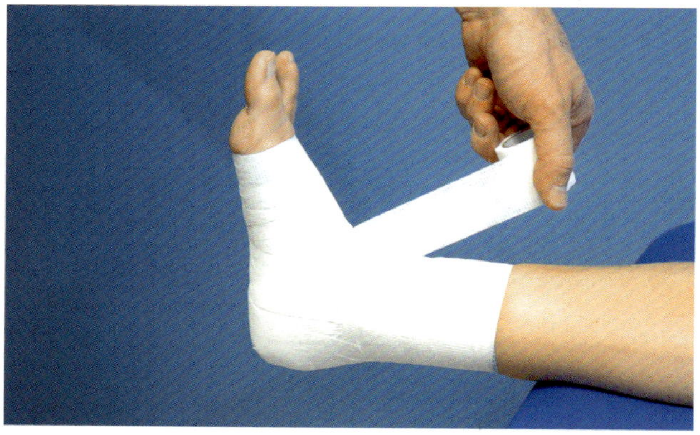

14

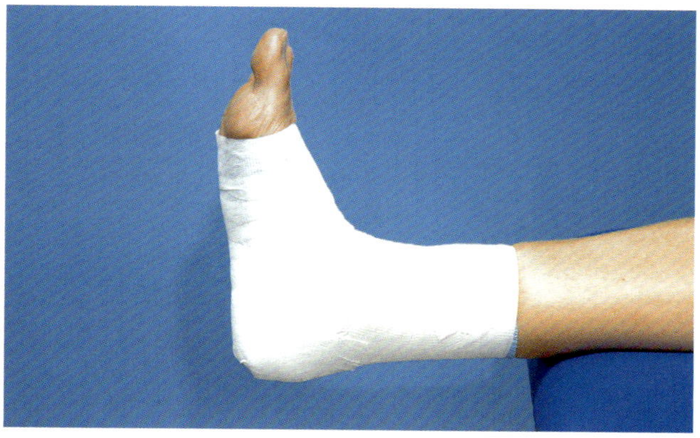

15

Limitation of inversion and eversion

9 The bandage is brought to wrap the plantar arch.

10 Next, the bandage runs over the dorsum of the foot, covering the tibiotarsal joint.

11 Having made a complete wrap around the axis of the lower leg, the bandage is diagonally brought down toward the lateral area of the heel.

12 The bandage is again brought below the plantar arch and then directed toward the dorsum of the foot, covering the tibiotarsal joint.

13 A wrap of bandage is made around the axis of the lower leg, and the bandage is diagonally brought toward the heel to cover the medial area.

14-15 Next, the heel is covered and the bandage is brought toward the lower leg, where it is cut and secured to the bandaging.

TIBIOTARSAL JOINT

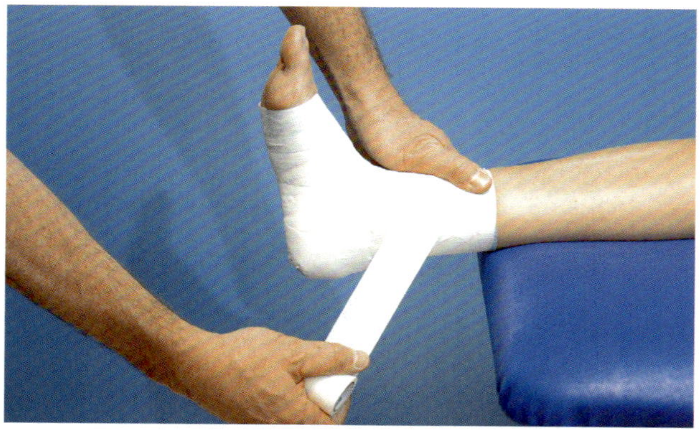

16

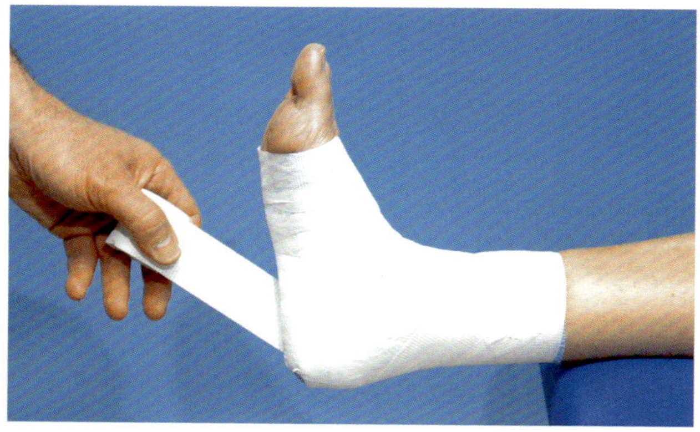

17

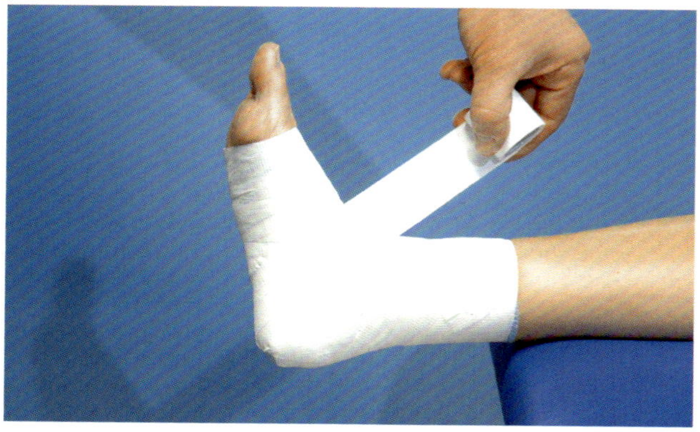

18

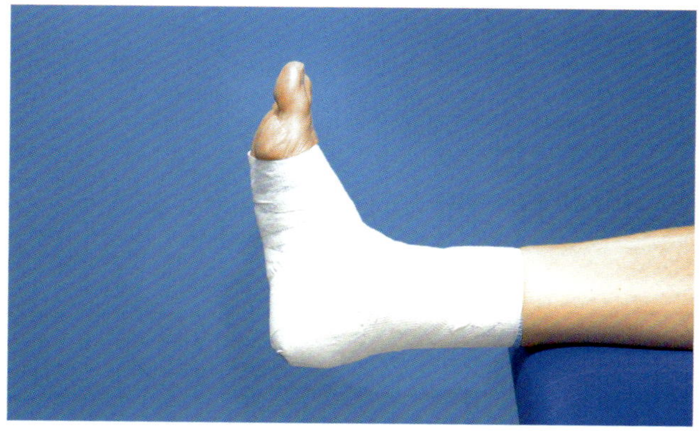

19

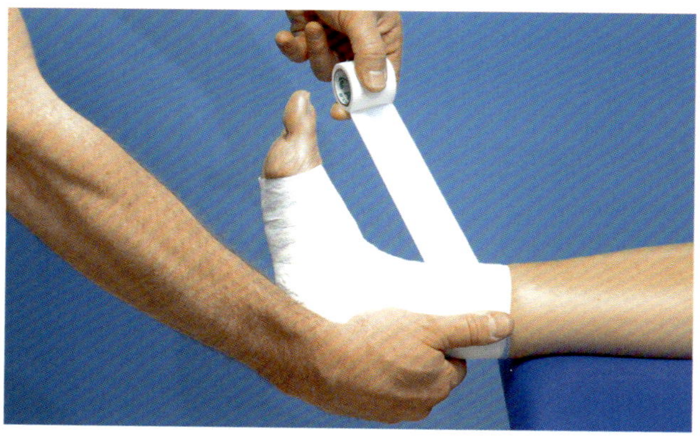

20

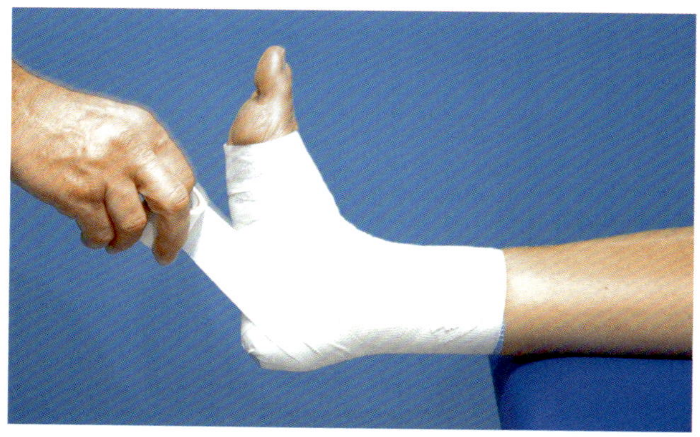

21

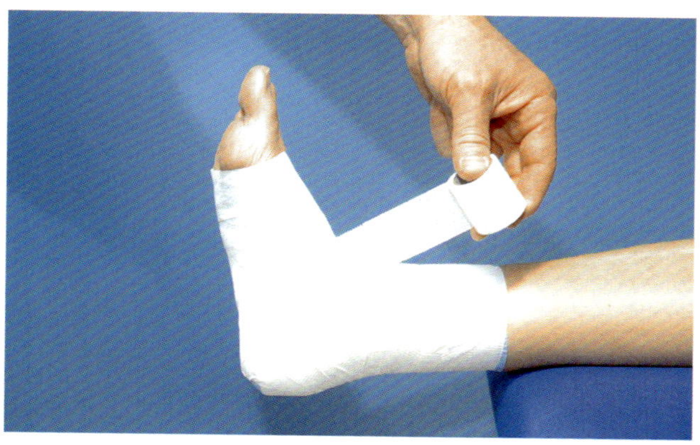

22

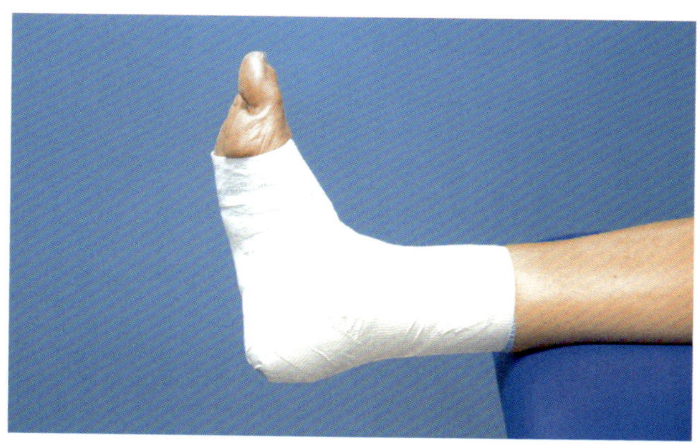

23

Limitation of inversion and eversion

16-17 The hindfoot is additionally stabilized with the application of two strips of bandage that pass lateral to the heel. The first strip is applied with a pulling force laterally to medially, then is passed behind the Achilles tendon to wrap the lateral part of the heel.

18 From here, the bandage passes below the plantar arch and is directed toward the dorsum of the tibiotarsal joint.

19 The bandage is now cut and adhered to the bandaging.

20 The second strip of bandage is applied with a pulling force medially to laterally.

21 Once it has passed behind the Achilles tendon, the bandage covers the medial part of the heel.

22 The bandage crosses the plantar arch and runs toward the dorsum of the tibiotarsal joint, where it is finally cut and adhered to the bandaging.

23 Bandaging is complete.

INDICATIONS

- ✓ *Posttraumatic conditions*
- ✓ *Preventative sports treatment*

TIBIOTARSAL JOINT

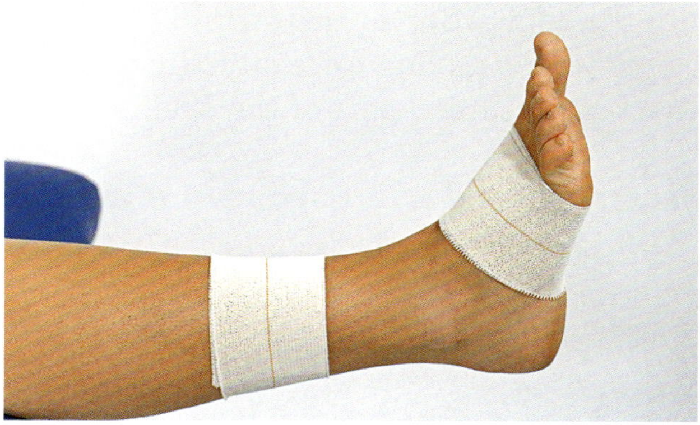

1

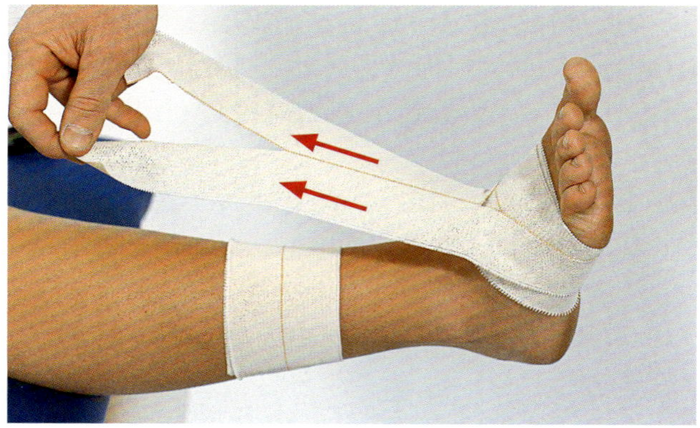

2

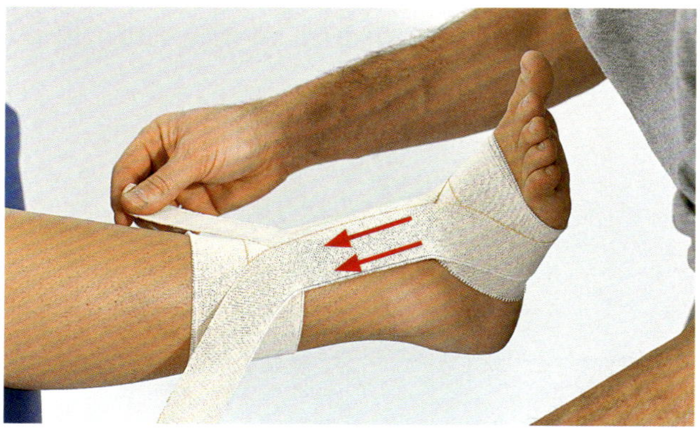

3

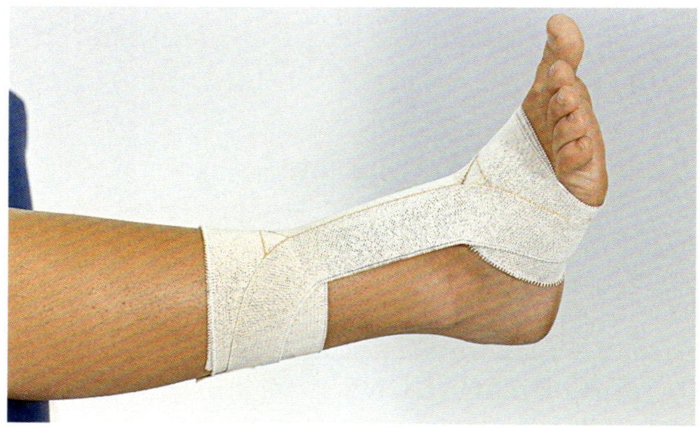

4

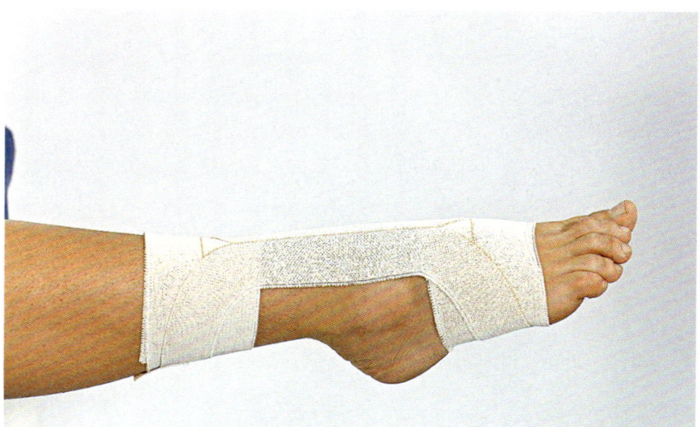

5

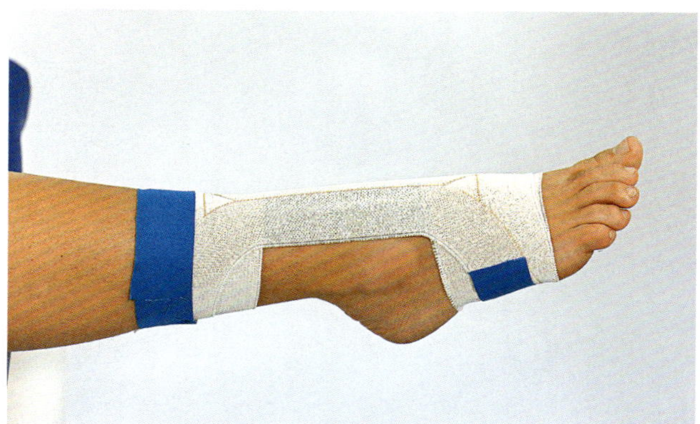

6

Unloading and limitation of plantar flexion

MATERIAL

- ✓ Cotton fabric porous elastic adhesive bandage that can be stretched lengthwise, 7.5 cm in width
- ✓ Inelastic adhesive tape for affixing the bandage

APPLICATION

1 The subject is in the supine position with the foot kept in dorsal flexion and the lower leg off the end of the table. With a full wrap of bandage, the proximal anchoring point is applied at the distal third of the lower leg and the distal anchoring point is applied, covering the forefoot at the metatarsal heads.

2 An X-shaped bandage is prepared by longitudinally cutting an elastic adhesive strip from both ends. The pieces from one end are applied to the distal anchoring point.

3-4 The bandage is pulled distal to proximal. The still-free parts are applied to the proximal anchoring point.

5-6 Finally, the bandage is adhered to the skin and the bandaging is refined with secure anchor points made of inelastic adhesive tape.

INDICATIONS

- ✓ *Reeducation of dorsal flexion motion*

ACHILLES TENDON

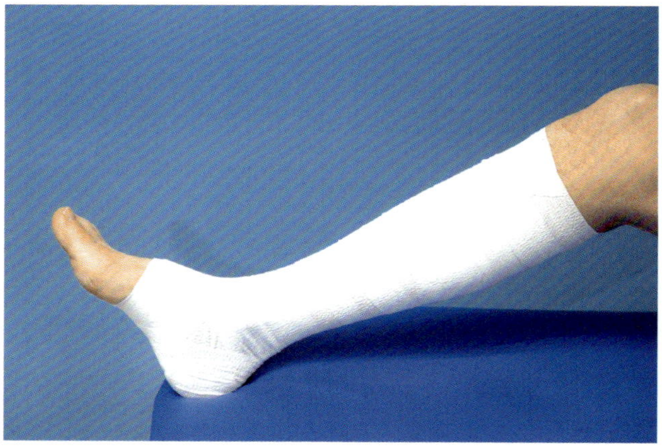

1

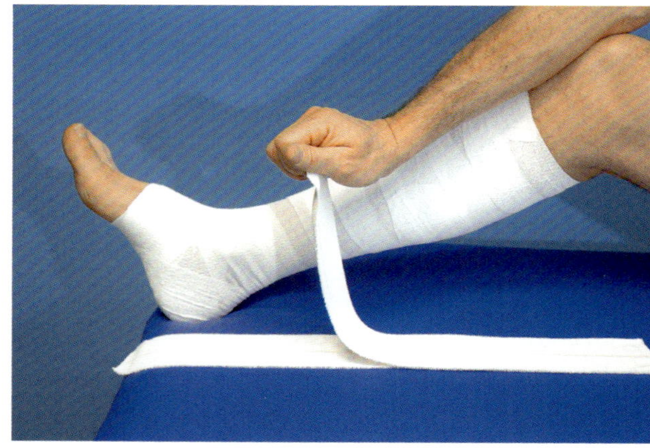

2

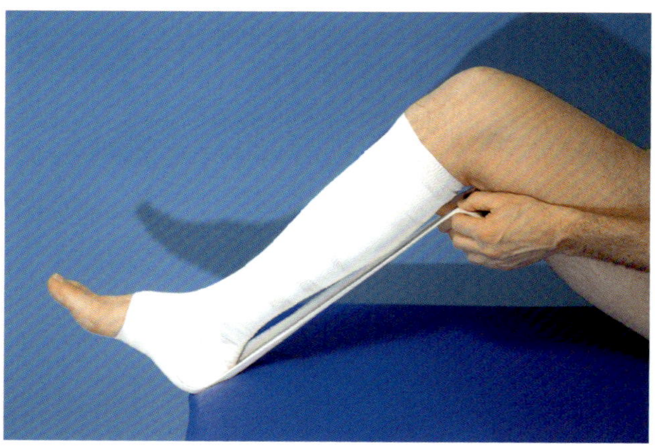

3

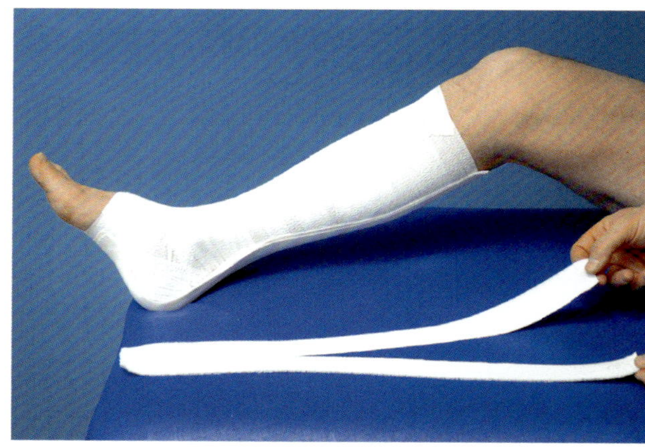

4

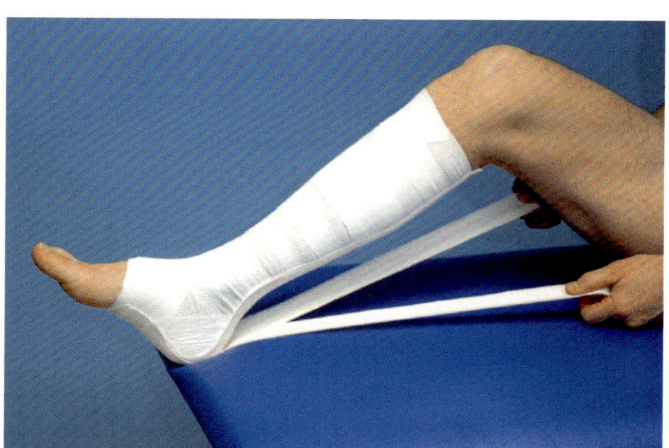

5

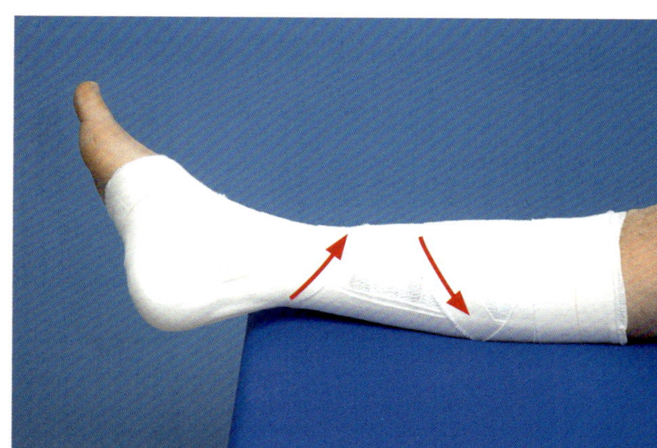

6

Preventative bandaging

MATERIAL

- ✓ 7.5 cm wide elastic cohesive bandage for base bandaging
- ✓ Cotton fabric porous elastic adhesive bandage that can be stretched lengthwise, 7.5 cm in width

APPLICATION

1 Base bandaging is made with the cohesive bandage, beginning from the midfoot and covering the lower leg up to the proximal third.

2 A reinforced fastener is prepared using two to three strips of mono-extensible adhesive elastic bandage overlapping one another.

3 With the foot in plantar flexion, the reinforced elastic fastener is applied under the plantar arch to cover the heel and then is put under tension along the skin projection of the Achilles tendon and adhered to the base bandaging.

4 Using another mono-extensible adhesive elastic bandage, a Y-shaped bandage of the proper length is prepared.

5 The single end of the Y-bandage is applied under the heel, while the other two ends, still free, are placed under tension.

6 The lower leg is covered with the two arms of the Y-bandage, which is then secured with two full wraps of bandage around the proximal third of the lower leg and the midfoot.

INDICATIONS

- ✓ *Preventative sports treatment*
- ✓ *Posttraumatic preventative treatment*
- ✓ *Inflammation*

ACHILLES TENDON

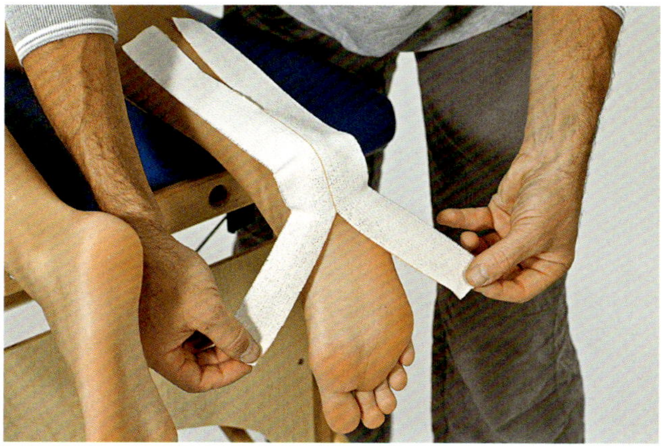

1

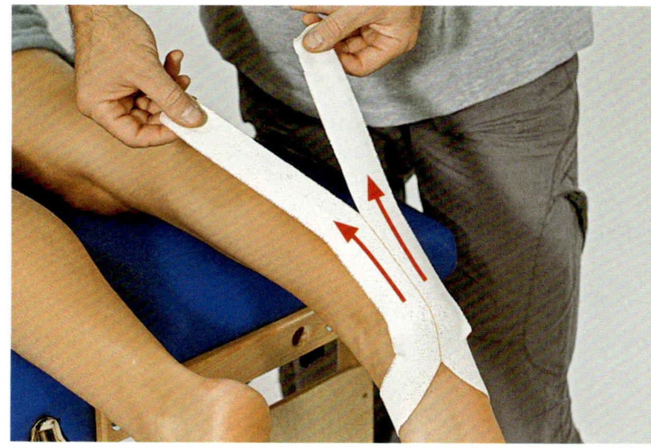

2

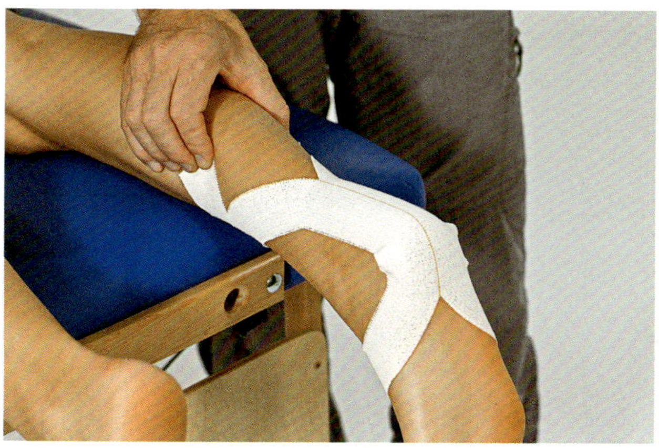

3

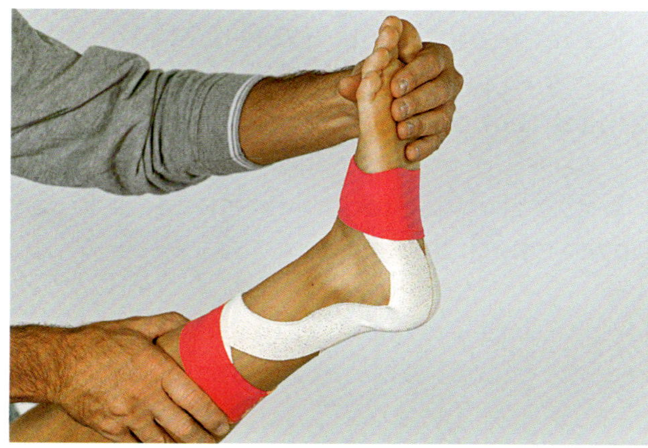

4

Unloading with X-shaped bandage, limitation of dorsal flexion

MATERIAL

- ✓ Cotton fabric porous elastic adhesive bandage that can be stretched lengthwise, 7.5 cm in width
- ✓ Inelastic adhesive tape for affixing the bandage

APPLICATION

1 The subject lies prone and keeps the foot in slight plantar flexion. A bandage of the proper length must be cut lengthwise from both ends in order to make an X. The central part of the bandage is applied in such a way as to cover the heel.

2 The distal parts of the bandage are secured, covering the midfoot.

3 The proximal parts of the bandage are placed under tension longitudinal to the axis of the Achilles tendon and adhered to the distal third of the lower leg, covering the skin projection of the myotendinous junction of the gastrocnemius.

4 Bandaging ends with the application of several affixing strips made of inelastic adhesive material, or with a full wrap of adhesive elastic bandage.

INDICATIONS

- ✓ *Inflammation of the Achilles tendon*
- ✓ *Preventative sports treatment*
- ✓ *Inflammation of the paratenon*

ACHILLES TENDON

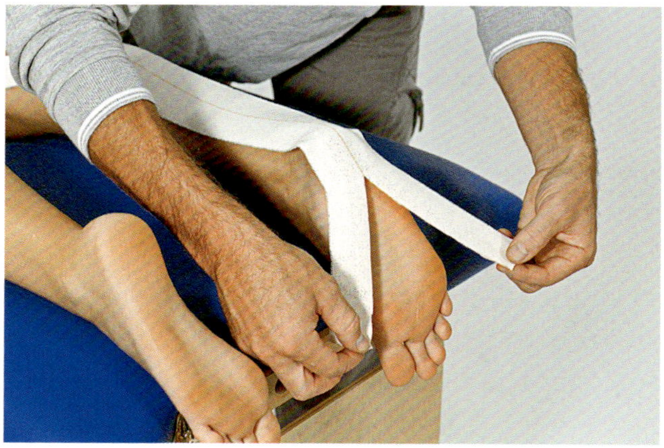

1

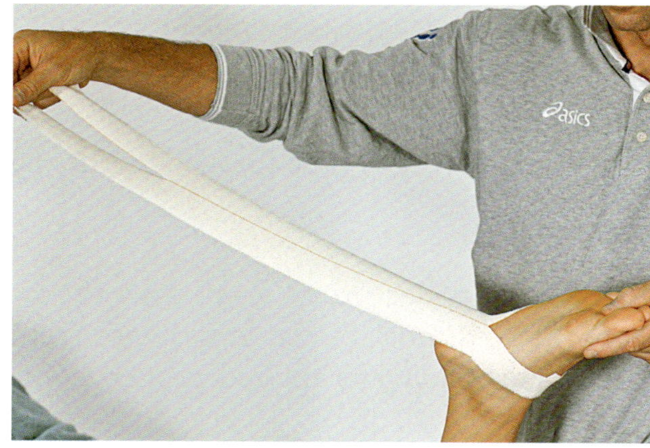

2

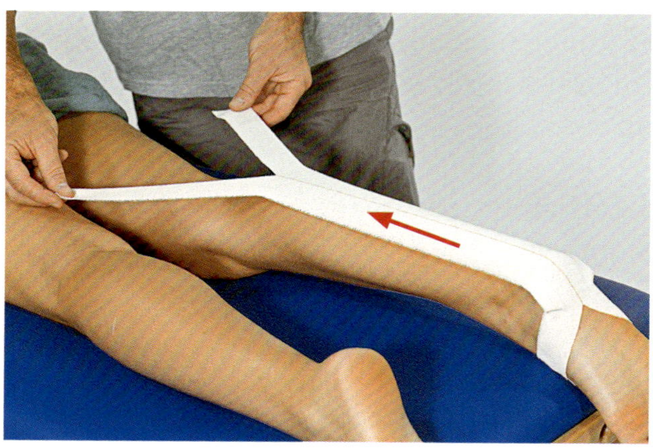

3

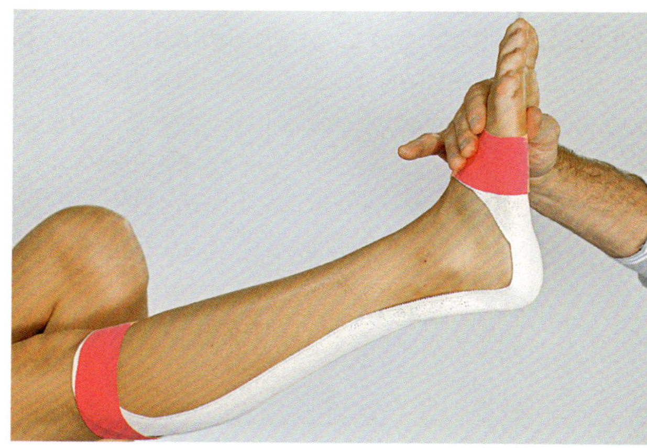

4

Musculotendinous unloading, limitation of dorsal flexion

MATERIAL

✓ Cotton fabric porous elastic adhesive bandage that can be stretched lengthwise, 7.5 cm in width
✓ Inelastic adhesive tape for affixing the bandage

APPLICATION

This type of bandaging is recommended for dysfunction of the muscles of the posterior compartment of the lower leg.

1 The subject lies prone and keeps the foot in slight plantar flexion. A bandage of the proper length must be cut lengthwise from both ends in order to make an X. The central part of the bandage is placed longitudinal to the axis of the lower leg, starting from the heel and proceeding to the proximal third of the tibia and fibula.

2 The distal parts of the bandage are secured, covering the midfoot.

3 The proximal parts of the bandage are put under tension, longitudinal to the direction of the Achilles tendon, and are adhered after covering the proximal third of the lower leg.

4 The bandaging is secured and finished with the application of several strips of inelastic adhesive material.

INDICATIONS

✓ *Inflammation of the Achilles tendon*
✓ *Preventative sports treatment*
✓ *Inflammation of the paratenon*
✓ *Tendinous inflammation resulting from contracture of the gastrocnemius*

ACHILLES TENDON

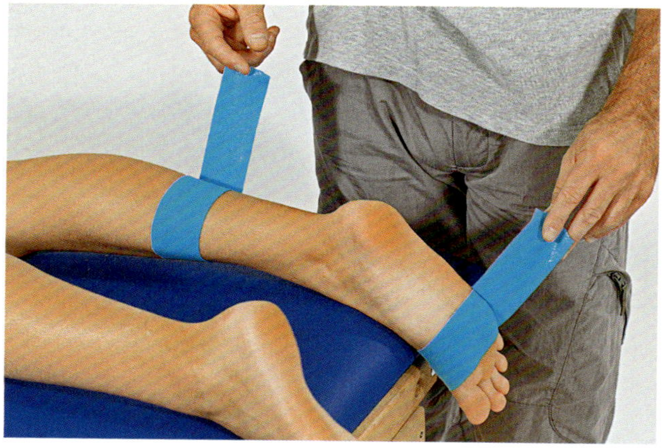
1

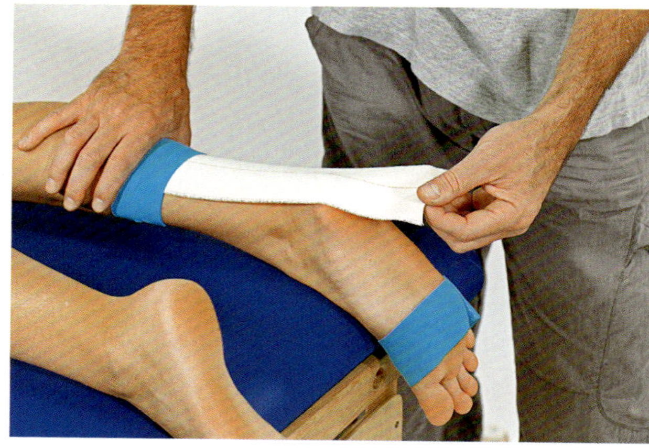
2

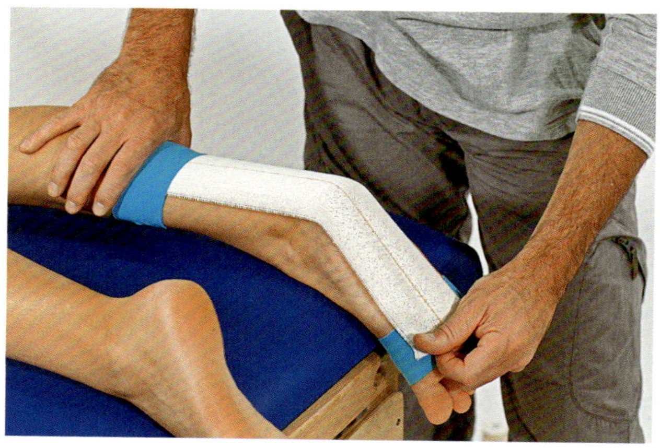
3

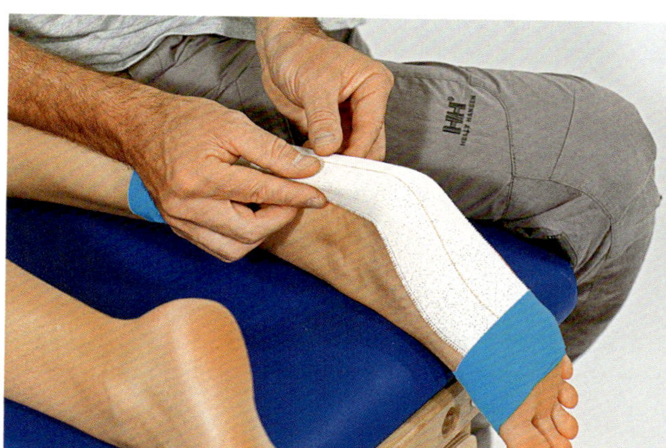
4

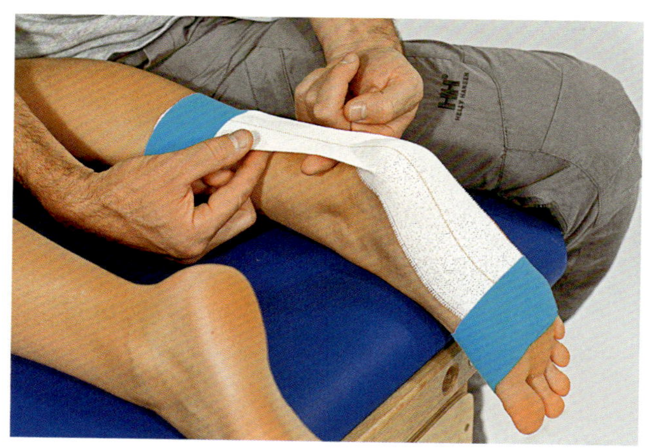
5

Unloading bandaging

MATERIAL

- ✓ Cotton fabric porous elastic adhesive bandage that can be stretched lengthwise, 7.5 cm in width
- ✓ Elastic adhesive tape, 5 cm in width

APPLICATION

1 The subject lies prone and keeps the foot in plantar flexion. To begin, the distal anchoring point is prepared by wrapping the forefoot at the metatarsals, and the proximal anchoring point at the myotendinous junction of the gastrocnemius, with a wrap of elastic adhesive tape. The wrap of tape is left open.

2 Next, a strip of elastic adhesive bandage of the proper length is applied starting from the proximal anchoring point, which is then secured.

3 The bandage is placed under tension and applied on the distal anchoring point, which is then closed.

4-5 The portion of bandage located at the Achilles tendon is folded over on itself in order to create a reinforcement for the tendon itself.

It is possible to reinforce the anchoring points with the semicircular application of several strips of inelastic adhesive tape.
The bandaging may be completed with the application of a cohesive bandage with several spiral wraps in the distal to proximal direction.

INDICATIONS

- ✓ *Preventative sports treatment*
- ✓ *Tendinous inflammation*
- ✓ *Inflammation of the paratenon*

ACHILLES TENDON

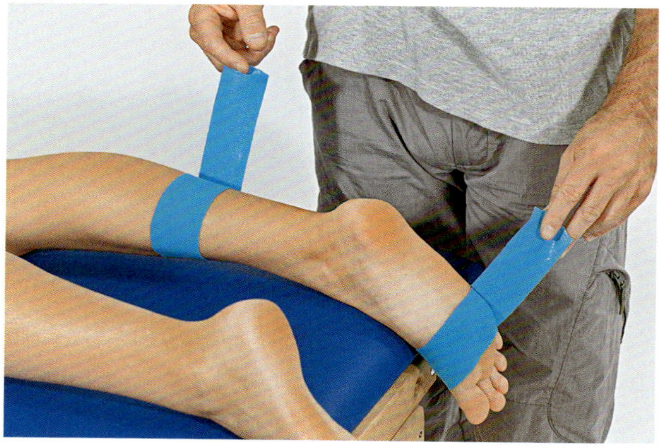

1

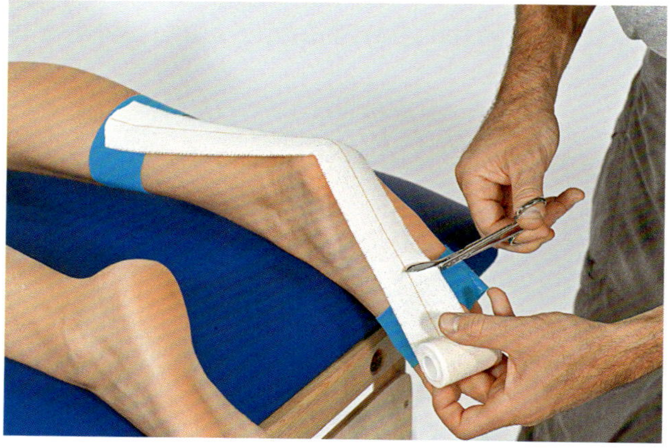

2

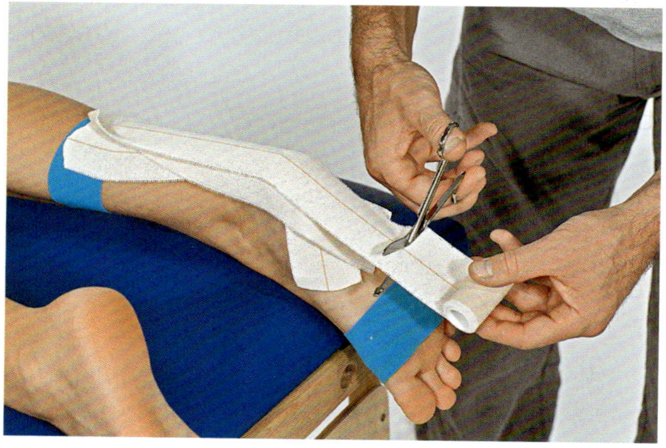

3

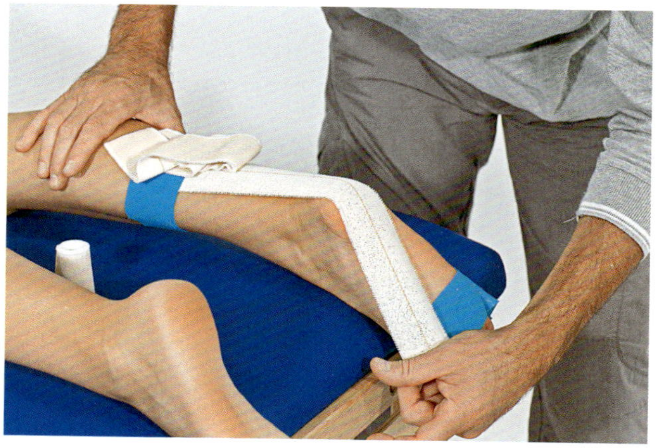

4

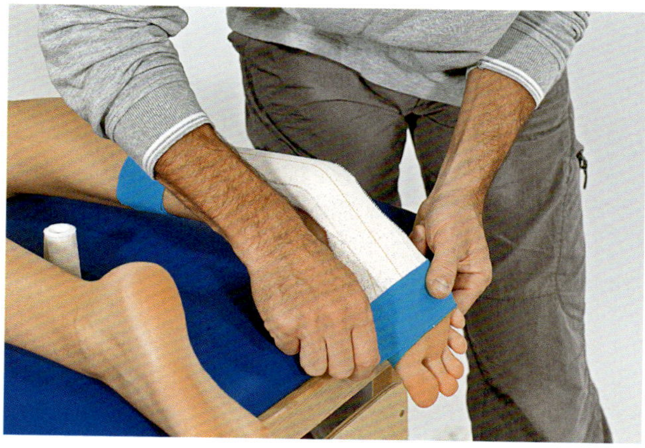

5

Unloading with stabilization of the hindfoot

MATERIAL

- ✓ Cotton fabric porous elastic adhesive bandage that can be stretched lengthwise, 7.5 cm in width
- ✓ Elastic adhesive tape, 7.5 cm in width
- ✓ Inelastic adhesive tape, 5 cm in width

APPLICATION

1 The subject lies prone and keeps the foot in plantar flexion. To begin, the distal anchoring point is prepared by wrapping the forefoot at the metatarsals, and the proximal anchoring point at the myotendinous junction of the gastrocnemius with a wrap of elastic adhesive tape. The wrap of tape is left open.

2-3 Three strips of porous elastic adhesive bandage are prepared and applied one by one, starting from the proximal third of the lower leg until reaching the heel, where the bandages are cut around the halfway point of the plantar arch. The first strip is placed in the medial region of the proximal third of the lower leg, the second is placed in the lateral region, and the third in the central region overlapping the first two.

4-5 After securing the three strips, the bandages are pulled proximal to distal and affixed one by one to the distal anchoring point using the piece of elastic adhesive tape previously left free as the proximal anchoring point. The first is brought to laterally wrap the heel and later is applied at the plantar projection of the first metatarsal head. The second, after medially wrapping the heel, is affixed at the plantar projection of the fifth metatarsal head. The third, finally, passes over the central area of the heel and ends by covering the previous bandages.

ACHILLES TENDON

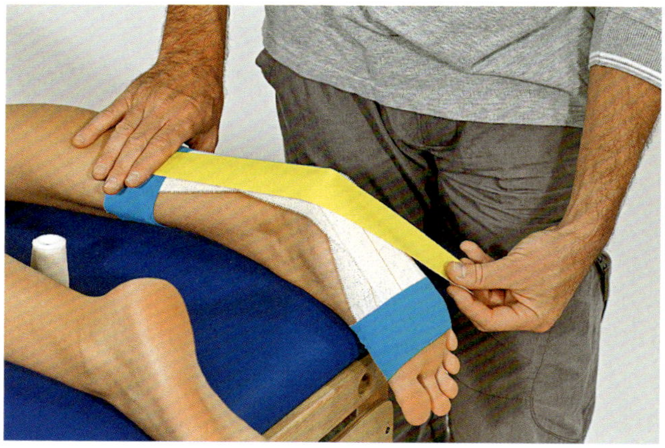

6

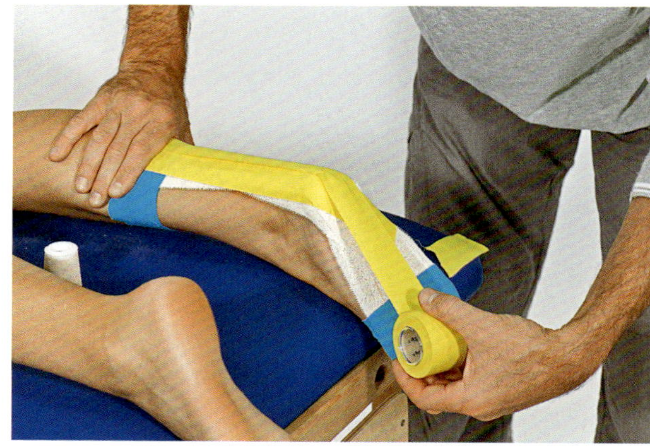

7

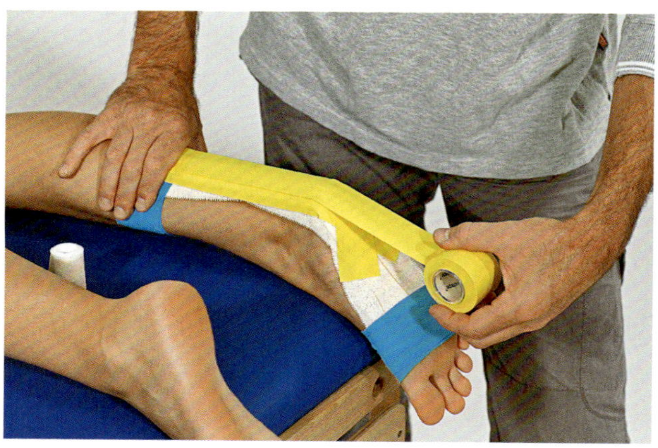

8

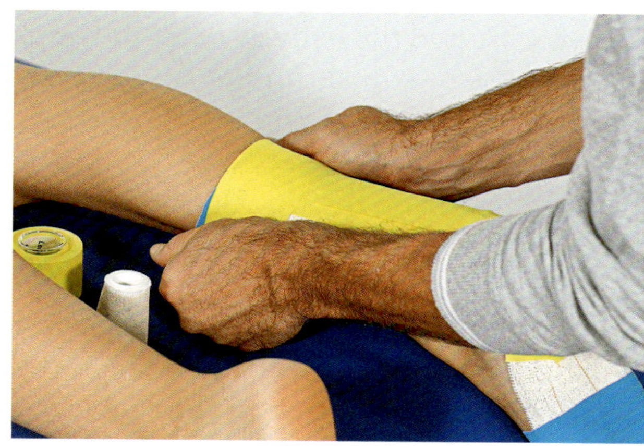

9

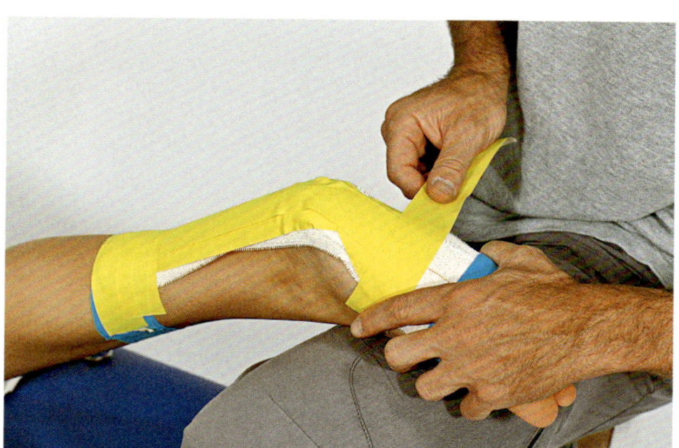

10

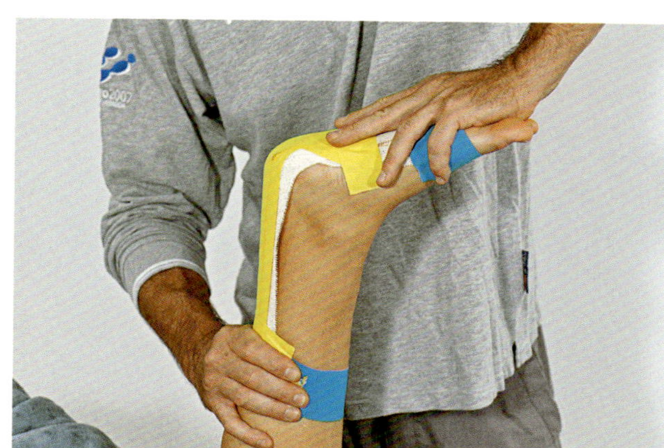

11

Unloading with stabilization of the hindfoot

6-7-8 Several strips of inelastic adhesive tape are applied in order to additionally reduce the dorsal flexion of the tibiotarsal joint and the tensing of the Achilles tendon. The strips are placed in an analogous way to that done with the mono-extensible elastic adhesive bandages.

9-10-11 The bandaging concludes, having several strips of inelastic adhesive material adhered to the proximal and distal anchoring points perpendicular to the longitudinal axis of the lower leg.

The direction of the three strips of inelastic adhesive tape applied to stabilize the hindfoot and reduce the tension of the Achilles tendon is shown well in these images, where the pieces of tape are shown one at a time.

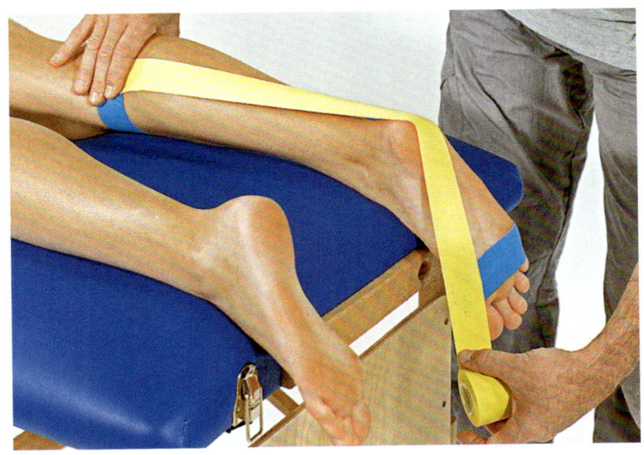

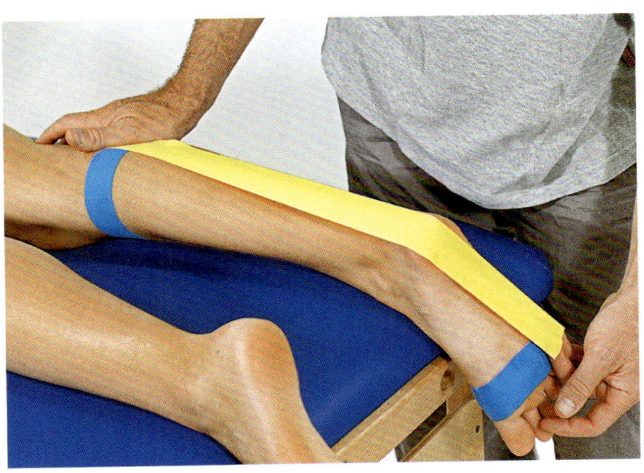

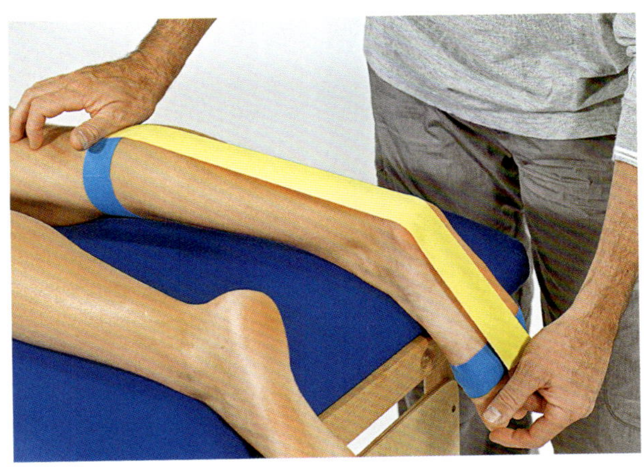

INDICATIONS

- ✓ *Unloading of the Achilles tendon for inflammation without muscular involvement*
- ✓ *Effects of sprain of the ankle with instability of the hindfoot*

ACHILLES TENDON

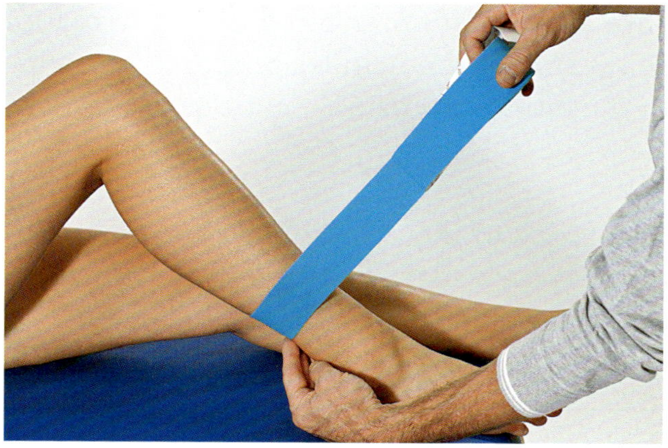

1

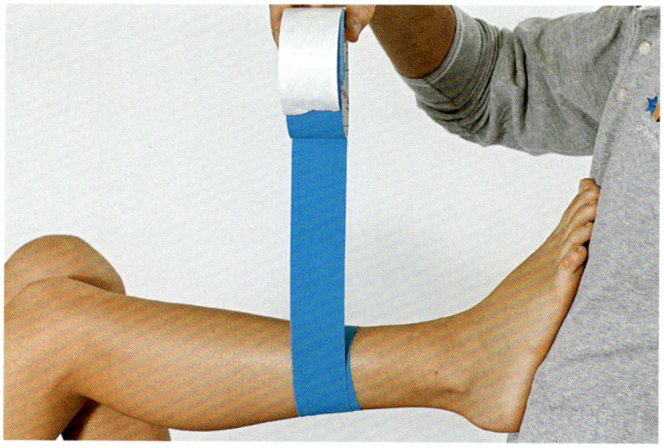

2

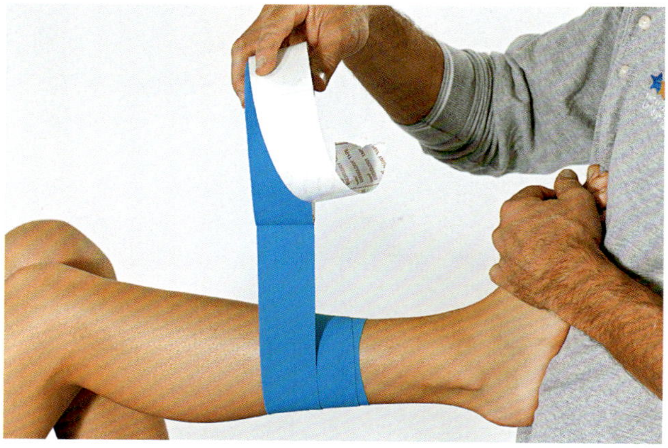

3

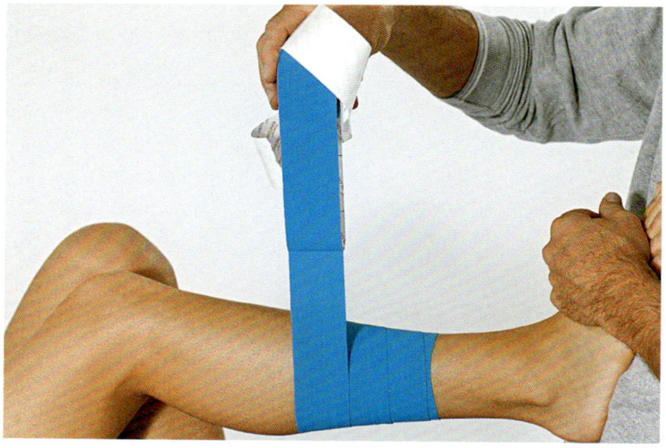

4

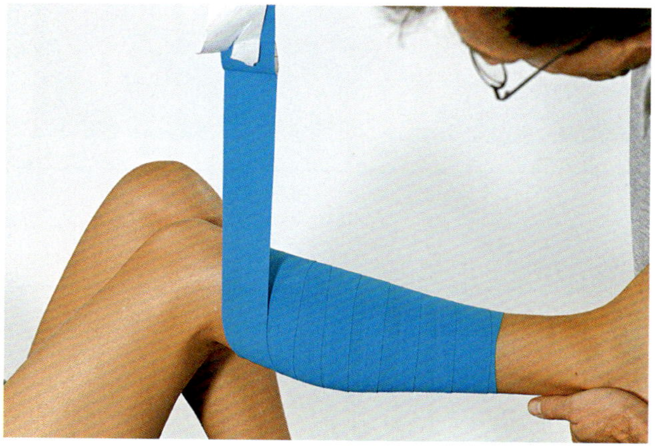

5

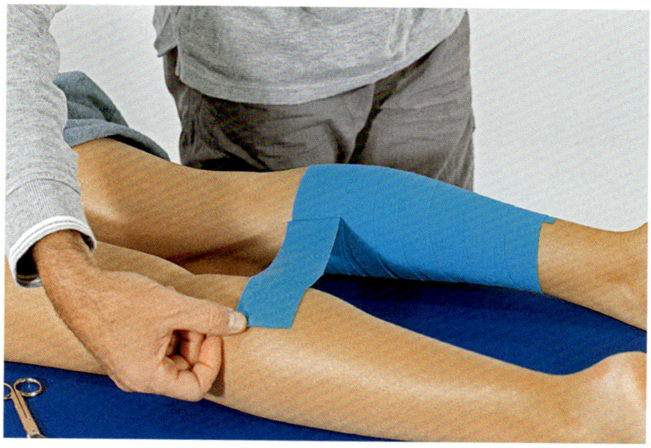

6

Musculotendinous unloading with stabilization of the hindfoot

MATERIAL

✓ Elastic adhesive tape, 5 cm in width
✓ Cotton fabric porous elastic adhesive bandage that can be stretched lengthwise, 7.5 cm in width
✓ Inelastic adhesive tape, 5 cm in width

APPLICATION

1 The subject lies in supine position with the knee flexed. The first complete wrap of elastic adhesive tape is applied below the skin projection of the myotendinous junction of the gastrocnemius.

2-3-4-5 Next, a complete bandaging of the lower leg is done, with spiral tape wraps overlapping by 50% moving in the distal to proximal direction.

6 The subject lies prone and keeps the foot in plantar flexion. The end of the elastic adhesive tape is left free in order to later use it as a proximal anchoring point.

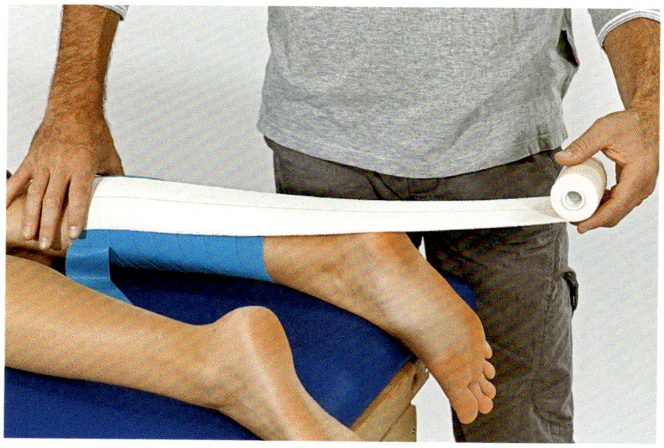

7

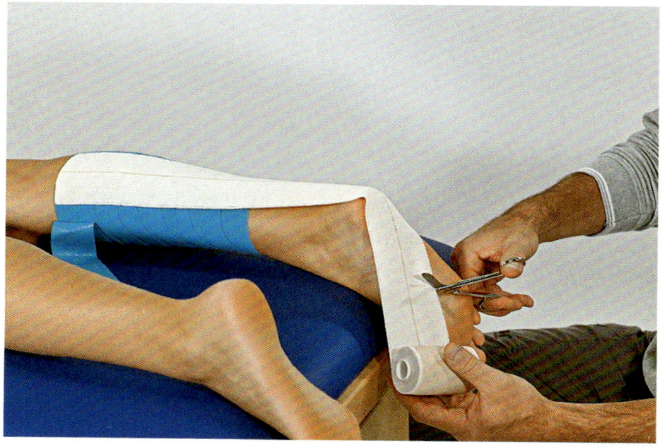

8

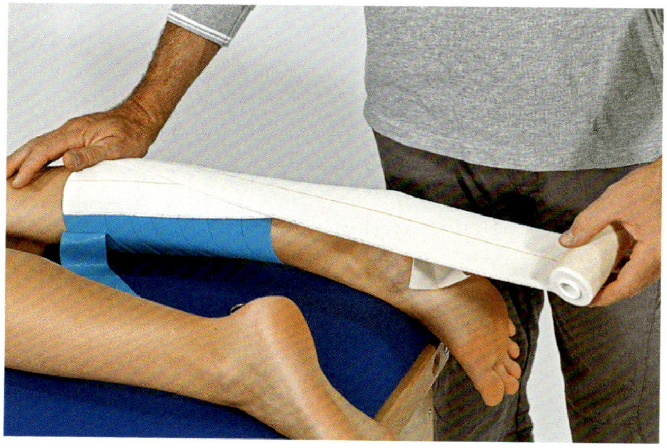

9

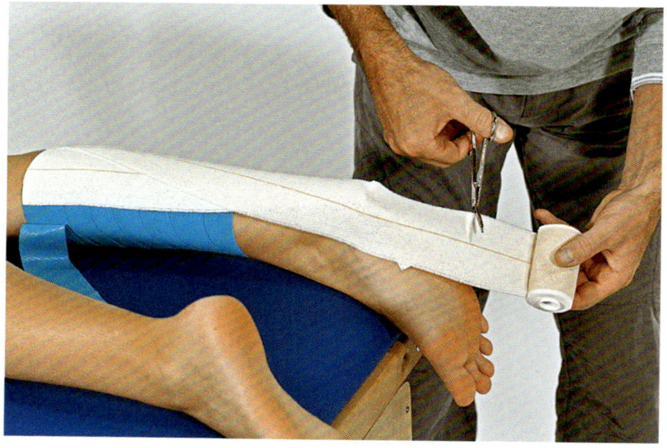

10

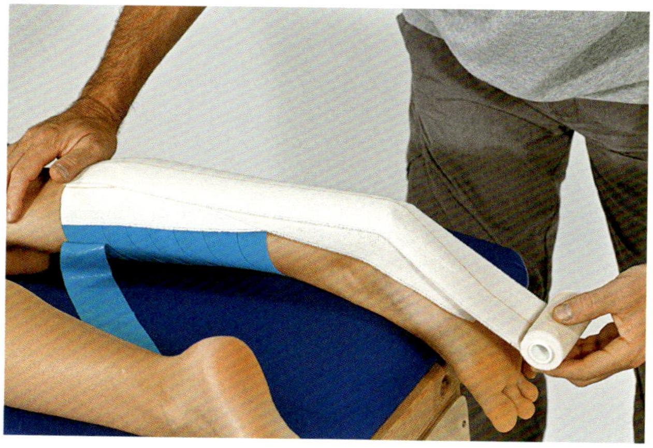

11

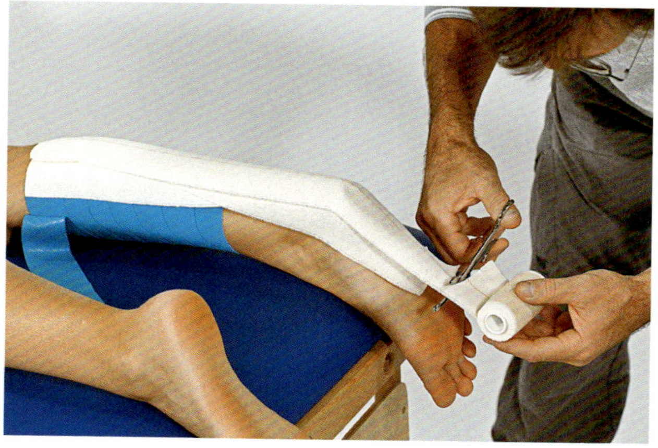

12

Musculotendinous unloading with stabilization of the hindfoot

7-8 The first strip of porous elastic adhesive bandage is prepared and applied starting from the medial part of the proximal third of the lower leg until reaching the lateral region of the heel. Here, the bandage is cut around the halfway point of the plantar arch.

9-10 The second strip is applied in a similar way to the first, starting from the lateral part of the proximal third of the lower leg until reaching the medial region of the heel, where it is cut around the halfway point of the plantar arch.

11-12 The last strip of elastic adhesive bandage starts from the central portion of the proximal third of the lower leg and, covering the two preceding bandages by 50%, proceeds to the central region of the heel, where the bandage is cut around the halfway point of the plantar arch.

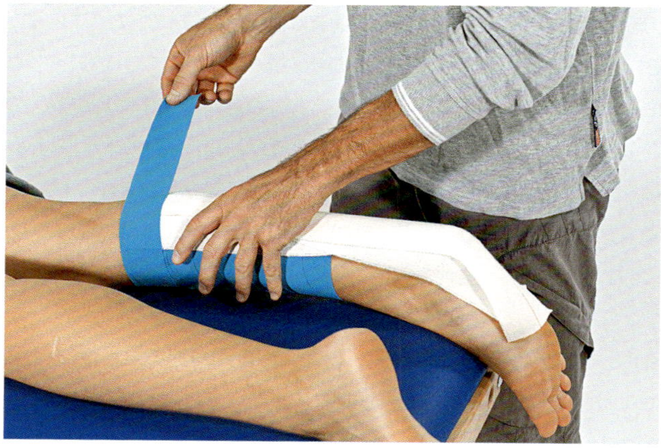
13

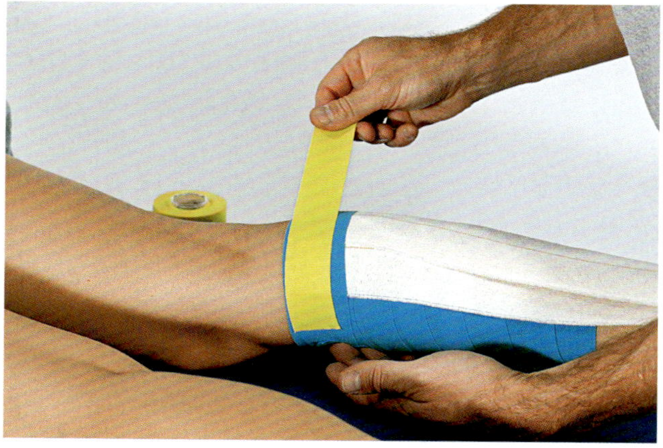
14

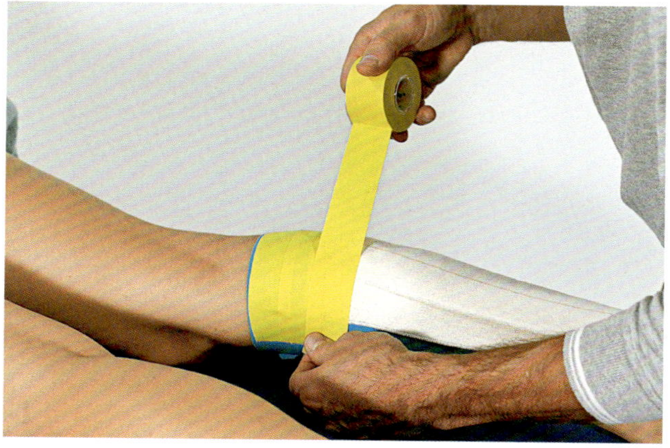
15

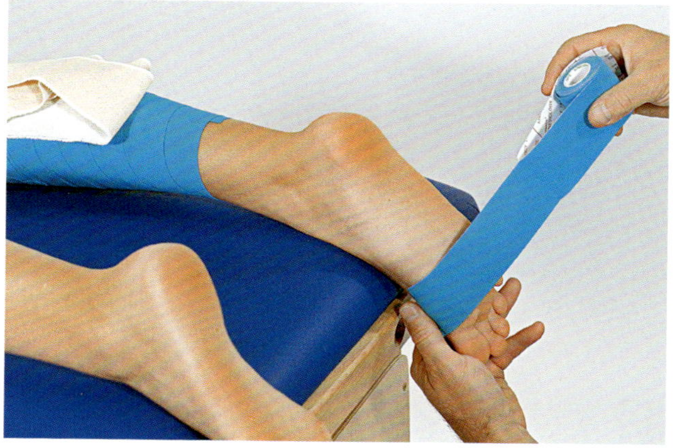
16

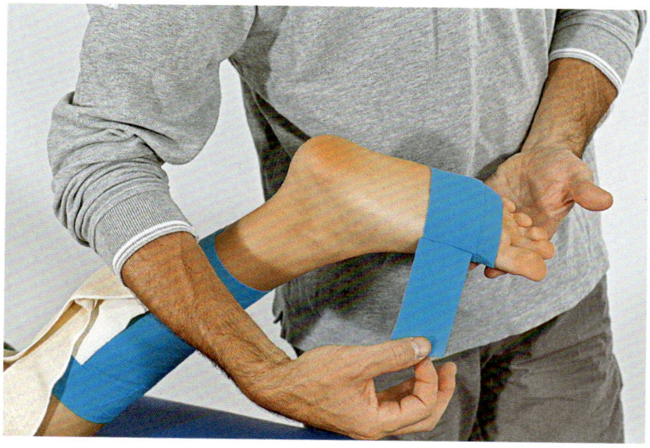
17

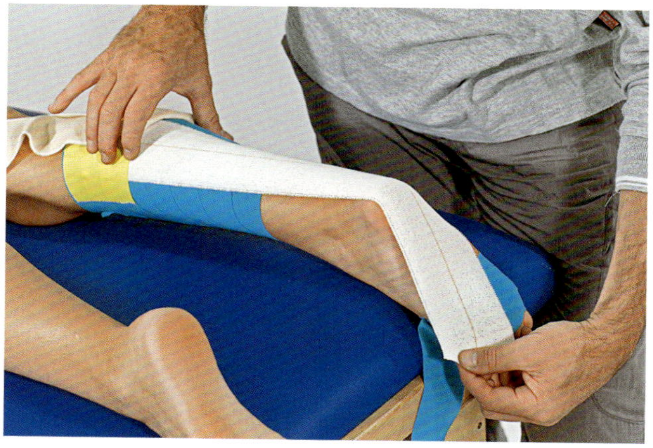
18

Musculotendinous unloading with stabilization of the hindfoot

13 The three bandages are secured with the piece of elastic adhesive tape previously left free.

14-15 The proximal anchoring point is now reinforced with the application of several strips of inelastic adhesive tape in a semicircle.

16-17 For the distal anchoring point, the forefoot is wrapped at the metatarsal heads with two complete wraps of elastic adhesive tape, leaving the final piece free.

18 After turning the three strips of porous elastic adhesive bandage backward, the first is pulled in the proximal to distal direction to laterally cover the heel, and then applied at the plantar projection of the first metatarsal head.

ACHILLES TENDON

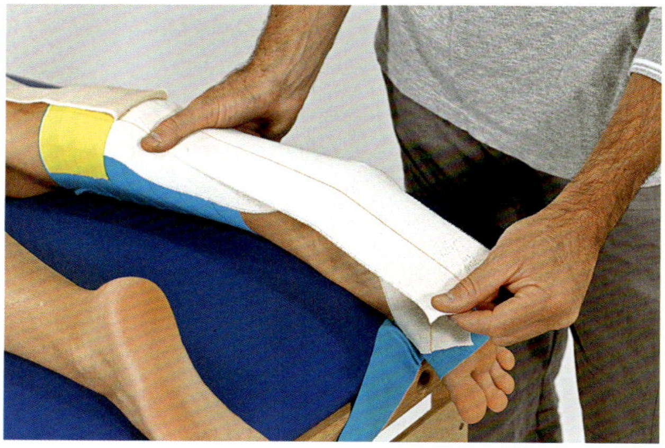
19

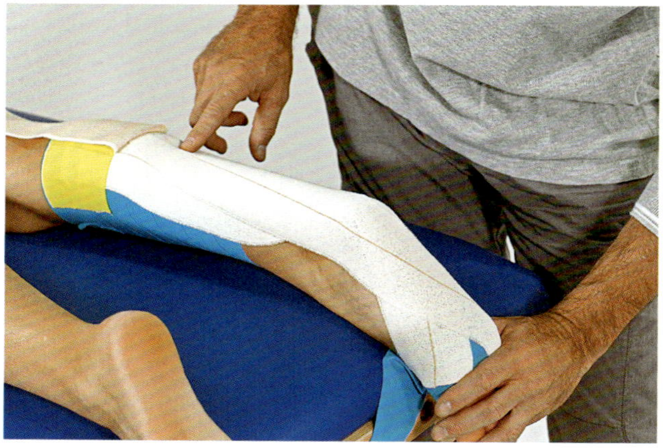
20

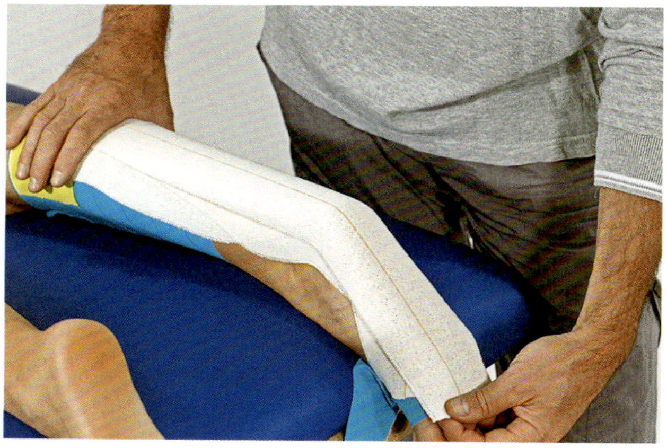
21

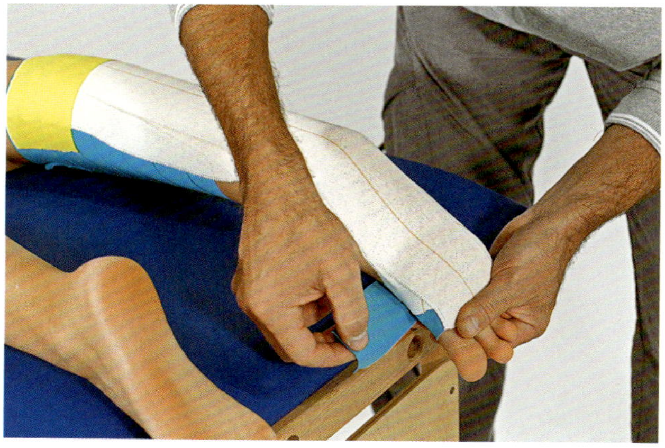
22

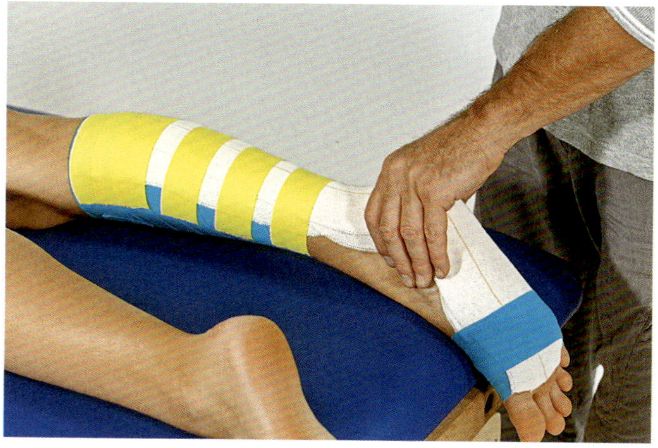
23

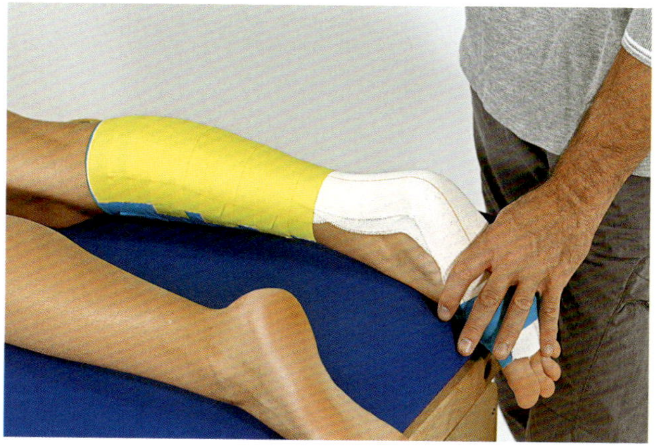
24

Musculotendinous unloading with stabilization of the hindfoot

19-20 Now the second strip of bandage is also pulled in the proximal-distal direction, bringing it to medially cover the heel and applying it at the plantar projection of the fifth metatarsal head.

21 The third strip of bandage, finally, covers the central area of the heel and ends covering the previous bandages.

22-23-24 The bandaging is now secured using both the piece of elastic adhesive tape left free as a distal anchoring point and strips of inelastic material positioned along the entire lower leg, perpendicular to its longitudinal axis.

In order to increase the tendon's unloading, a 0.5 cm wide foam rubber pad may be placed under the heel before bandaging.

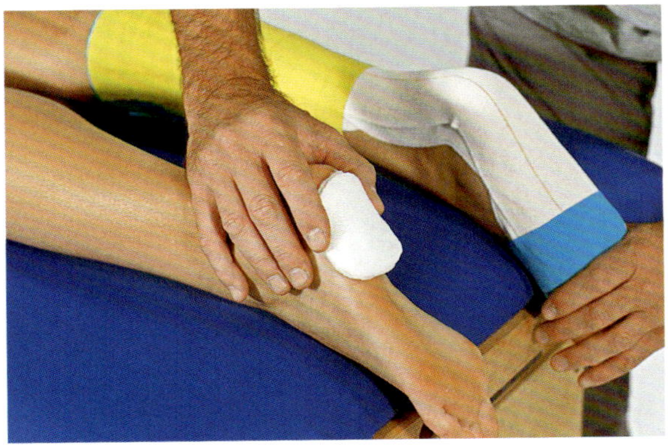

INDICATIONS

- ✓ *Inflammation of the Achilles tendon*
- ✓ *Postsurgical effects on the Achilles tendon*
- ✓ *Effects of sprain with instability of the hindfoot*
- ✓ *Effects of muscular trauma involving the Achilles tendon*
- ✓ *Effects of partial injury of the Achilles tendon*
- ✓ *Effects of muscular injury with load-taking of the satellite joint (tibiotarsal)*

ACHILLES TENDON

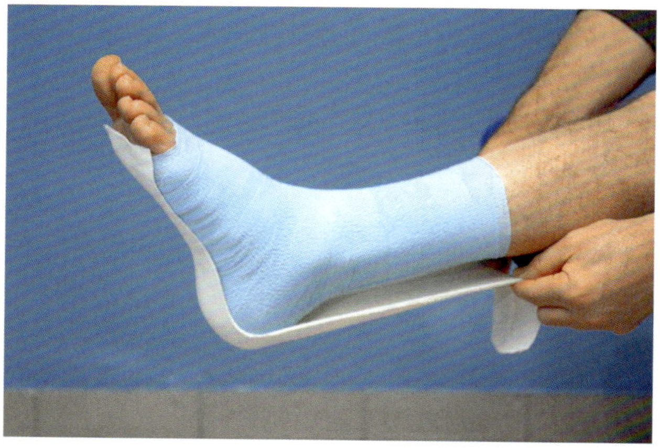

1

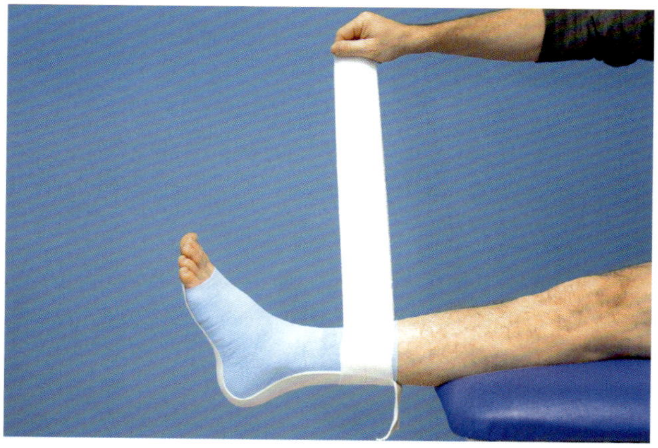

2

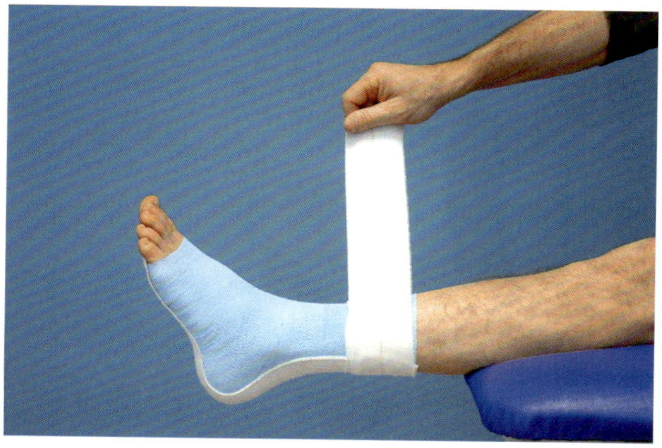

3

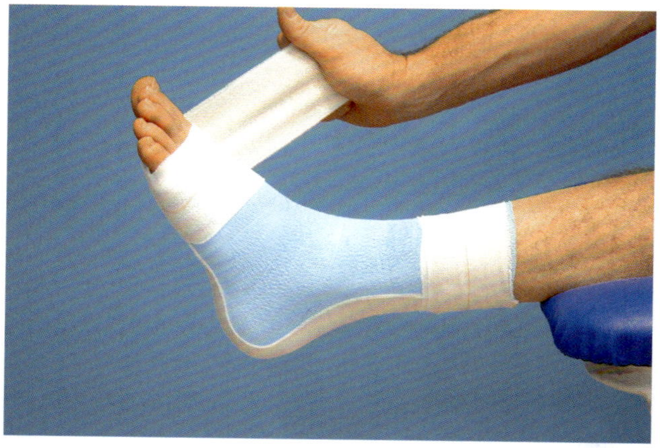

4

Unloading and support with elastic bandage

MATERIAL

- ✓ Elastic cohesive bandage, 7.5 cm in width
- ✓ Cotton fabric porous elastic adhesive bandage that can be stretched lengthwise, 7.5 cm in width
- ✓ Inelastic cohesive tape, 2 cm in width

APPLICATION

1 The subject, in the supine position, places the foot off the end of the table and flexes it at 20 degrees. The foot is prepared by applying base bandaging with a cohesive elastic bandage (see pages 184-185). A reinforced and pre-tensed elastic bandage is then placed on the plantar surface of the foot, covering the metatarsal heads. The bandage, placed under tension, is adhered to the base bandaging along the skin projection of the Achilles tendon.

The reinforced elastic bandage is prepared by overlapping three strips of adhesive elastic bandage. Then, on the tensed bandage, with the ulnar side of the hand, repeated passes are made with the aim of pre-tensioning it and having the adhesive affix well.

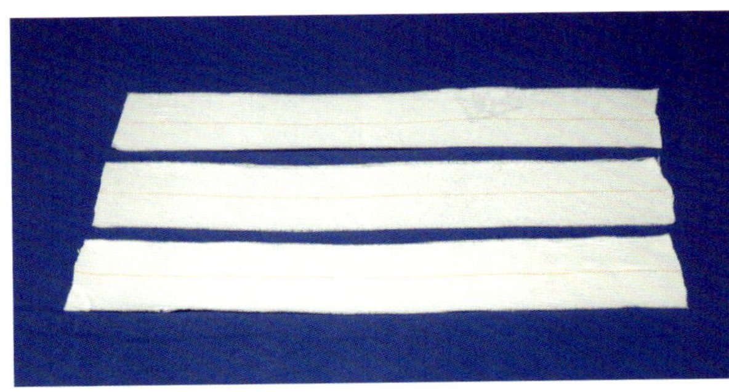

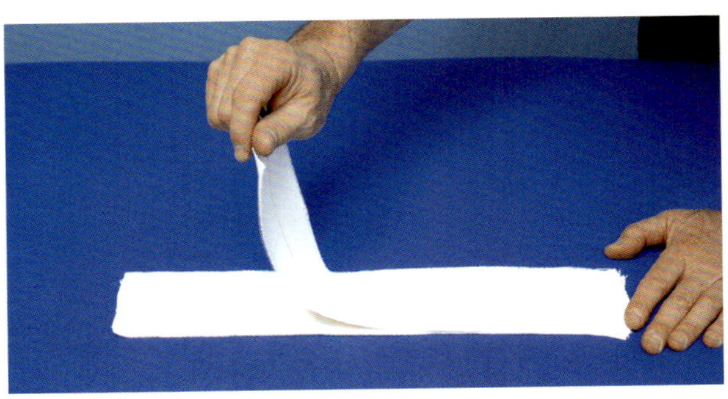

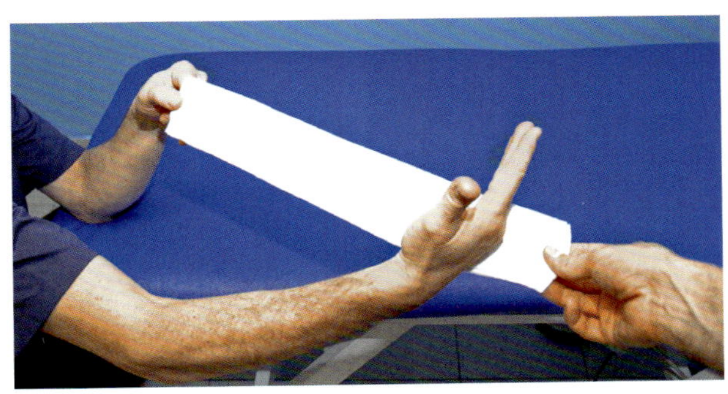

2 The reinforced fastener is affixed with a wrap of elastic adhesive bandage around the axis of the lower leg in the proximal portion of the base bandaging.

3 The excess part of the fastener is folded over itself and held in place with another wrapping of the bandage.

4 The reinforced fastener must be affixed with a wrap of elastic adhesive bandage that covers the metatarsal heads in the distal portion of the base bandaging.

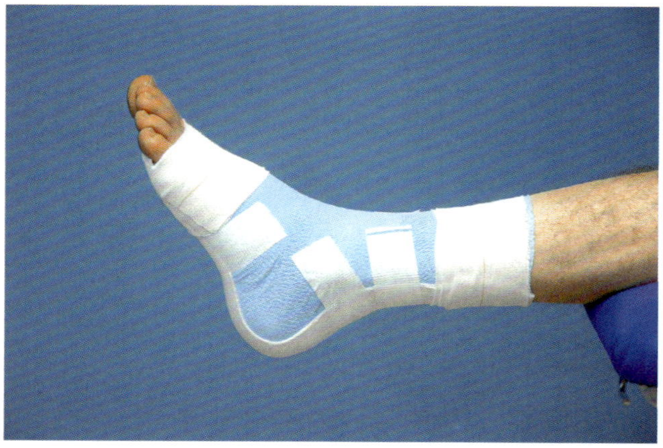

5

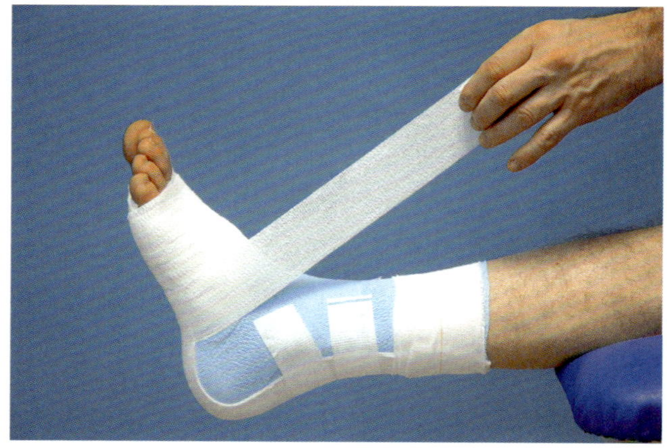

6

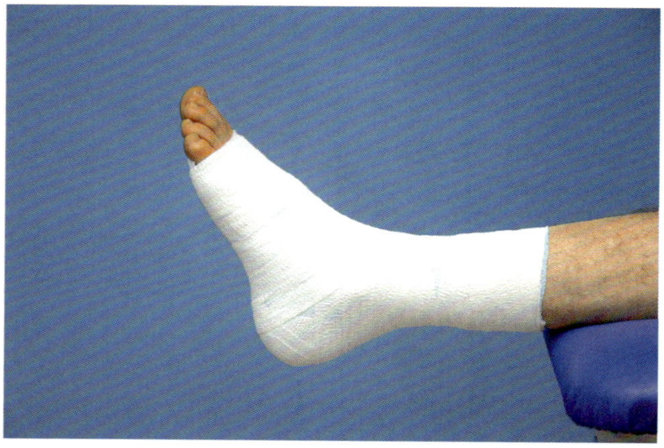

7

Unloading and support with elastic bandage

5 Next, several strips of inelastic bandage are applied to further secure the fastener.

6 With the cohesive bandage, the bandaging is secured, finished, and reinforced with several spiral wraps in the distal to proximal direction.

7 Bandaging is complete.

INDICATIONS

✓ *Posttraumatic conditions*
✓ *Preventative sports treatment*

ACHILLES TENDON

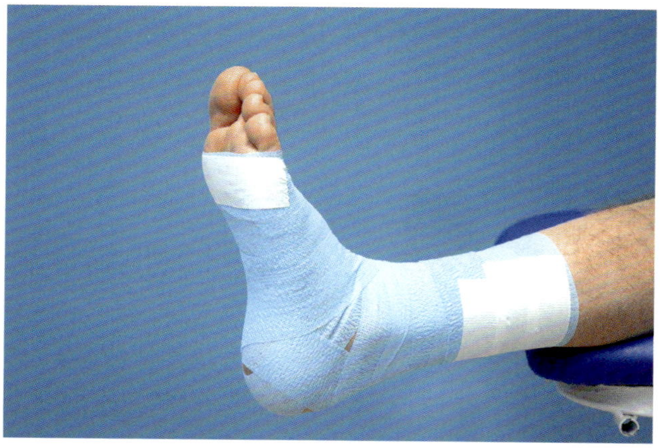

1

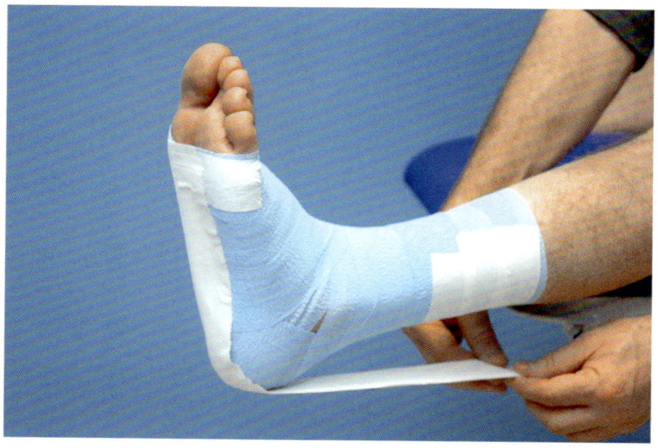

2

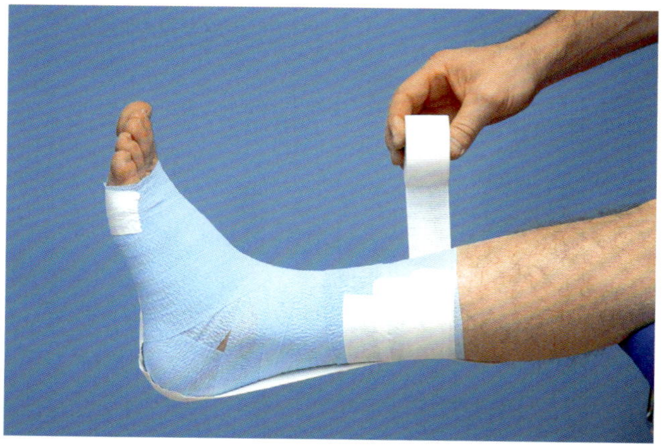

3

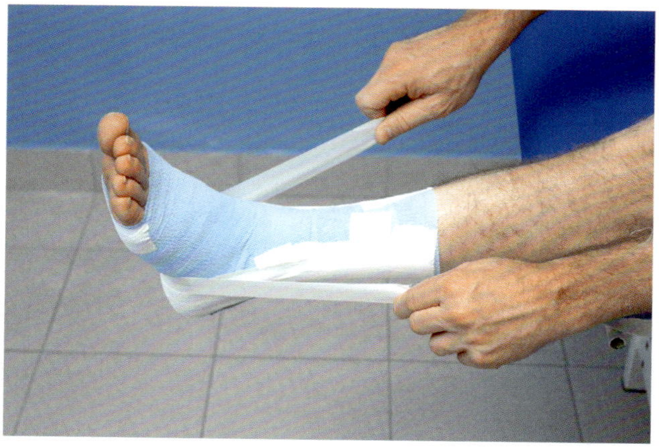

4

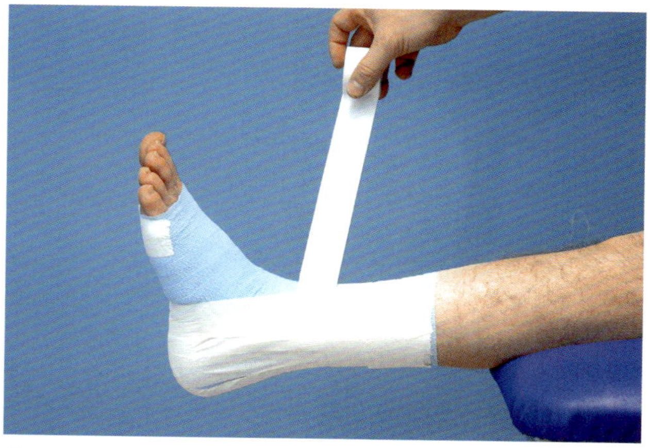

5

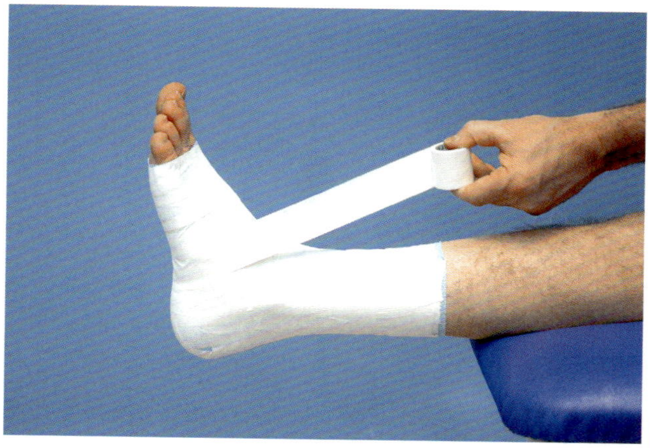

6

Unloading, support, and stabilization with inelastic bandage

MATERIAL

✓ Elastic cohesive bandage, 7.5 cm in width
✓ Inelastic cohesive tape, 2 cm in width

APPLICATION

1 The subject, in the supine position, places the foot off the end of the table. The proximal and distal anchoring points are prepared on the base bandaging made with cohesive elastic bandage (see pages 184-185), using an inelastic bandage applied in a semicircle.

2 The subject puts the foot in plantar flexion at an angle of inclination of 10-20 degrees. A reinforced fastener made of inelastic material is affixed to the distal anchoring point, then adhered to the cohesive bandage following the line of the plantar fascia, wraps around the heel, and is directed toward the skin projection of the Achilles tendon.

The reinforced fastener is prepared by overlapping four strips of inelastic cohesive bandage.

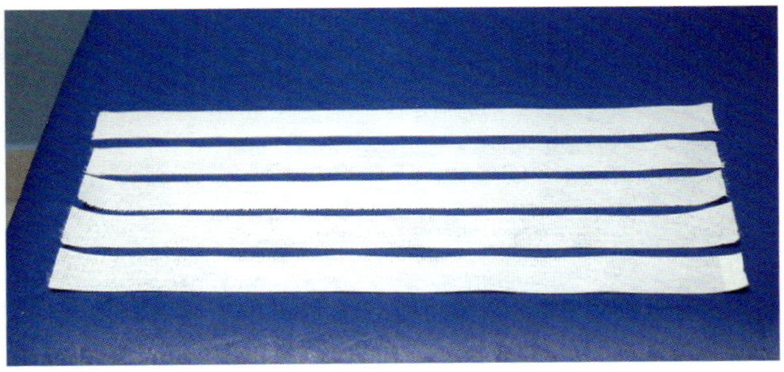
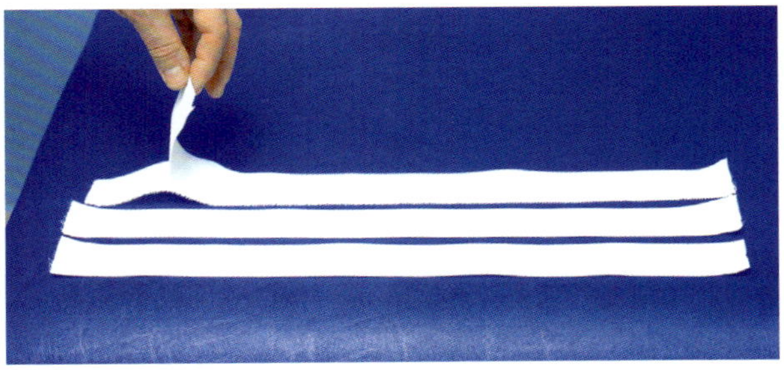

3 The tape is affixed to the proximal anchoring point with several strips of bandage applied in a semicircle.

4 Bandaging proceeds with four stabilization fasteners applied in horseshoe fashion, passing them under the heel and over the skin projections of the fibular and tibial malleoli to then adhere to the proximal anchoring point.

5 The support fasteners are secured with several complete wraps of bandage, wrapping around the distal third of the lower leg, the heel, the midfoot, and the forefoot.

6 Bandaging is completed using the inelastic band to stabilize the hindfoot with two figure-eight wraps that obliquely pass over the medial and lateral areas of the heel. The bandage begins from the medial malleolus, wraps around the plantar arch, and runs over the dorsum of the foot.

ACHILLES TENDON

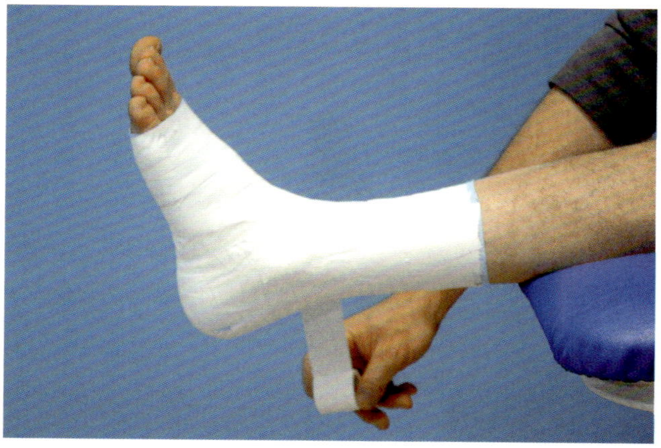

7

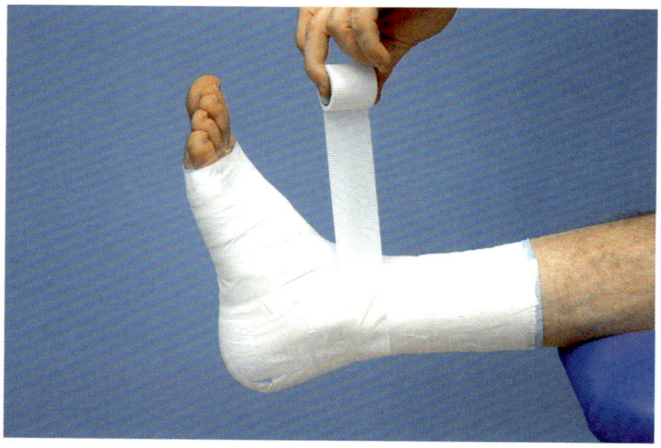

8

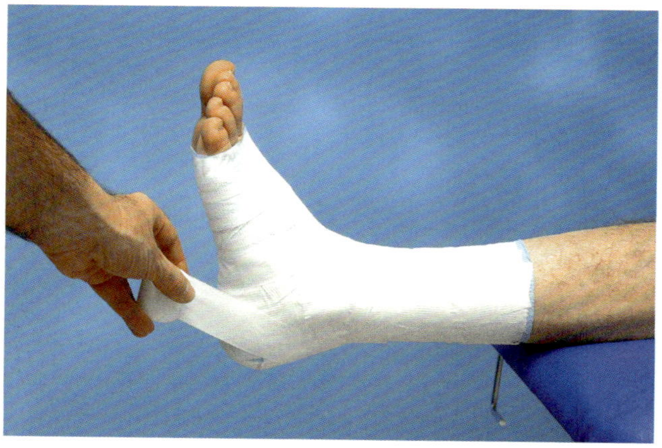

9

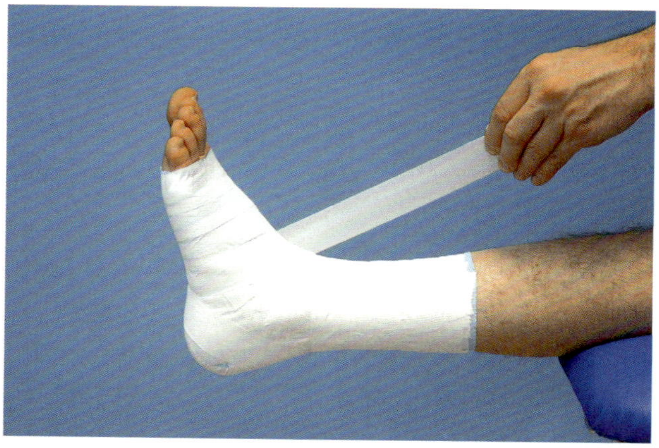

10

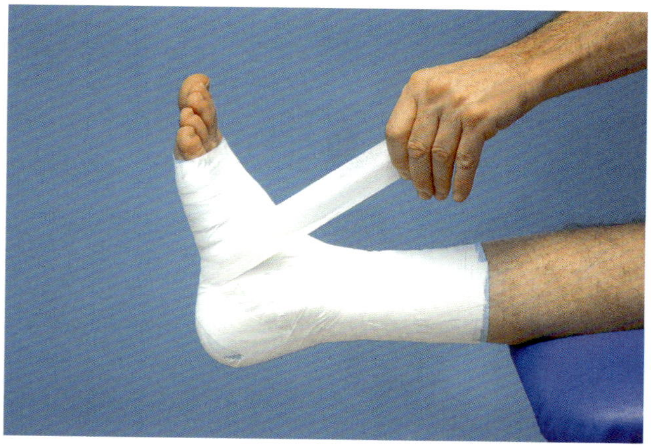

11

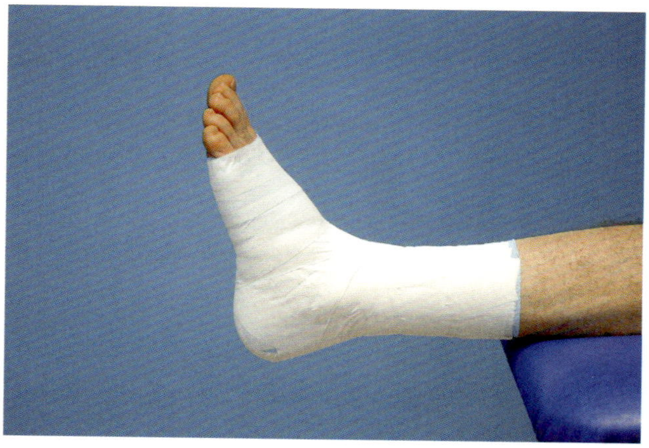

12

Unloading, support, and stabilization with inelastic bandage

7 The bandage covers the tibiotarsal joint.

8 A wrap of bandage is made around the axis of the lower leg.

9 The bandage obliquely crosses the lateral compartment of the heel.

10 The bandage is again brought below the plantar arch and then directed toward the dorsum of the foot, covering the tibiotarsal joint.

11 A wrap of the bandage is made around the axis of the lower leg and the bandage is diagonally brought toward the heel to cover the medial compartment, then goes around the heel and runs toward the lower leg, where it is cut and secured over the bandaging.

12 Bandaging is complete.

INDICATIONS

✓ *Posttraumatic conditions*

PLANTAR APONEUROSIS

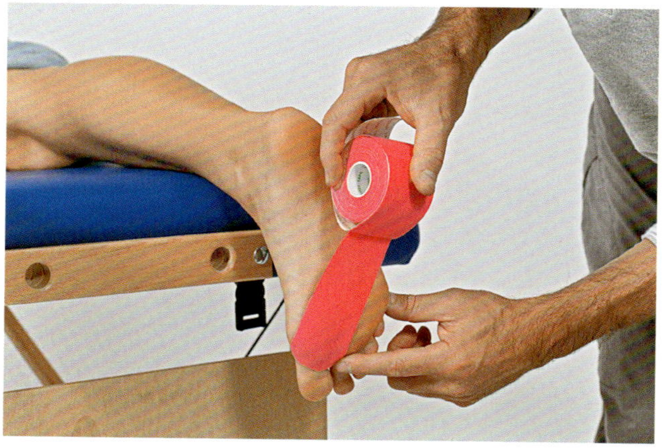

1

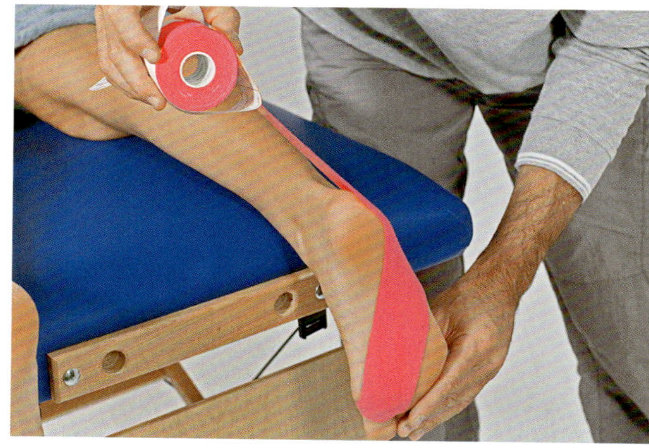

2

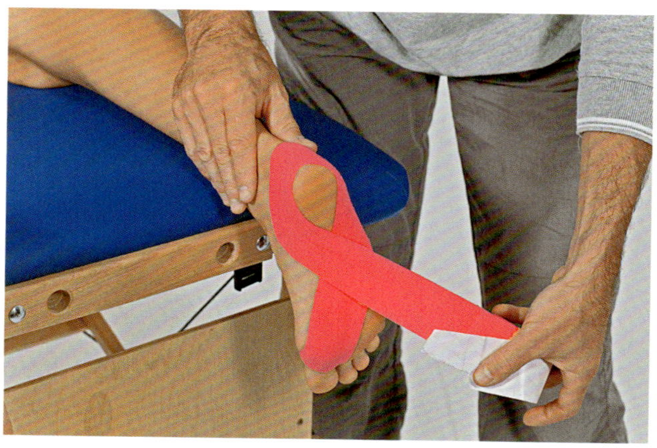

3

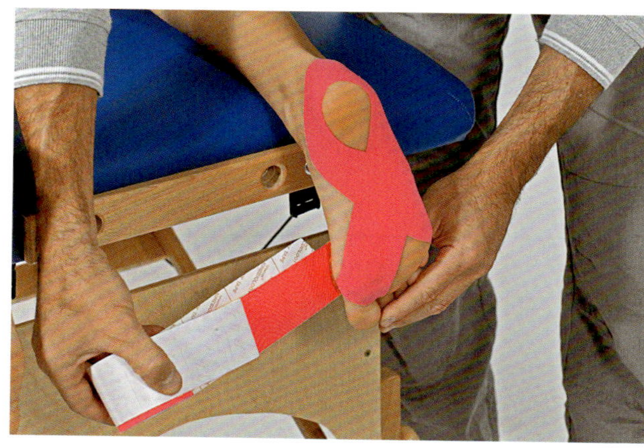

4

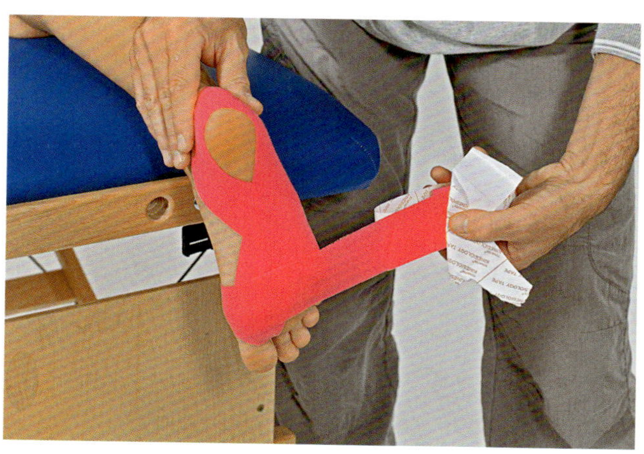

5

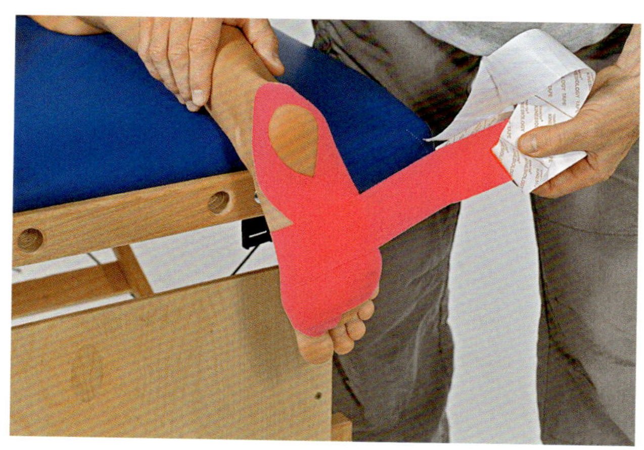

6

Unloading with elastic adhesive tape

MATERIAL

✓ Elastic adhesive tape, 5 cm in width

APPLICATION

1 The end of the elastic adhesive tape is shaped by cutting its corners so as to be able to apply it without difficulty at the plantar skin projection of the first metatarsal head.

2-3 The tape is pulled and directed toward the skin projection of the heel. Once the heel has been wrapped, the tape is directed toward the skin projection of the base of the fifth metatarsal head.

4-5-6 Bandaging concludes by making several spiral wraps of tape with an overlap of 30% in a distal to proximal direction so as to wrap the metatarsal heads and the midfoot.

INDICATIONS

✓ *Plantar fasciitis*
✓ *Dysfunction of the plantar fascia or arch*

PLANTAR APONEUROSIS

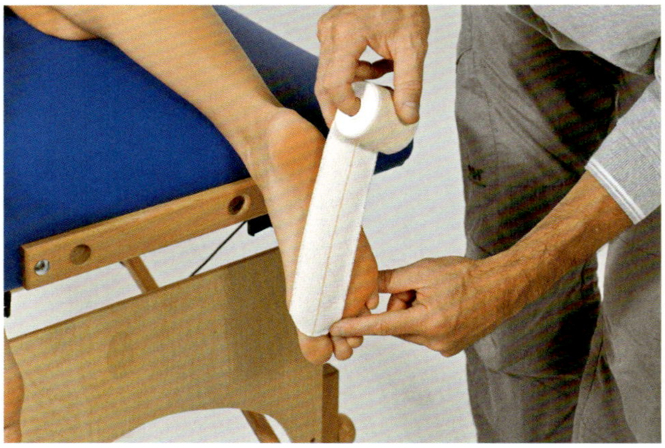

1

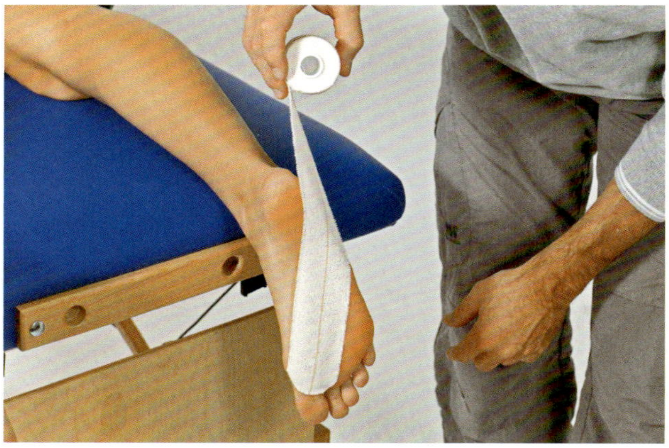

2

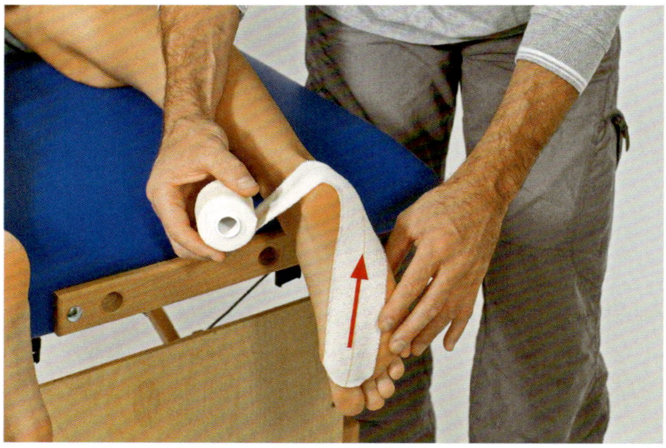

3

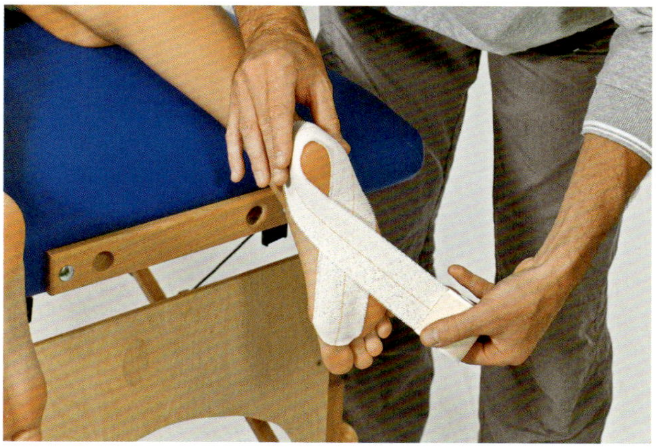

4

Unloading with reinforcement

MATERIAL

- ✓ Cotton fabric porous elastic adhesive bandage that can be stretched lengthwise, 5 cm in width
- ✓ Inelastic adhesive tape, 5 cm in width

APPLICATION

1 The end of the mono-extensible elastic adhesive bandage is applied at the plantar skin projection of the first metatarsal head.

2-3 The bandage is placed under tension and brought toward the skin projection of the lateral border of the heel.

4 The bandage, after wrapping around the heel, is pulled in the direction of the fifth toe, crossing the previous path under the plantar arch.

The end of the mono-extensible porous elastic adhesive bandage must be shaped by cutting its corners so as to be able to apply it without difficulty at the plantar skin projection of the first metatarsal head.

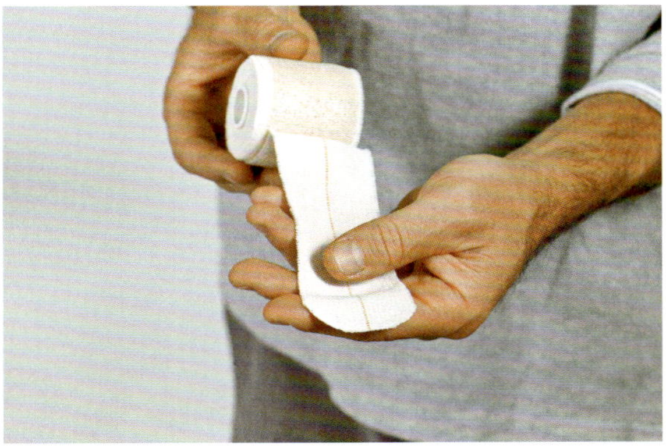

PLANTAR APONEUROSIS

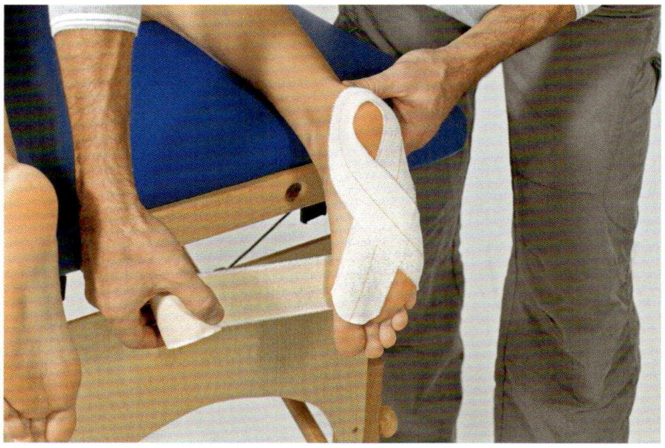

5

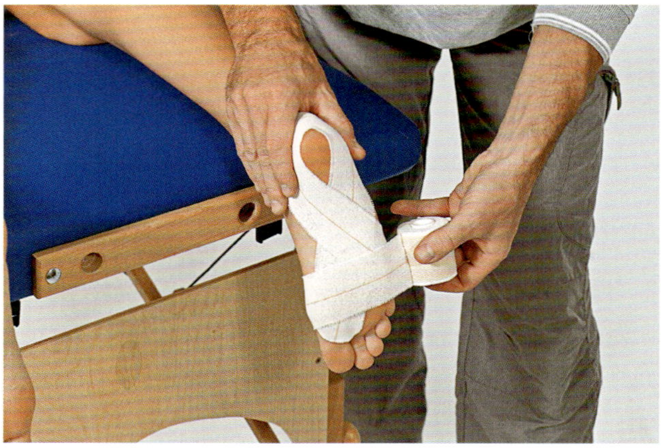

6

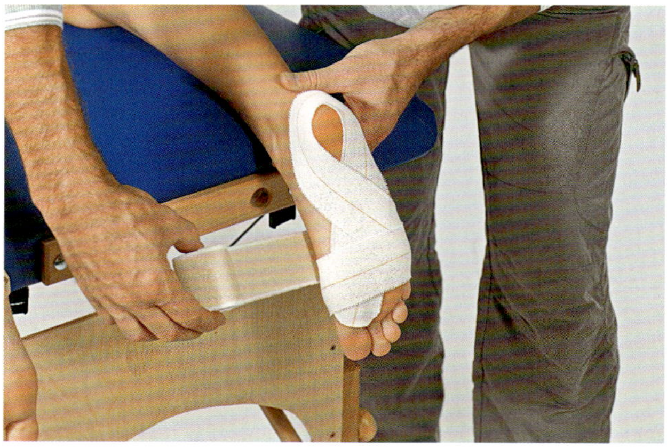

7

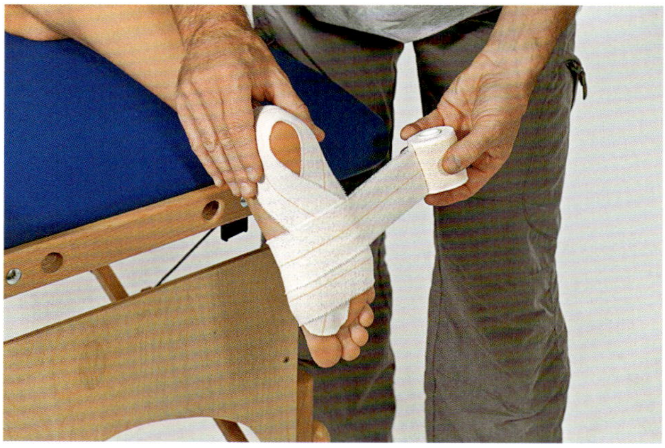

8

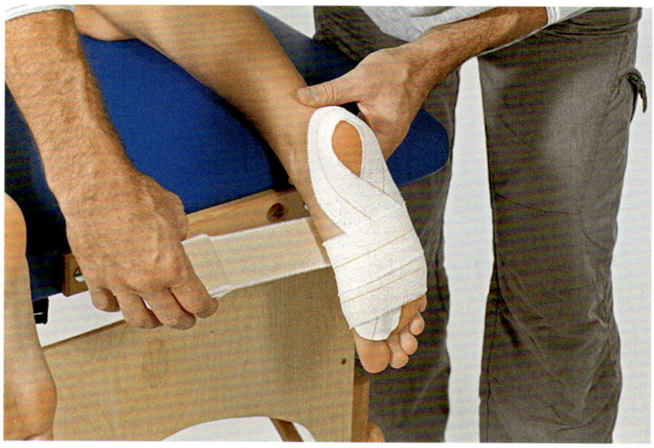

9

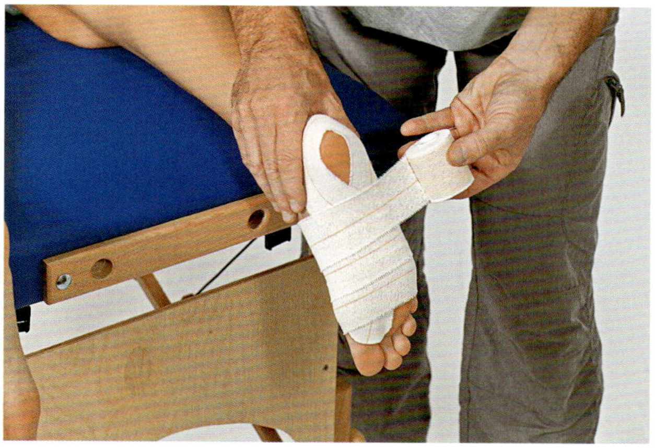

10

Unloading with reinforcement

5-6-7-8-9-10 Bandaging proceeds by making several spiral wraps of bandage with an overlap of 30% in a distal to proximal direction so as to wrap the metatarsal heads and the midfoot.

The adhesive material and the cotton fabric of the porous elastic adhesive bandage confer optimal elasticity to this bandaging, reducing the glue's strength acting on the skin.

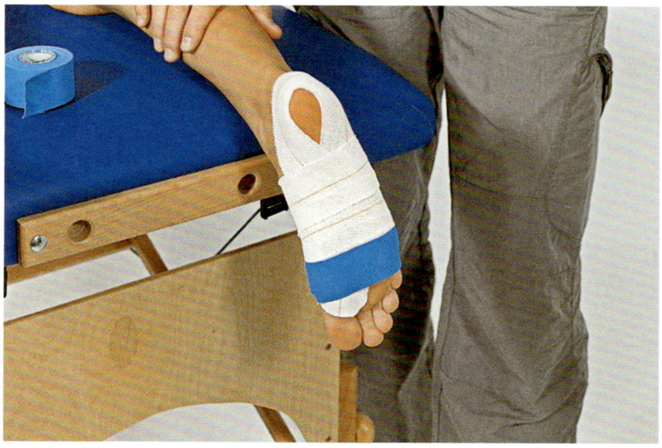

11

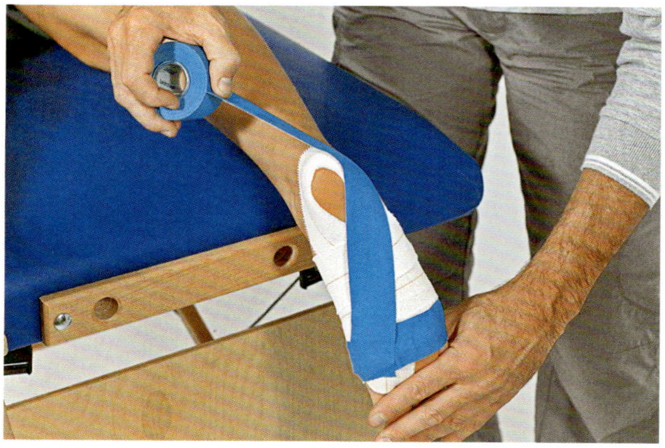

12

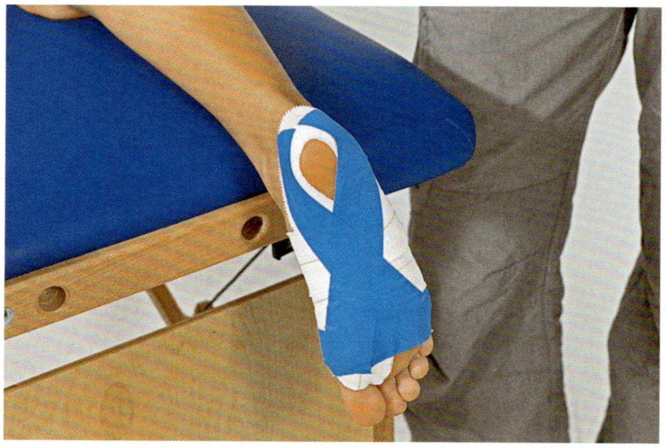

13

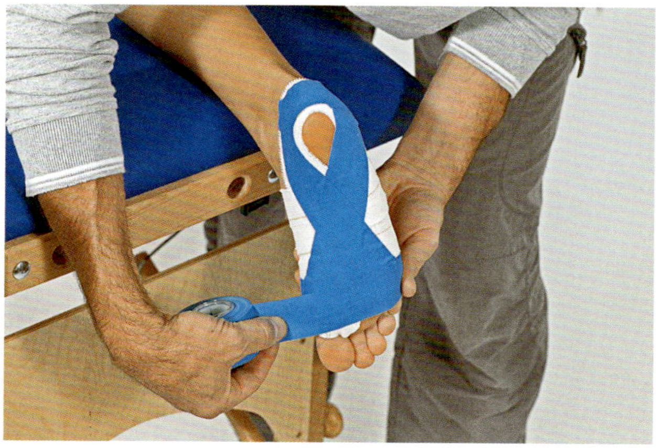

14

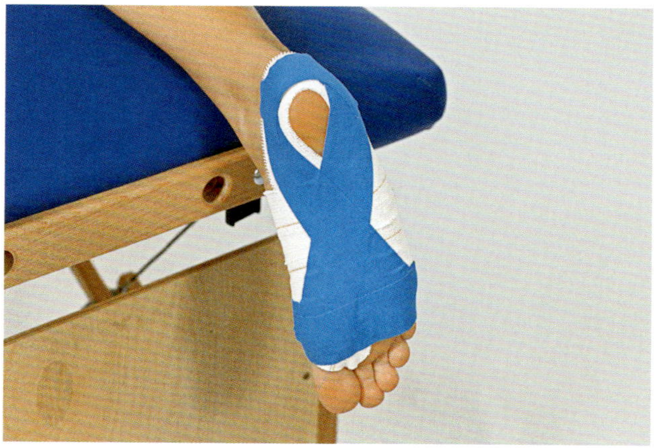

15

Unloading with reinforcement

11 A distal anchoring point is prepared by using inelastic adhesive tape applied at the metatarsal heads.

12-13 Two strips of inelastic adhesive tape are adhered to the base bandaging, crossing at the plantar arch.

14-15 The bandaging concludes with the securing of the distal and proximal anchoring points.

INDICATIONS

✓ *Plantar fasciitis*
✓ *Dysfunction of the plantar fascia or arch*

PLANTAR APONEUROSIS

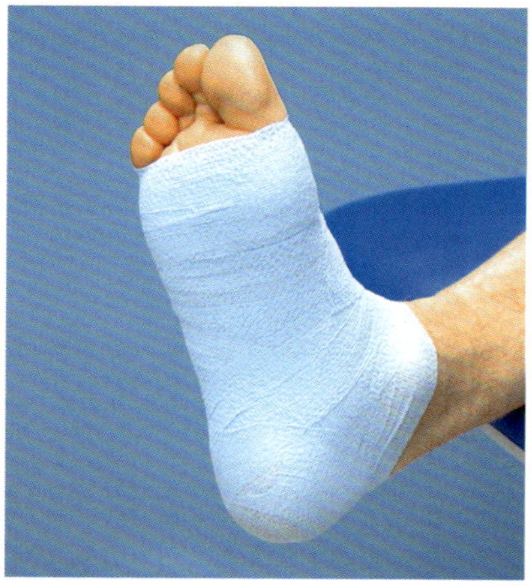

1

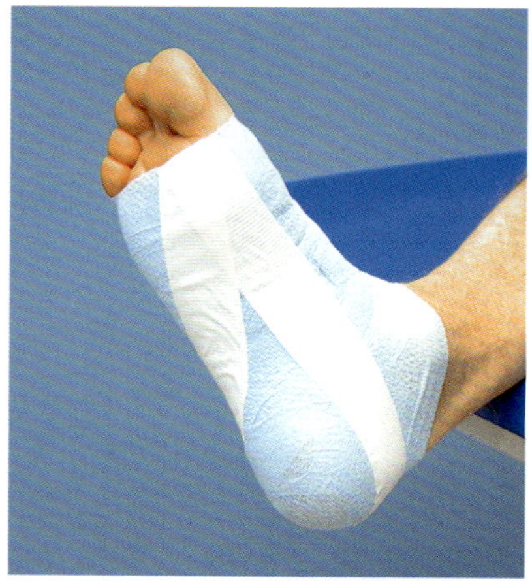

2

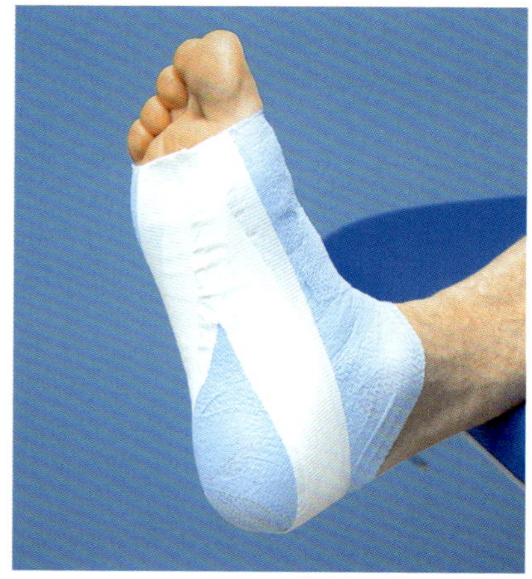

3

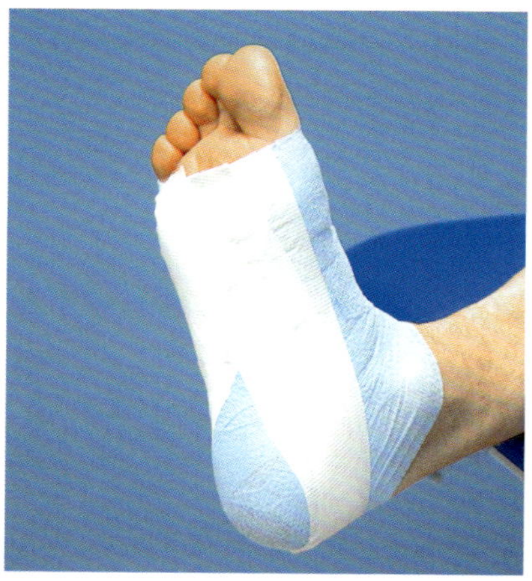

4

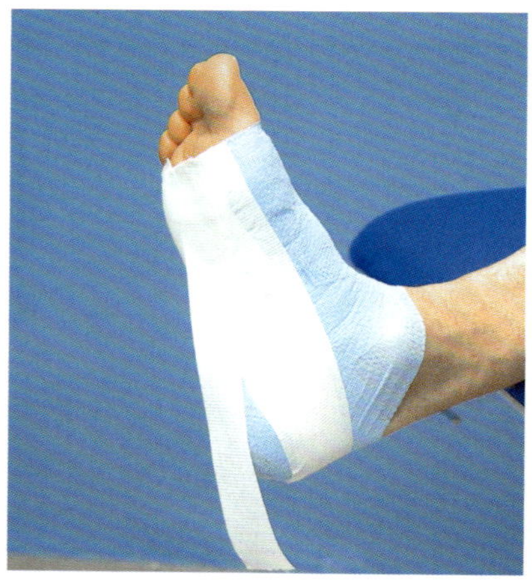

5

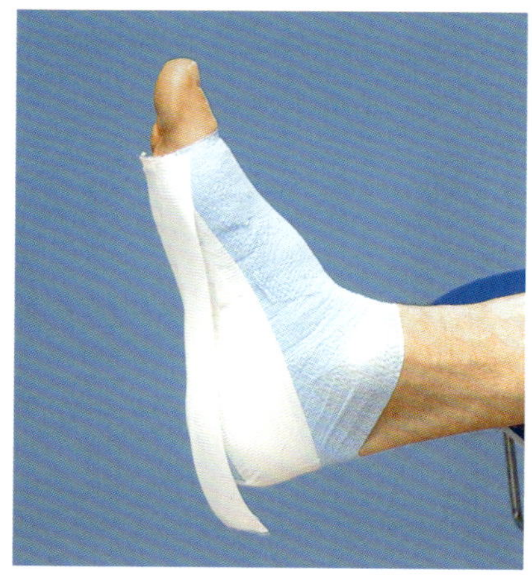

6

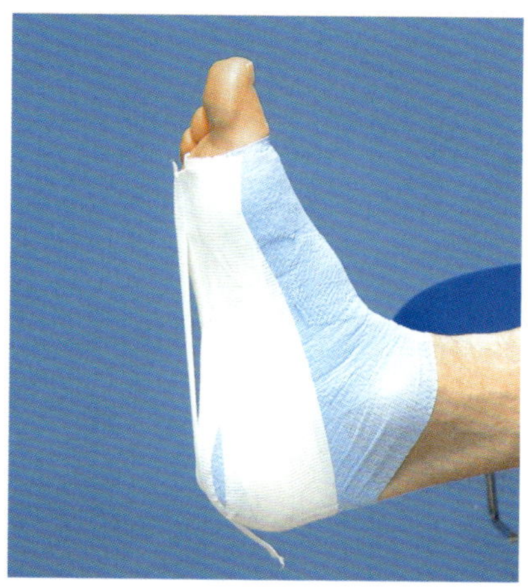

7

Support of the foot and the plantar arch

MATERIAL

- ✓ Elastic cohesive bandage, 2.5 cm in width
- ✓ Inelastic cohesive tape, 1 or 2 cm in width

APPLICATION

1 The subject, in the supine position, places the foot off the end of the table and keeps it in the neutral position. With a cohesive elastic bandage, base bandaging is prepared to cover the plantar arch, making several wraps of bandage around the forefoot, midfoot, and hindfoot.

2 In order to support the plantar arch, three fasteners of inelastic material are placed passing posterior to the heel. The first fastener starts from the skin projection of the first toe and arrives at that of the second toe.

3 The second fastener starts from the skin projection of the second toe and arrives at that of the third toe.

4 The third fastener starts from the skin projection of the fourth toe and arrives at that of the fifth toe.

5 Bandaging proceeds by placing three fasteners made of inelastic material that cover the plantar arch. The first fastener starts over the skin projection of the second and third toes.

6 The second fastener starts over the skin projection of the first toe.

7 The third fastener starts over the skin projection of the fourth and fifth toes.

PLANTAR APONEUROSIS

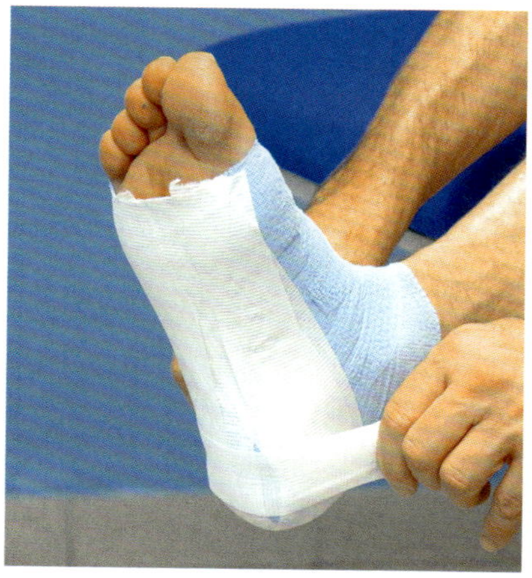
8

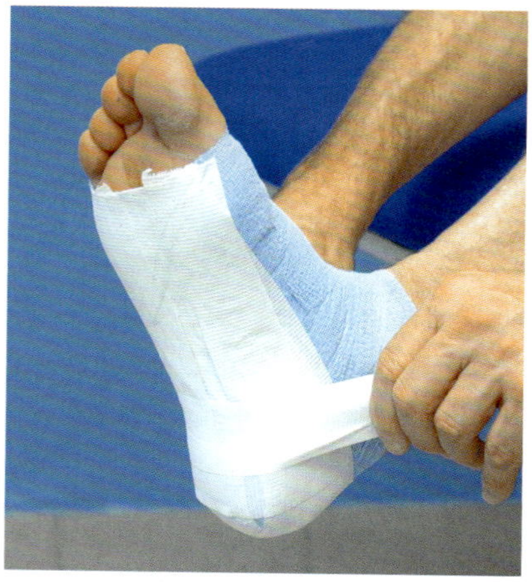
9

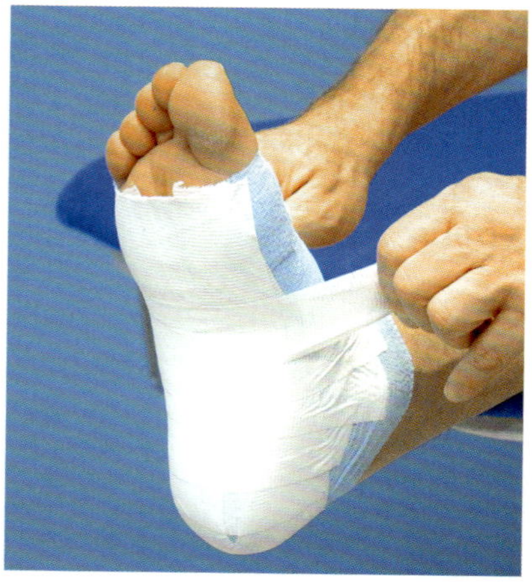
10

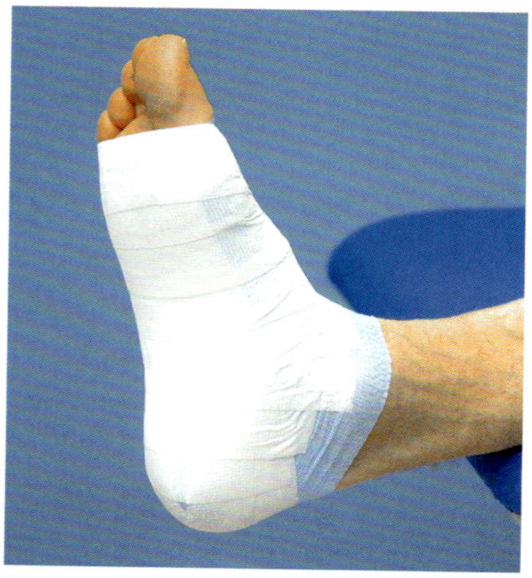
11

Support of the foot and the plantar arch

8-9-10 All three fasteners are adhered to the plantar arch and on the posterior portion of the heel, to then be secured with several transverse closing fasteners wrapped around the heel, the plantar arch, and the metatarsal heads.

11 Bandaging is complete.

INDICATIONS

- ✓ *Preventative sports treatment*
- ✓ *Posttraumatic conditions*

METATARSOPHALANGEAL JOINTS

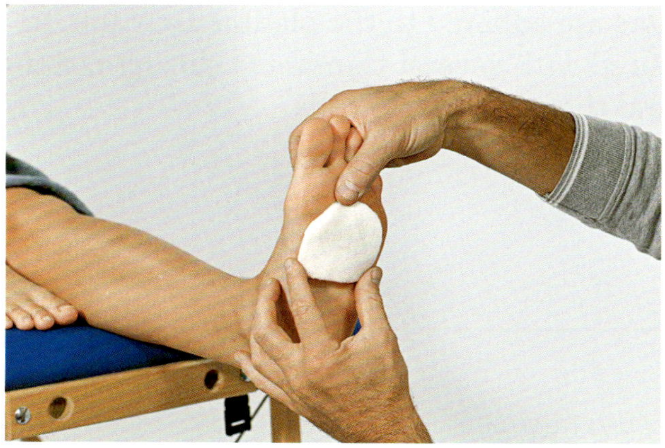

1

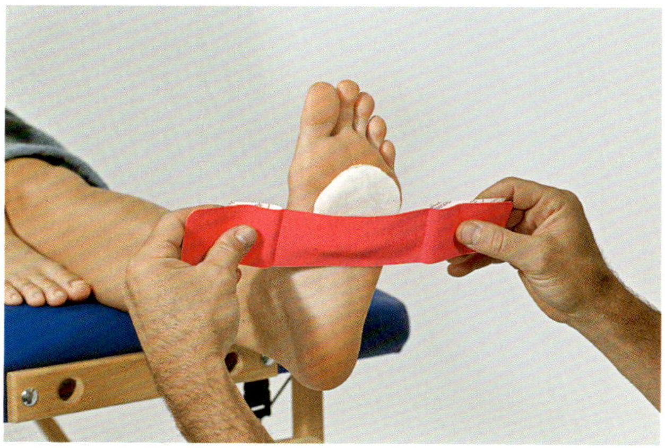

2

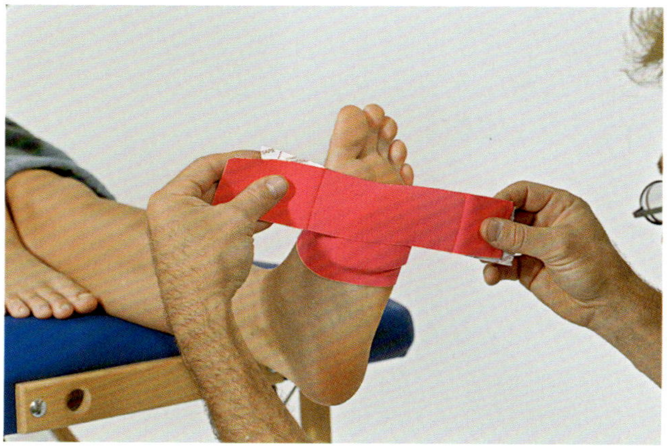

3

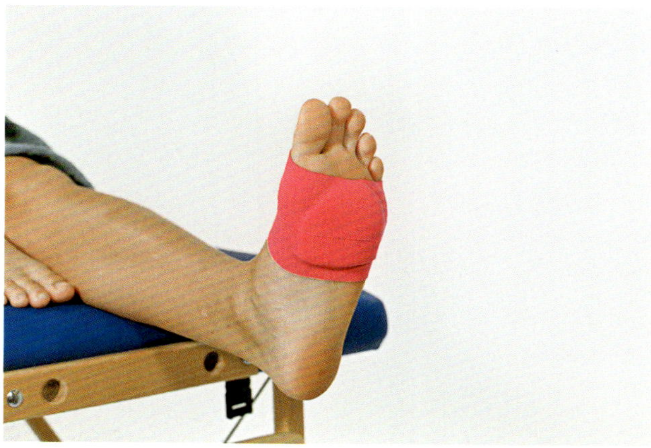

4

Unloading with pad

MATERIAL

✓ Foam rubber or pre-tape compress for creating an unloading pad
✓ Elastic adhesive tape, 5 cm in width

APPLICATION

1 The unloading compress must be placed at the base of the metatarsal heads.

2-3 The unloading compress is secured with the application of several strips of partially overlapping elastic adhesive tape in a semicircle.

4 Bandaging is complete.

INDICATIONS

✓ *Metatarsalgia*

METATARSOPHALANGEAL JOINTS

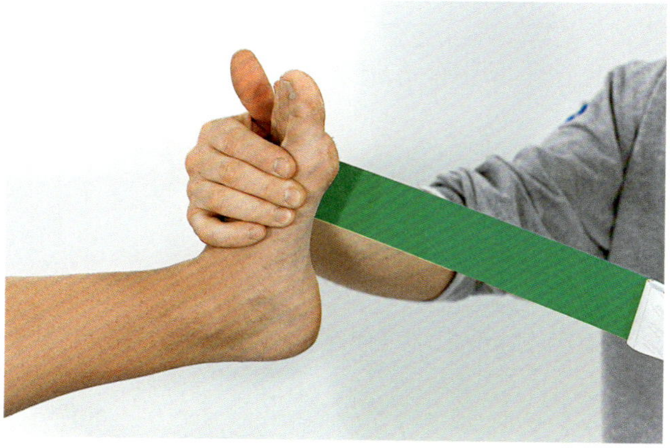

1

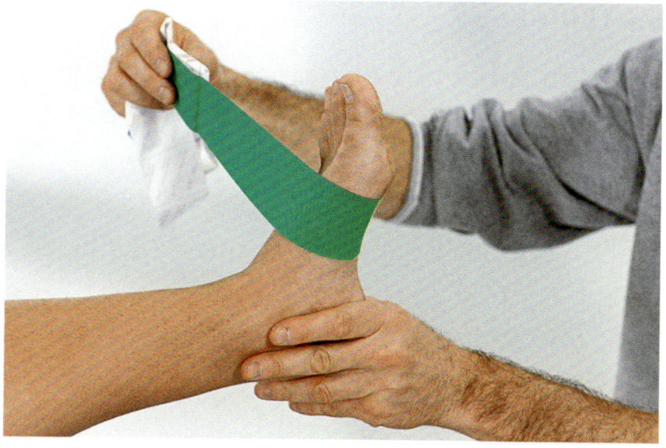

2

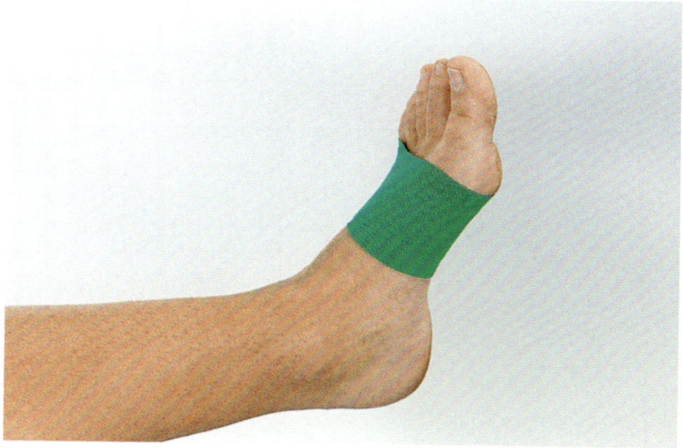

3

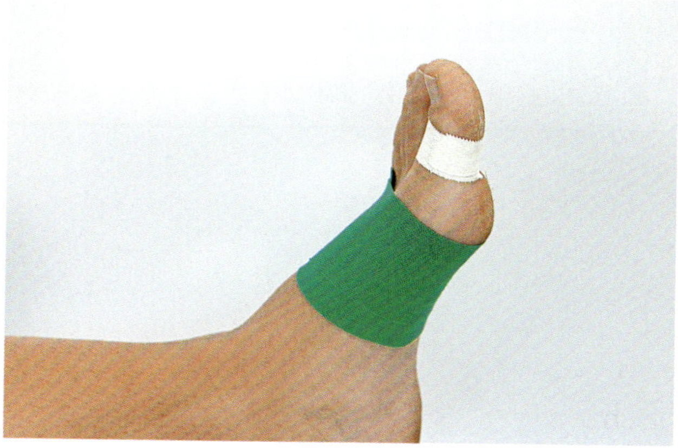

4

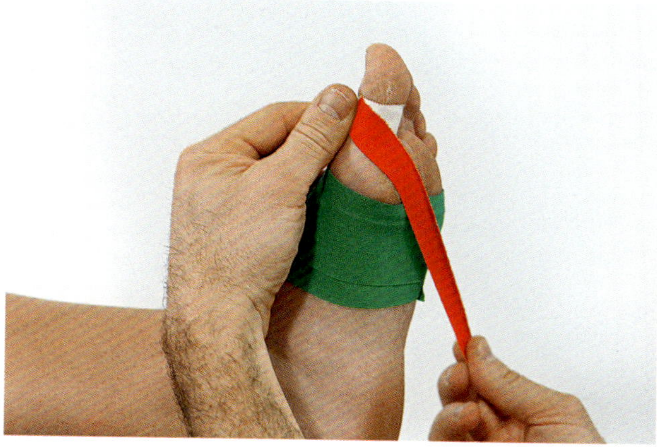

5

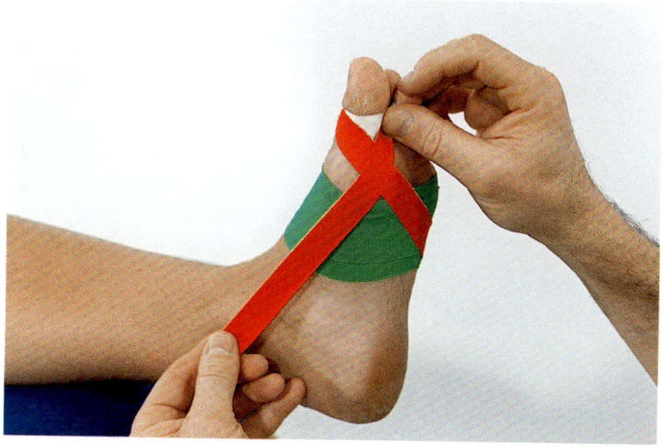

6

Stabilization of the joint of the great toe

MATERIAL

- ✓ Elastic adhesive tape, 5 cm in width
- ✓ Inelastic adhesive tape, 1 cm in width
- ✓ Inelastic adhesive tape for affixing the bandage

APPLICATION

1-2-3 Two wraps of elastic adhesive tape are applied as proximal anchoring point beginning from the skin projection of the ray of the fifth toe and going on to wrap around the forefoot.

> *Alternatively, for the proximal anchoring point, a 5 cm wide longitudinally extensible porous elastic adhesive bandage may be used; in this case, it is sufficient to apply a single wrap of bandage for an anchoring point.*

4 Next, a distal anchoring point is prepared with a wrap of inelastic adhesive tape applied at the phalanx of the first digit.

5 Beginning over the distal anchoring point from the medial edge of the phalanx, a strip of 1 cm wide inelastic adhesive tape is applied and brought over the plantar surface of the foot, where it is secured over the proximal anchoring point at the ray of the fifth digit.

6 A second strip of inelastic adhesive tape of the same dimensions begins over the distal anchoring point from the lateral edge of the phalanx of the first digit.

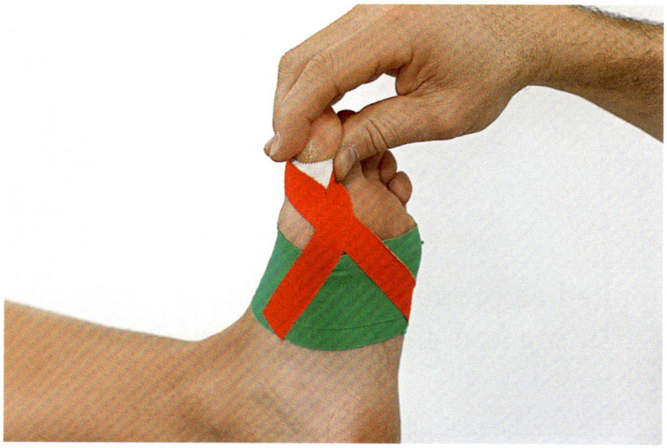

7

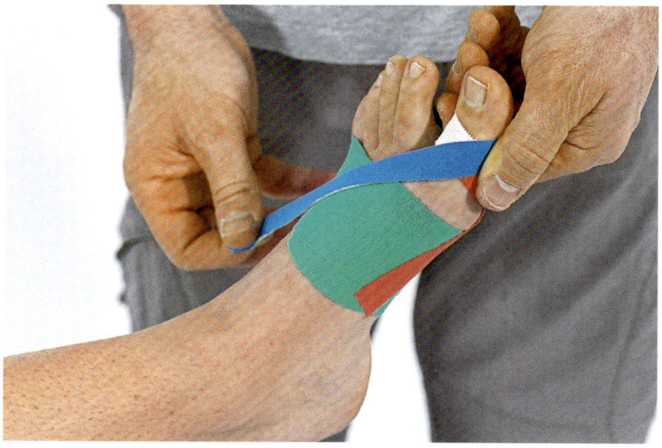

8

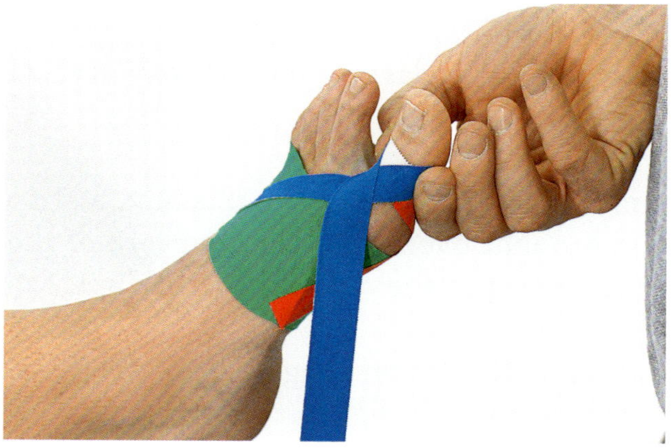

9

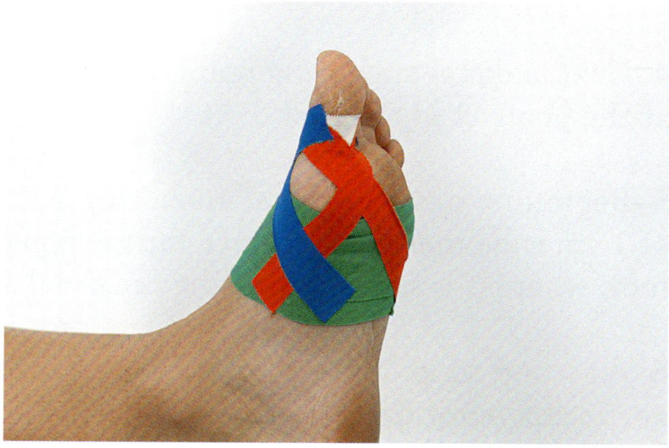

10

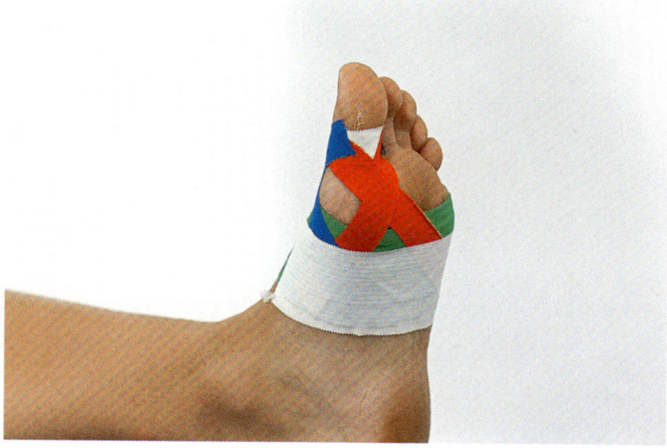

11

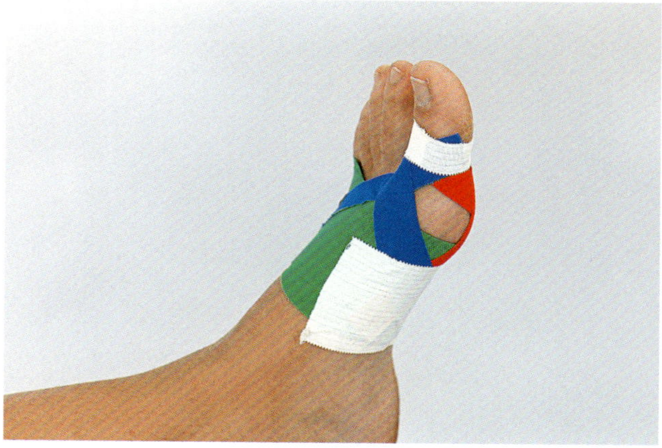

12

Stabilization of the joint of the great toe

7 The strip is adhered over the plantar surface in order to end over the proximal anchoring point at the ray of the first digit.

8 Bandaging proceeds by applying another strip, still made of inelastic material, beginning at the distal anchoring point over the medial edge of the first digit. The tape is then brought over the dorsal surface of the foot and is adhered over the proximal anchoring point at the ray of the fifth digit.

9-10 A final strip, beginning from the lateral border of the first digit, is adhered over the dorsal surface of the foot in order to end over the proximal anchoring point at the ray of the first digit.

11-12 Bandaging finishes by applying two pieces of securing tape in a semicircle.

INDICATIONS

✓ *Effects of sprain of the great toe*

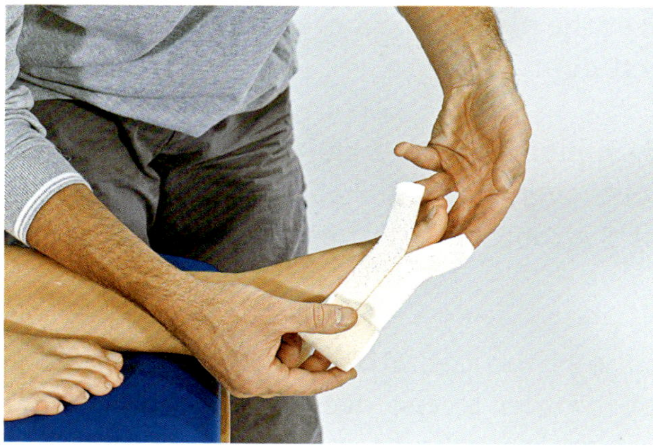

1

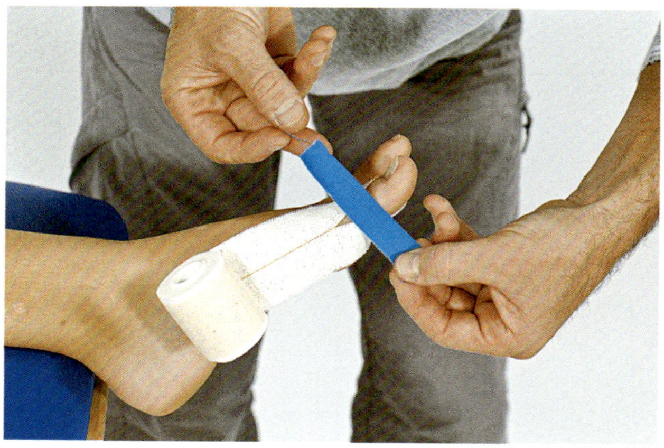

2

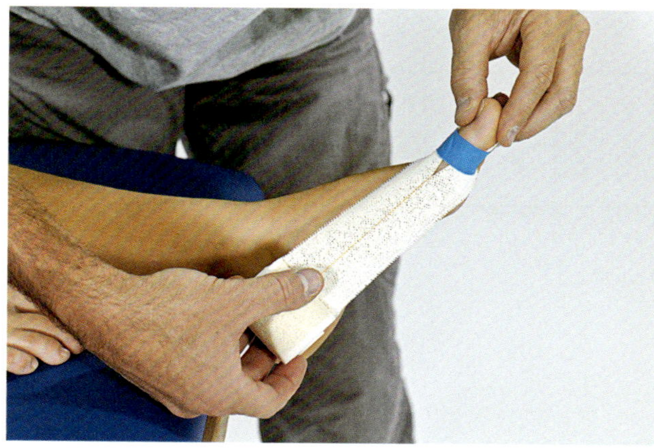

3

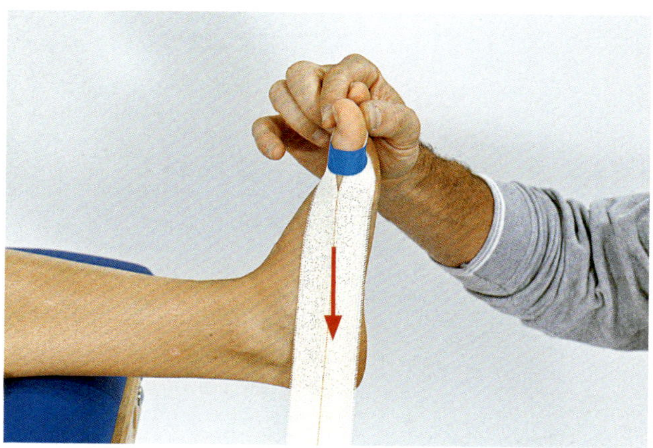

4

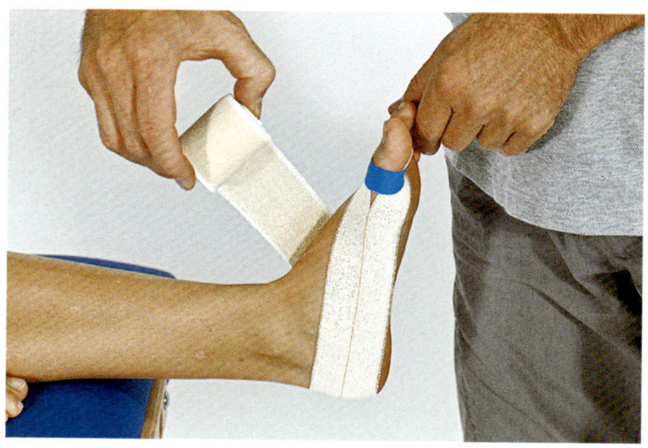

5

Unloading of the metatarsophalangeal joint of the great toe

MATERIAL

- ✓ Cotton fabric porous elastic adhesive bandage that can be stretched lengthwise, 5 cm in width
- ✓ Inelastic adhesive tape, 2.5 or 4 cm in width
- ✓ 1 cm wide inelastic adhesive tape to affix bandaging

APPLICATION

1 The adhesive elastic bandage is divided into two parts with a longitudinal cut and applied so as to wrap around the phalanx of the first digit above the metatarsophalangeal joint.

2-3 The first anchoring point is secured with a wrap of 1 cm wide inelastic adhesive tape.

4-5 The tibiotarsal joint is kept flexed at 90 degrees. The bandage is pulled distal to proximal to wrap around the heel and also posteriorly.

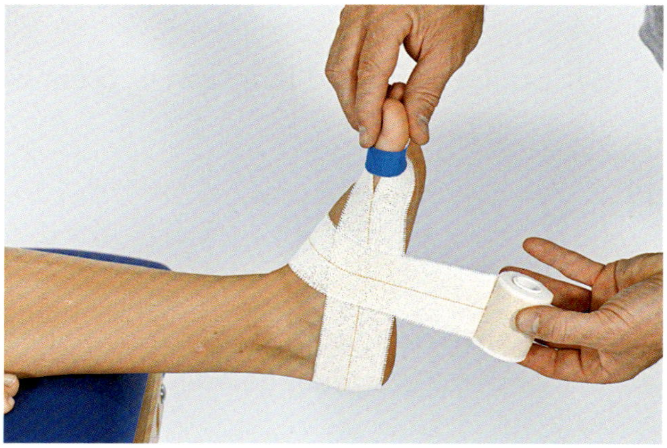

6

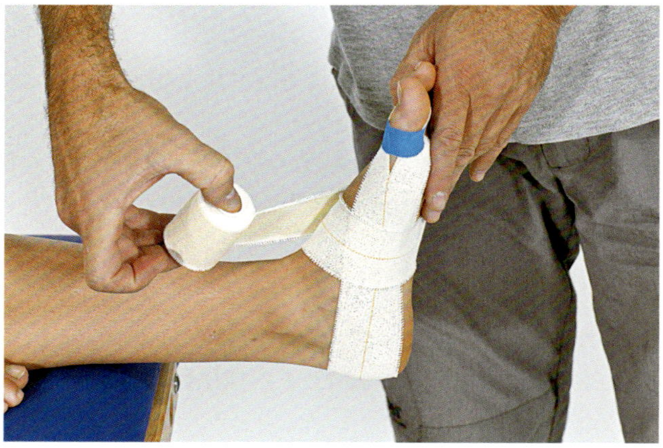

7

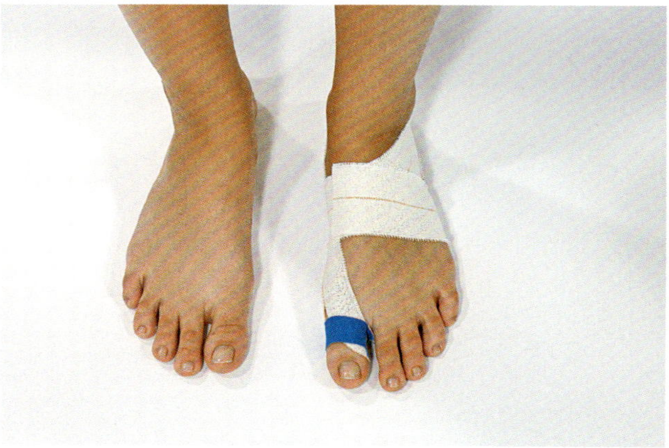

8

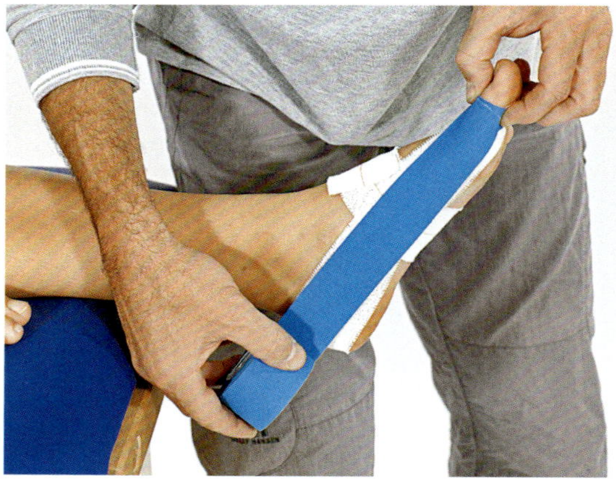

9

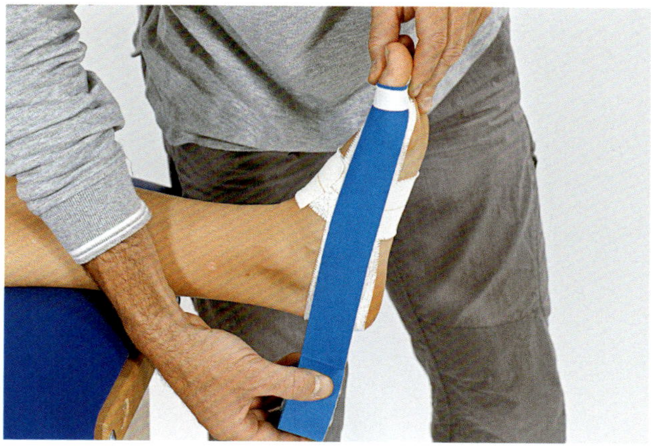

10

Unloading of the metatarsophalangeal joint of the great toe

6-7-8 With a wrap of bandage that perpendicularly crosses the first path, the midfoot is now wrapped, passing the bandage over the dorsal and plantar surface of the foot.

9-10 The base bandaging is reinforced with several strips of inelastic adhesive tape, varying between 2.5 and 4 cm. The first strip is secured with an anchoring point at the phalanx of the first digit and is then applied following the course of the porous elastic adhesive bandage in order to posteriorly wrap around the heel.

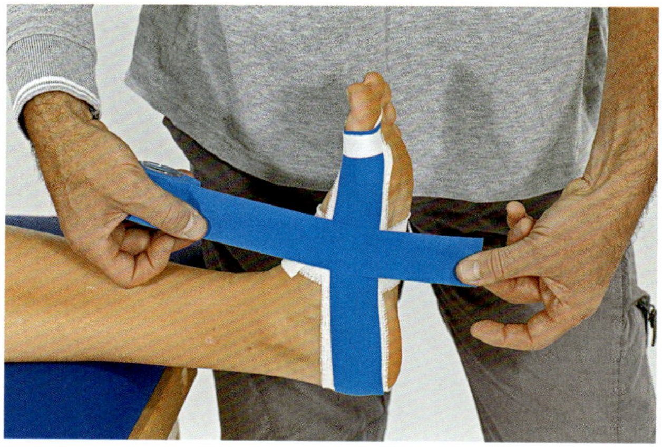
11

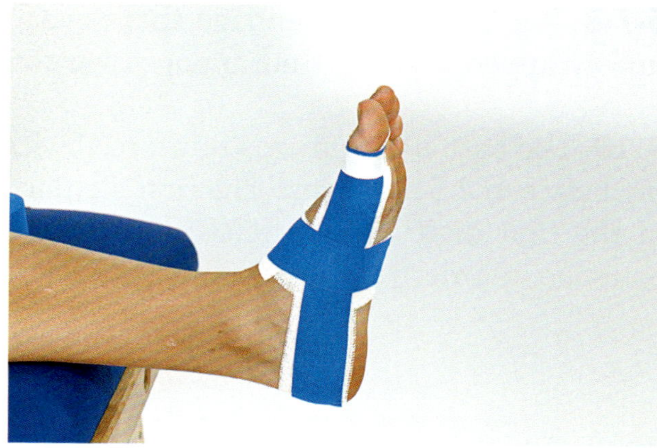
12

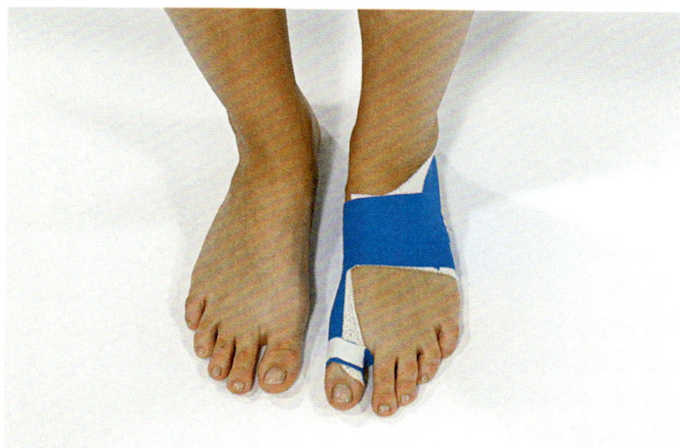
13

Unloading of the metatarsophalangeal joint of the great toe

11-12 The second strip of inelastic adhesive tape is applied perpendicular to the first so as to wrap around the midfoot and reinforce the retention of the bandaging.

13 Bandaging is complete.

INDICATIONS

- ✓ *Hallux valgus*
- ✓ *Inflammation of the metatarsophalangeal joint of the first digit*

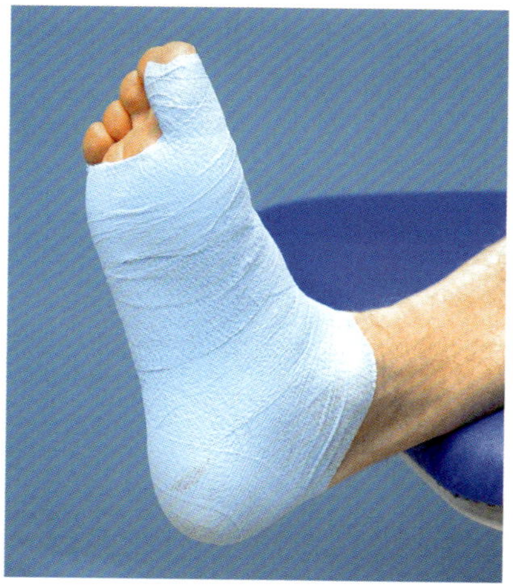
1

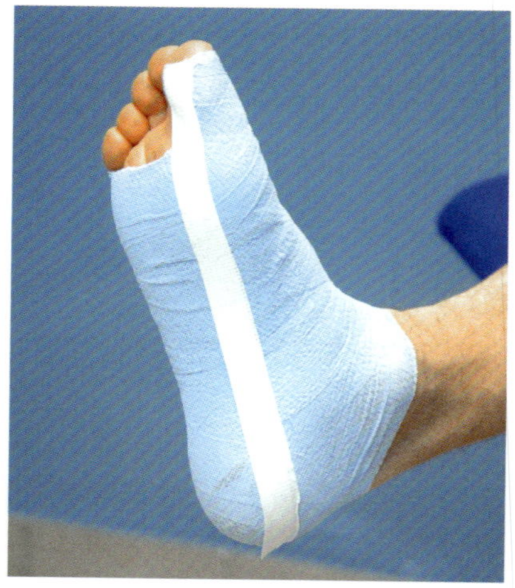
2

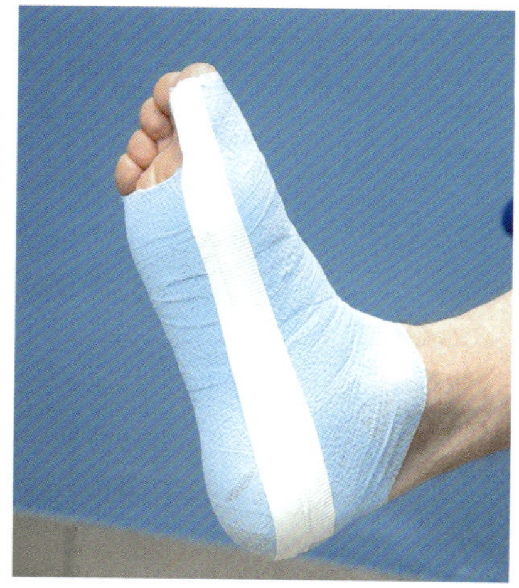
3

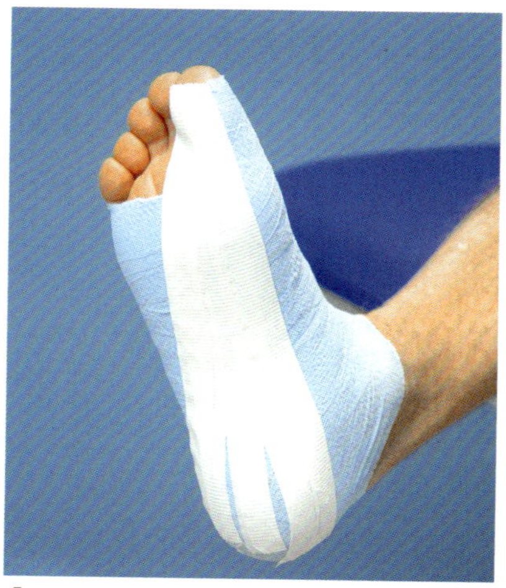
4

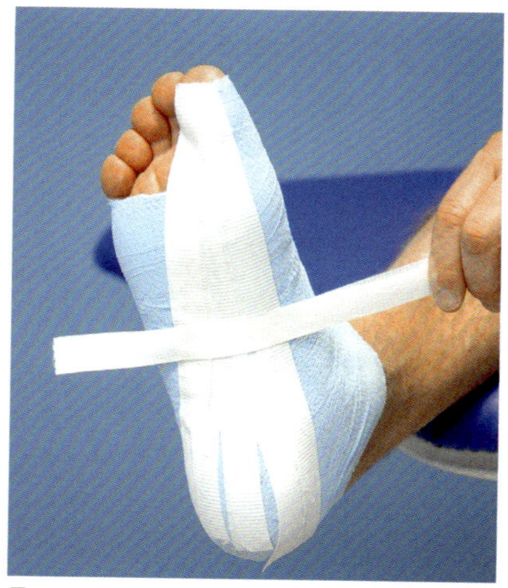
5

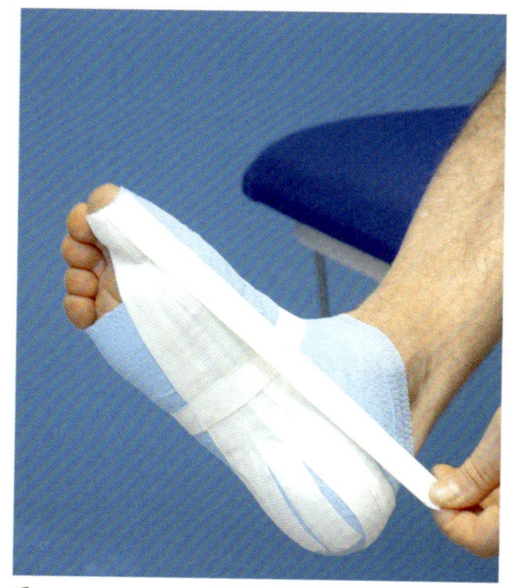
6

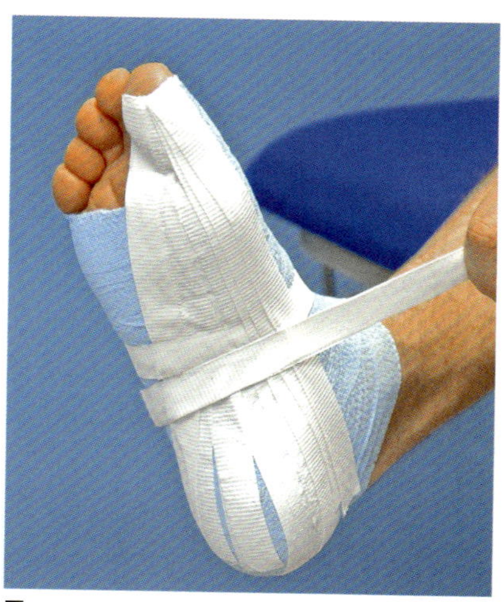
7

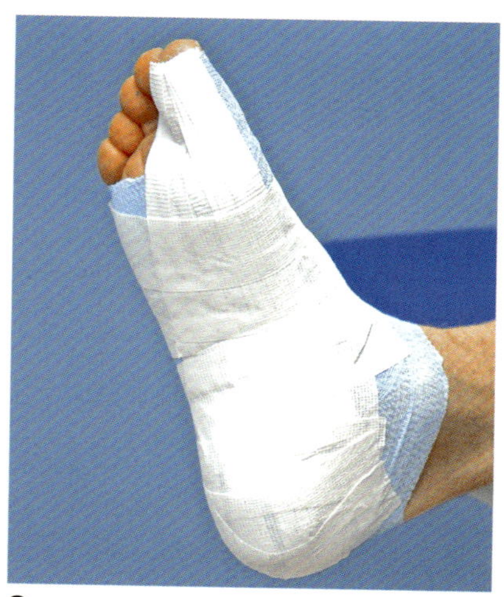
8

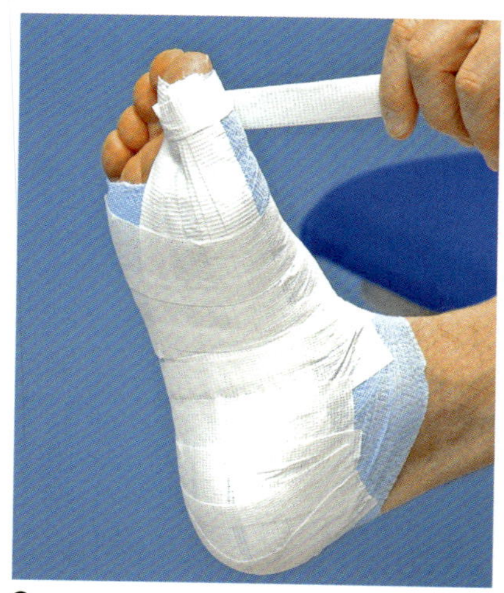
9

Support of the great toe, limitation of hyperextension and abduction

MATERIAL

✓ Cohesive elastic bandage for base bandaging, 2.5 cm wide
✓ Inelastic cohesive tape, 1 or 2 cm in width

APPLICATION

1 The subject, in the supine position, places the foot off the table. Base bandaging is done with the cohesive bandage, making several full wraps around the first digit and the entire plantar arch.

2 With the great toe flexed at 10 degrees, the support fasteners are placed using an inelastic bandage. The first fastener is applied starting from the first digit until reaching the heel.

3-4 Bandaging proceeds with the application of the support fasteners, always beginning from the first digit in order to then fan out and cover the heel.

5 A transverse closing fastener is placed at the midfoot.

6 The bandaging is reinforced with the application of another three fasteners that run from the first digit in the direction of the medial portion of the heel.

7-8 The base of the foot, from the heel to the metatarsal heads, is completely covered with several transverse closure fasteners.

9 Bandaging is completed with several full wraps of bandage around the phalanx of the first digit.

INDICATIONS

✓ *Posttraumatic conditions*
✓ *Prevention in sports of stress during hyperextension and abduction*